GREAT ISSUES FOR MEDICINE IN THE TWENTY-FIRST CENTURY

ETHICAL AND SOCIAL ISSUES ARISING OUT OF ADVANCES IN THE BIOMEDICAL SCIENCES

ANNALS OF THE NEW YORK ACADEMY OF SCIENCES
Volume 882

GREAT ISSUES FOR MEDICINE IN THE TWENTY-FIRST CENTURY

ETHICAL AND SOCIAL ISSUES ARISING OUT OF ADVANCES IN THE BIOMEDICAL SCIENCES

Edited by Dana Cook Grossman and Heinz Valtin

The New York Academy of Sciences
New York, New York
1999

The softcover edition of this book shows ancient (a Sumerian prescription) and modern (genetic) texts.

Library of Congress Cataloging-in-Publication Data

Great issues for medicine in the twenty-first century : ethical and
social issues arising out of advances in the biomedical sciences /
edited by Dana Cook Grossman and Heinz Valtin.
        p.   cm. — (Annals of the New York Academy of Sciences, ISSN
0077-8923 ; v. 882)
    Includes bibliographical references and index.
    ISBN 1-57331-143-X (cloth : alk. paper). — ISBN 1-57331-144-8
(paper : alk. paper)
    1. Medical ethics—Forecasting Congresses.   2. Social medicine—
Forecasting Congresses.   3. Twenty-first century—Forecasts
Congresses.   4. Medical sciences—Forecasting Congresses.
I. Grossman, Dana Cook.   II. Valtin, Heinz.   III. Series.
    [DNLM: 1. Delivery of Health Care.   2. Ethics, Medical.
3. Genetic Engineering.   4. Genome, Human.   W1 AN626YL v.882 1999 /
W 84 G786 1999]
Q11.N5   vol. 882
[R724]
500 s—dc21
[174'.2]
DNLM/DLC
for Library of Congress   99-30118
                                                             CIP

GYAT / PCP
Printed in the United States of America
ISBN 1-57331-143-X (cloth)
ISBN 1-57331-144-8 (paper)

ANNALS OF THE NEW YORK ACADEMY OF SCIENCES
Volume 882
June 30, 1999

GREAT ISSUES FOR MEDICINE IN THE TWENTY-FIRST CENTURY

ETHICAL AND SOCIAL ISSUES ARISING OUT OF ADVANCES IN THE BIOMEDICAL SCIENCES[a]

Editors
DANA COOK GROSSMAN AND HEINZ VALTIN

CONTENTS

[a]This volume comprises the proceedings of a conference entitled **Great Issues for Medicine in the Twenty-first Century: A Consideration of the Ethical and Social Issues Arising Out of Advances in the Biomedical Sciences** held by the Dartmouth Medical School in Hanover, New Hampshire, on September 5–7, 1997.

Neuroscience Session:
Intelligence—The Origin and Substrate of Thinking

Health Care Session: The Issues—For Whom and By Whom?

Special Address

World Population Session: The Crisis of Human Crowding

Closing Session: The Future—Through the Looking Glass

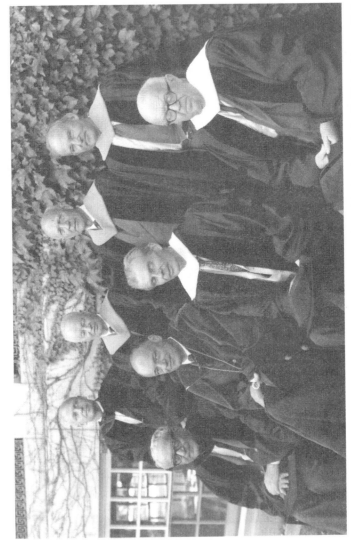

Dartmouth Medical School's 1960 "Great Issues" symposium was chaired by René Dubos (not pictured). Pictured here with two Dartmouth administrators are the six foreign speakers, on whom honorary degrees were conferred at the closing ceremonies. From left to right, seated, are Mahomedali Chagala, Indian Ambassador to the United States and Mexico; John Sloan Dickey, then president of Dartmouth College; writer Aldous Huxley; and writer and scientist Sir Charles (C.P.) Snow. Standing are Marsh Tenney, then dean of Dartmouth Medical School; Brock Chisholm, director-general of the World Health Organization; neurosurgeon Wilder Penfield; and Sir George Pickering, the Regius Professor of Medicine at Oxford University. Photo credit: Dartmouth College Archives.

Preface

In selecting a title for Dartmouth Medical School's Bicentennial Symposium, the Symposium Planning Committee continued a Dartmouth tradition of contemplating the large issues of the time. In 1947—exactly 50 years before the September 1997 Bicentennial Symposium that is represented in this volume—Dartmouth College President John Sloan Dickey initiated a course for undergraduates called "Great Issues." This course brought leading personages to Dartmouth to discuss the major issues of the day.

Then in 1960, Dartmouth Medical School held an international symposium to mark what has since been called the "refounding" of the School. Taking a lead from the undergraduate course, that symposium was called "Great Issues of Conscience in Modern Medicine," referring to the period in biomedicine—the late 1940s and the 1950s—when it became possible for physicians to maintain life by artificial means, a development that raised important philosophical questions.

It seemed fitting, therefore, to title the 1997 symposium "Great Issues for Medicine in the 21st Century." But tradition was not the determining factor in that choice. Rather, it was the fact that biomedicine continues to face ethical and social problems that are every bit as compelling today, at the dawn of the 21st century, as were those of earlier decades. In fact, the Symposium Planning Committee was struck that the overpopulation of our planet, which was identified as the number-one problem at the 1960 symposium, remains so today. The Committee chose the three other topics—genetics, neuroscience, and health care—not only because they are at the forefront of biomedical research, but equally because each raises major moral questions. In a sense, then, these proceedings are a record of some of the most significant problems confronting biomedicine at the turn of the century.

In editing this volume, we have tried to preserve and convey the congenial, informal atmosphere that prevailed during the Symposium. Therefore, most of the contributions appear here in the form of carefully edited transcripts of the speakers' presentations rather than as formal papers. We have also kept the temporal references as the speakers delivered them — that is, with the present being September 1997 — and have interposed a reminder of that fact in square brackets as appropriate. In addition, we have augmented the presentations themselves with a commentary on each of the four topical sessions of the Symposium, written by a member of the Dartmouth faculty eminent in that discipline. These commentaries provide critical annotations to the presentations, summarizing the main points made by each speaker, relating the presentations to each other and to other work in the field, and bringing in any pertinent historical issues.

On behalf of the Symposium Planning Committee, Dartmouth Medical School, and Dartmouth College, we extend a final, deep thanks to Drs. Michael Brown and Joseph Goldstein for cochairing the Symposium, as well as to the speakers who agreed to explore these topics at the event and who helped to extend the discourse beyond those three days with their gracious willingness to participate in this published proceedings.

—DANA COOK GROSSMAN
—HEINZ VALTIN

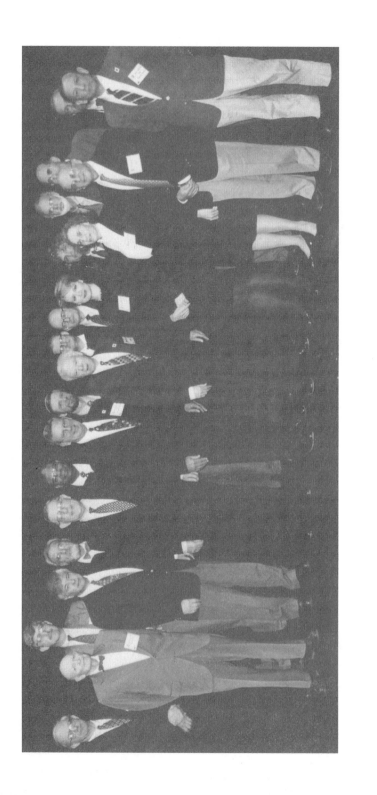

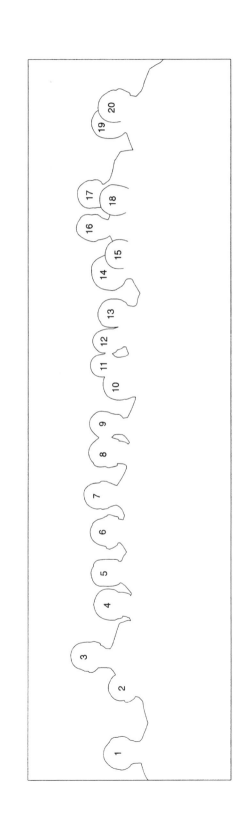

Speakers at the Dartmouth Medical School Symposium, September 5–7, 1999. (1) Michael S. Teitelbaum, (2) S. Marsh Tenney, (3) Francis S. Collins, (4) Michael S. Brown (Symposium Co-chair), (5) C. Everett Koop, (6) James O. Freedman, (7) Lonnie R. Bristow, (8) Andrew G. Wallace, (9) Nils M.P. Daulaire, (10) Joseph L. Goldstein (Symposium Co-chair), (11) Robert G. Evans, (12) Gerald M. Edelman, (13) Susan G. Dentzer, (14) Steven Pinker, (15) Hania Zlotnik, (16) Marcus E. Raichle, (17) Richard Axel, (18) Pasko T. Rakic, (19) Philip Kitcher, (20) Heinz Valtin. *Not pictured*: David Botstein, Daniel J. Callahan, Thomas Homer-Dixon, Ruth B. Purtilo, William L. Roper, Sir David Weatherall, and Nancy Wexler. Photo courtesy of Flying Squirrel Graphics.

ACKNOWLEDGMENTS

The Symposium on which this volume is based was the result of three years' work by the Dartmouth Medical School Bicentennial Symposium Planning Committee. Its members were: Heinz Valtin (chair); Barbara T. Blough (vice chair); Jane A. Auger; Alfred A. Blum, Jr. (*ex officio*); George F. Cahill, Jr.; Alfonso Caramazza; Peter Chin; James O. Freedman (*ex officio*); Ronald M. Green; Dana Cook Grossman; Leslie P. Henderson; Marta Hristova; R. Peter Mogielnicki; Colette Roberts-Finn; James C. Strickler; Jeffrey S. Taube; S. Marsh Tenney; Pamela S. Van Siclen; Andrew G. Wallace (*ex officio*); and John H. Wasson.

We extend many thanks to George Cahill and Rosemary Lunardini for help with editing the session on genetics; to Megan McAndrew Cooper for preparing the biographies of the presenters; to the New York Academy of Sciences' Bill Boland for agreeing to publish these proceedings as an *Annals* volume and Justine Cullinan for shepherding the book through production; and to Deborah A. Donovan for her secretarial help.

And our deep gratitude goes to the following individuals and organizations for their generous financial support of the Symposium itself: Glaxo Wellcome, Inc.; the Kettering Family Foundation; the Offices of the President and the Provost of Dartmouth College; James C. Strickler; Peggy Y. Thomson and the late Andrew Thomson, Jr.; the Tuscarora Foundation, Inc.; and Mr. and Mrs. James D. Vail III.

—D.C.G. and H.V.

[*Dana Grossman and Heinz Valtin coedited these proceedings. Grossman is director of publications for the Medical School and editor of its quarterly magazine,* Dartmouth Medicine, *and was a member of the Symposium Planning Committee. Valtin, former chair of Dartmouth Medical School's Department of Physiology and now the Vail and Hampers Professor of Physiology Emeritus, chaired the Bicentennial Symposium Planning Committee.*]

Two Hundred Years of Medicine at Dartmouth

BARBARA T. BLOUGH AND DANA COOK GROSSMAN

Dartmouth Medical School, Hanover, New Hampshire 03755, USA

Like the fabled phoenix, Dartmouth Medical School has endured crisis after crisis, reinventing itself and surviving each time with renewed strength and spirit. The story starts in 1796 with Nathan Smith,[a] a young, Harvard-trained physician from Cornish, New Hampshire, whose patients were spread the length and breadth of the Upper Connecticut River Valley. Dr. Smith (FIG. 1) found that the distances among the scattered settlements made it hard to reach the sick when he was needed, and he reasoned that a medical school at the new college in Hanover would bring more physicians and improved medical care to the area.

That was essentially the argument Smith made in a letter of August 25, 1796, to the Trustees of Dartmouth College. Today it seems inconceivable that Dartmouth, itself poor and struggling for survival, would agree to start a school of medicine far from the sources of support enjoyed by the three existing schools—the University of Pennsylvania (founded in 1765) in Philadelphia, King's College [Columbia] (1767) in New York, and Harvard (1782) in Boston. But in an extraordinary leap of faith, the Trustees did just that, commencing more than 200 years of continuous medical education at Dartmouth. The Board may have been swayed by Smith's promises to prepare himself by studying at his own expense in Edinburgh, Scotland (then the world's center of medical knowledge), to contribute his own laboratory and classroom equipment to the effort, and to teach all the courses himself.

Although the Trustees delayed his formal faculty appointment for nearly two years, Dr. Smith moved swiftly and began lecturing on November 22, 1797. For the first two years, he taught in a rented house; in 1799, the College gave him a room in Dartmouth Hall. Such were the Medical School's beginnings—one man, one room, and, at the outset, a handful of students.

But Nathan Smith was a gifted teacher, ahead of his time in medical theory and practice, and passionately committed to a scientific approach to medicine. Within a few years, as his reputation spread, he had all the students he could handle. He also continued his practice, taking students along with him on horseback as he treated his far-flung patients. In addition, his lectures were so popular with undergraduates (among them, Daniel Webster) that he is credited with introducing science into the College's curriculum; the 1806 catalog lists 45 medical students and 36 undergraduates in his classes.

Finances were a problem from the beginning. The College, chronically underfunded itself, could provide little help until 1805, when Dr. Smith was offered a salary of $200. Earlier, at Smith's request, the New Hampshire legislature had given

---

[a]The first truly full-scale biography of Nathan Smith was published shortly after the Bicentennial Symposium, as another of the School's anniversary observances. Titled *Improve, Perfect, & Perpetuate: Dr. Nathan Smith and Early American Medical Education,* it was written by Oliver S. Hayward, M.D., and Constance E. Putnam and published by University Press of New England (Hanover, NH, 1998).

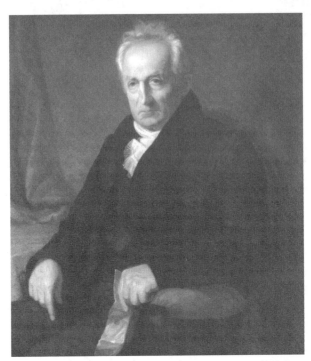

FIGURE 1. Nathan Smith, who single-handedly founded Dartmouth Medical School, played a role in the founding of three other schools, leading historians to dub him the "Johnny Appleseed of American medicine." Courtesy of the Hood Museum of Art, Dartmouth College.

him $600 for medical equipment, so when the space in Dartmouth Hall became clearly inadequate he turned to the state again. Recognizing the value of a medical school to the state, the legislature awarded him $3,450 towards construction of a three-story building. Completed in 1811, the "New Medical House" was one of the first buildings in the nation constructed specifically for the purpose of medical education (FIG. 2).

For 13 years, Nathan Smith carried the full burden of planning, administration, and teaching; then, in 1810, the Trustees hired a second faculty member. With a little breathing room, Smith turned his attention to upgrading the level of medical education. In 1812, he revised the curriculum and qualified the School to award the M.D. degree in place of only a bachelor of medicine, following Harvard in this move by one year.

This achievement was essentially the last in Smith's extraordinary career at Dartmouth. He left in 1813 to play a role in the founding of a medical school at Yale, returned briefly in 1816, and left again to help found two more medical schools—at Bowdoin and the University of Vermont. He died in 1829, a legend in his own time. Described by William Welch as "one of the most interesting and important figures in American medicine," Smith has also been called "the Johnny Appleseed of Amer-

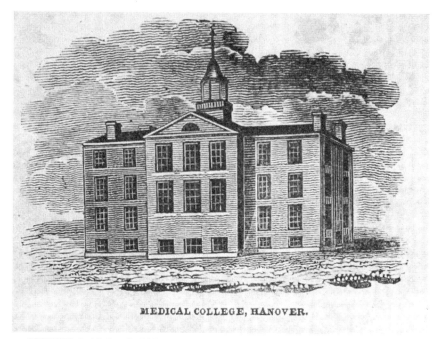

MEDICAL COLLEGE, HANOVER.

FIGURE 2. Nathan Smith's "New Medical House," built in 1811, served as Dartmouth Medical School's primary building for more than 150 years.

ican medicine" for his unmatched role in the establishment of no less than four medical schools.

Most of the faculty who succeeded Smith at Dartmouth were former students of his, including, in 1838, Dr. Dixi Crosby, a multitalented dynamo who gave the community its first hospital, a converted house called simply "Dr. Dixi's Hospital." Another new arrival in 1838 was the eminent poet-physician, Dr. Oliver Wendell Holmes, who during his two years on the Dartmouth faculty introduced the study of histology and the use of the stethoscope to the U.S. medical curriculum. Unlike Holmes, who returned to Boston in 1840, Dr. Crosby spent his entire career in Hanover. When he retired in 1870, his hospital closed, leaving a void that was not filled for 23 years. He had, however, established a new level in the interrelationship between patient care and teaching.

Selected to replace Dr. Crosby was Dr. Carlton Pennington Frost, an 1857 graduate of Dartmouth Medical School (DMS) and a leader very much in the Smith mold. Under his administration, the old lecture-apprenticeship system of instruction was changed to a full four-year program of combined academic and clinical instruction. Dr. Frost not only brought the School abreast of the times academically but was largely responsible for founding Mary Hitchcock Memorial Hospital. Shortly after Dr. Dixi's Hospital closed, Frost and his faculty formed the Dartmouth Hospital Association and set about acquiring land and funding. It was 19 years, however, before Frost persuaded his friend Hiram Hitchcock, a wealthy New York hotelier with a

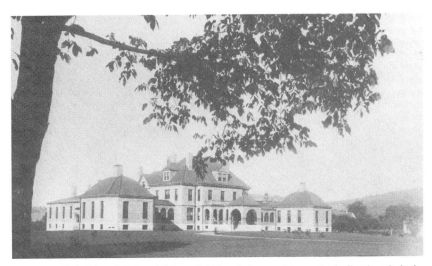

FIGURE 3. Mary Hitchcock Memorial Hospital, one of the nation's first hospitals designed on the pavilion plan, opened with 36 beds in 1893.

home in Hanover, to underwrite the project. Finished in 1893, the thoroughly modern 36-bed hospital was one of the first in the country built on the pavilion plan and was, from the beginning, intimately associated with the Medical School and its teaching program (FIG. 3).

A few years later, a significant contribution to American medicine emerged from Hanover. In February of 1896, just weeks after Wilhelm Roentgen had announced his discovery of X-rays, the first diagnostic use of the new technology in America was made in a laboratory at Dartmouth by Dr. Gilman Frost and his physicist brother, Edwin—both of them sons of Carlton.

By the turn of the century, there were 150 medical schools in the United States (compared to 125 today), and Dartmouth's was considered one of the best, its graduates consistently placing in the first rank on examinations. For a hundred years Dartmouth had been a leader in the continuing effort to improve medical education. It was ironic, therefore, that soon a drive to strengthen clinical teaching would affect Dartmouth adversely.

A national study begun in 1908 by the Carnegie Foundation looked at medical education in terms of the new emphasis on bedside teaching, which required large numbers of patients and varieties of illnesses. Concluding that the patient pool of this remote and thinly populated area was insufficient for clinical training, the Foundation's Flexner Committee recommended that Dartmouth abandon the M.D. program and merely offer preclinical instruction.

This was a bitter pill for the College and the Medical School, but the justice of the Committee's criticism could not be denied and, on April 26, 1913, the Trustees voted that "the clinical years of the course in Medicine be *suspended for the present*" and that resources be concentrated "upon the first two years of the course, *which may be elected by undergraduates of the College.*" The wording (emphasis added) clearly indicated the College's desire to eventually reinstate the M.D. program and its commitment to a continuing relationship between the medical and the undergraduate programs.

The Class of 1914 was the last (until 1973) to receive the M.D. degree; subsequent students, upon finishing the two-year program in the medical sciences, transferred for the two clinical years to other schools, primarily Harvard, Cornell, Penn, and a few others. Dartmouth Medical School had entered a new phase with its reputation for excellence intact and the intense loyalty of its students preserved.

As the clinical faculty gradually left, the Hospital began to have difficulty recruiting well-trained physicians and specialists because it was unable to offer positions with academic appointments. In 1927, Dr. John Bowler arrived from the Mayo Clinic to become dean of the Medical School and moved quickly to remedy this problem. He and four colleagues formed the Hitchcock Clinic, a group practice arrangement then relatively new; it soon reversed the Hospital's talent drain and raised the quality of medical care for the entire region.

Dr. Bowler, in addition to directing the Clinic, remained as dean until 1945, when he was succeeded by Dr. Rolf Syvertsen, a 1923 graduate of DMS. "Dr. Sy," as he was known to students and townspeople alike, concentrated all his attention on his 48 students, whom he had known as Dartmouth premedical advisees and had personally chosen for admittance to DMS. He was a stern but affectionate surrogate parent to his "boys," and alumni from his era still tell humorous and reverential "Sy stories." Dr. Syvertsen died in an automobile accident in 1960, just as the Medical School was confronting another challenge.

Since 1914, through two world wars and the Depression, the Medical School had had a superb record for the caliber of its two-year program, with graduates consistently distinguishing themselves at their transfer schools. But changes were again taking place in medical education, putting the School at yet another crossroads.

Since the end of World War II, medical education had slowly but inexorably reflected increasing emphasis on research. Dartmouth had come in for criticism because the faculty was small and had little interest in research and because the student body came almost entirely from Dartmouth College. These complaints eventually led the Association of American Medical Colleges and the Council on Medical Education to place the School on "confidential probation" in 1956. Once again, the Trustees were faced with a major decision.

Actually, the College, recognizing the handwriting on the wall, had already begun to make plans for revitalizing the Medical School and now restated its commitment to medical education and to securing new capital for expansion of DMS's faculty, facilities, and programs. In 1956, the Trustees authorized the "refounding" of DMS and invited Dr. S. Marsh Tenney, a 1944 graduate of the Medical School and a physiologist renowned for his research on human adaptation to high altitudes, to take on that herculean but overwhelmingly successful effort.

The transformation in the School affected both program and plant: In a span of just a few years, faculty and student body were more than doubled; women were admitted; new departments were added; and a medical sciences building, biomedical library, auditorium, and dormitory were constructed. The faculty was augmented by scientist-teachers with strong research capabilities, and enrollment was opened to the best candidates in the country, not just graduates of Dartmouth College. In addition, programs leading to the Ph.D. in several biomedical disciplines were introduced, in accord with the view that the Medical School and the College both had a good deal to gain by pooling their intellectual resources.

The refounding was celebrated in 1960 with a three-day symposium on which the 1997 Bicentennial Symposium was modeled. The 1960 event, whose honorary chair was René Dubos, brought to Hanover a slate of speakers that included Sir Charles (C.P.) Snow, Aldous Huxley, Sir George Pickering, and Brock Chisholm (see photo accompanying the Preface).

The refounding had restored the strength and vigor of Nathan Smith's vision but not yet the M.D. program. That was left to the next crisis, which was just around the corner. Once again, a nationwide change in medical education particularly affected Dartmouth. For some 50 years, the graduates of the two-year program had enjoyed easy access to the M.D. schools of their choice. But now the four-year schools, in response to a nationwide shortage of physicians and government incentives to increase the size of their entering classes, no longer had room for transfers. At the same time, educators determined that students should be introduced to patients early in their training and that basic science teaching should be reinforced throughout the entire program. These curricular revisions also worked against third-year transfers. The well-trained Dartmouth students began to find it hard to get accepted at top schools. It was obvious that the two-year school had a doubtful future.

Fortunately, changes in the surrounding community had been taking place as well. Mary Hitchcock Memorial Hospital had become a major referral center with over 400 beds, serving a population of 300,000 as one of only two academic medical centers in northern New England. The concept of the intensive care unit had been pioneered at Hitchcock in 1955 by Dr. William Mosenthal, a surgeon who still teaches anatomy to DMS students. The Veterans Administration Hospital in nearby White River Junction, Vermont, affiliated with the Medical School since 1945, provided another 224 beds. The Hitchcock Clinic was recording over 144,000 outpatient visits annually. All of these developments made a full-scale medical school once again quite possible.

So in April of 1968, the College Trustees voted to reinstate the M.D. program, "subject only to the development of the necessary funding." With a speed and commitment reminiscent of Nathan Smith, then-Dean Carleton Chapman and the faculty undertook massive fund-raising, construction, and curriculum-planning programs. New departments were created, additional faculty recruited, an M.D. curriculum designed, and, with the help of several major donors, the physical plant further expanded. Also during this period, the Medical School, the Hospital, and the Clinic began planning the formation of an overarching governing mechanism, leading to the birth of Dartmouth-Hitchcock Medical Center. In 1970, Dartmouth admitted its first M.D. candidates in 60 years and entered the modern era of its long history.

Today, just over a quarter of a century later, the Medical School is stronger than ever. It selects its first-year class of about 75 M.D. students from over 7,000 applicants and is recognized nationally for the excellence of its teaching. Several of its research programs have national reputations, and it ranks in the top 20% nationwide in federal research funding per basic science faculty member. Its Center for the Evaluative Clinical Sciences, directed by outcomes research pioneer Dr. John Wennberg, established the first graduate program in the country in the evaluative clinical sciences. DMS is also recognized for its emphasis on the art as well as the science of medicine and for its students' commitment to community service. In 1995, Dartmouth received the American Medical Student Association's Paul R. Wright Award for community service, and 80% of first- and second-year medical students do some sort of volunteer work in the region.

With about 300 M.D. students, 100 Ph.D. candidates (including several in an M.D./Ph.D. program), and 75 master's and doctoral candidates in the clinical evaluative sciences, DMS is of such a size that interdisciplinary collaborations can easily flourish. Its size also fosters close student-faculty relationships—a factor that is surely responsible in part for the fact that on a recent Association of American Medical Colleges survey of graduating medical students, 53% of DMS graduates professed themselves "very satisfied" with their education—compared to 35% nationally.

Through the mid and late 1990s, the School put in place the final phases of a comprehensive new curriculum known as "New Directions." Among its key facets are much small-group and interactive learning; greatly reduced lecture time; early and ongoing contact with patients through the Longitudinal Clinical Experience, which pairs each medical student from the first week of first year with a primary-care clinician in the region; and reinforcement of key scientific concepts in a fourth-year course called Advanced Medical Science. And long popular with students are clinical rotations in such diverse locations as the Navajo reservation in Arizona and the Indian Health Service hospital in Bethel, Alaska.

The Medical School also has a significant resource in its clinical partners in Dartmouth-Hitchcock Medical Center (DHMC)—a network of unusual breadth. The Hitchcock Clinic, one of the largest physician-managed group practices in the country, has practice sites spread through New Hampshire and parts of Vermont. And Mary Hitchcock Memorial Hospital has spearheaded a cooperative relationship—not a merger but a working affiliation—among a number of smaller health-care providers in northern New England under the Hitchcock Alliance. The White River Junction Veterans Affairs Hospital is also a key component in the Medical Center's research and teaching effort, and it is home to the VA's national centers for ethics, post-traumatic stress disorder, and quality improvement.

The three New Hampshire-based partners in DHMC boast a stunning new clinical and research facility in the Dartmouth-Hitchcock Medical Center complex opened in 1991 in Lebanon, New Hampshire. But the Center's focus is regionwide; its many outreach programs bring the highest quality care and latest technology into small communities throughout northern New England.

Conceived 200 years ago as a medical voice in the wilderness, strengthened by adversity, and looking to the future with confidence, Dartmouth Medical School clearly continues to be guided by the vision of Nathan Smith.

Opening Session

Welcoming Remarks

ANDREW G. WALLACE

Dean, Dartmouth Medical School, Hanover, New Hampshire 03755, USA

Friends of Dartmouth, faculty, students, and distinguished guests, I have the extraordinary privilege this morning of welcoming all of you to the Dartmouth campus and of declaring that Dartmouth Medical School's Bicentennial Symposium is hereby open.

Today, President Freedman and I enjoy a quite unusual position among university presidents and medical school deans. We are only the fourth such officers in our country's history to have the opportunity of presiding at a 200th birthday of one of her medical schools.

The pride we share in this historic event is exceeded by very few things, but certainly among them are the ambition conveyed by the title of our symposium, "Great Issues for Medicine in the 21st Century," plus the anticipation of engaging with speakers who have contributed so uniquely to what the future actually holds and who, in the true spirit of professionalism, possess special insight into the ethical and social issues arising out of advances in science.

Before I go any further, I want to pause a moment and express profound thanks from all of us to Heinz Valtin, professor of physiology emeritus at Dartmouth Medical School and chair of the Symposium Planning Committee; to Nobel Laureates Joseph Goldstein and Michael Brown, the co-chairs of this symposium; to Barbara Blough, vice chair of the Symposium Planning Committee; and to the rest of the team that has worked tirelessly for three years toward this meeting. This event, this theme, and the talent assembled to challenge all of us could not have happened without them. We are very, very grateful!

The history of Dartmouth Medical School has been told more than once this bicentennial year, and I will not recite it again here. However, I invite you to take a moment to travel back in time with me to the School's founding in 1797 and to reflect on that time and on what has transpired since.

George Washington completed his presidency in the winter of 1797, and John Adams was inaugurated as the second president of the United States. Thomas Jefferson, Adams's opponent in that election, won the second largest number of electoral votes and so, as was the custom, became vice president. Napoleon won a dazzling series of victories in Italy, bringing an end to the French Revolution. It was the year that composer Franz Schubert and author Mary Shelley were born. Edward Jenner had just reported immunity to smallpox among milkmaids who had been infected with cowpox, laying the foundation for inoculation therapy. Dartmouth College was 28 years old. John Wheelock, son of founder Eleazar Wheelock, was the College's president.

Nathan Smith, a physician from Cornish, N.H., had petitioned the College trustees the year before to allow him to start a medical school in Hanover. Smith began

1

his lectures in the fall of 1797. There were two medical students enrolled in his course, but undergraduates attended his lectures as well. Among them was Daniel Webster. From my perspective, the essential connectedness between the College and its medical school, which is one of the themes we celebrate here, began on that first day of classes.

Even the title of this symposium has its roots in Dartmouth history. Exactly 50 years ago, College President John Sloan Dickey initiated a course for undergraduates called "Great Issues." It was a course that brought distinguished individuals from outside Dartmouth to the campus to discuss and share their views on major issues of the day.

And in 1960, when Dartmouth Medical School was "refounded," an international symposium to mark the event was held in Hanover. It was called "Great Issues of Conscience in Modern Medicine."

When the planning committee conceived of this symposium, it returned again to the title "Great Issues"—this time "Great Issues for Medicine in the 21st Century." And they added a very important subtitle: "A Consideration of the Ethical and Social Issues Arising Out of Advances in the Biomedical Sciences."

As was true in President Dickey's day and in his course, and as was true at the 1960 symposium, we have an extraordinary array of speakers to challenge us. Many of these men and women have made profound contributions to our understanding of biology and medicine. Others have made equally profound contributions to our philosophical thinking about life on this planet and the place of science and medicine in our lives.

These are people who look at the world and ask how it might be better. They look at institutions and ask how they might be renewed. They have been risk-takers. One of the things they all share is that they are remarkable innovators.

It is with tremendous pride that I welcome all of you to this occasion, and with equal pride that I now introduce James O. Freedman, the 15th president of Dartmouth College, to add his welcome and his perspective on our theme.

Medical Education and the American Future

JAMES O. FREEDMAN

President, Dartmouth College, Hanover, New Hampshire 03755, USA

It is a very great pleasure to welcome this distinguished audience to the Bicentennial Symposium of Dartmouth Medical School, the fourth oldest medical school in the United States.

We gather at a time when medical education faces new and vigorous challenges, even as it is a time when it has become fashionable to cast doubt upon the very idea of progress. To some, progress is nothing but a fiction fabricated by white male imperialists to conceal the terrible realities of power and oppression. To others, progress is no more than a chimera of Enlightenment theory, its possibilities most typically thwarted by human selfishness and myopia. Without commenting on the more subtle permutations of these dubious views, I feel confident in declaring that the first 200 years of Dartmouth Medical School's existence provide indisputable evidence of the authenticity of progress in the sphere of medical education.

On August 25, 1796, Nathan Smith, a 33-year-old practitioner from Cornish, New Hampshire, petitioned Dartmouth's Board of Trustees to allow him to establish, in his own words, "a medical school in this college." Noting that New Hampshire was without such a school, Smith proposed that he travel to Edinburgh and "attend to the several branches of medicine as taught and practised there." Then, upon his return, he would, with the board's consent, teach the art and science of medicine at Dartmouth.

The Board of Trustees concurred, and in the following year, 1797, Nathan Smith, having duly studied at Edinburgh, founded Dartmouth Medical School. That initial year he lectured in a small, two-story house on College Street; his entire annual budget was $160. Two years later, the trustees assigned him Room 6 in Dartmouth Hall. In 1803, they gave Smith a second room, and the New Hampshire legislature granted him $600 for equipment.

The School, during those earliest days, was chronically underfinanced. But in 1811, Smith's lobbying efforts finally succeeded when the legislature appropriated $3,450 for a new building, provided Smith himself donate the land on which to erect the structure, as well as his own laboratory as equipment for the School. For its first 10 years, Nathan Smith was Dartmouth Medical School's only faculty member, and he taught the entire course of study.

Yet even under such austere conditions, Smith impressed the proper authorities. After attending one of Smith's lectures, Dartmouth's second president, John Wheelock, is said to have offered this prayer in the College chapel: "O Lord, we thank Thee for the Oxygen Gas; we thank Thee for the Hydrogen Gas; and for all the gases. We thank Thee for the Cerebrum; we thank Thee for the Cerebellum; and for the Medulla Oblongata. Amen."

I dare not attempt to live up to my predecessor's spiritual powers and rhetorical gifts, but I delight in being able to welcome you to a larger and better endowed Dartmouth Medical School, and I note that the title of this bicentennial symposium, "Great Issues for Medicine in the 21st Century," speaks to our shared commitment to the idea of progress. I say "commitment to" rather than "faith in" because all of us recognize that progress is not inevitable; it does not just happen. But we also recognize that it is possible and that it does occur, as the breathtaking scientific advances in modern medicine attest.

In celebrating this bicentennial, we commemorate achievements that are the result of a historical process of interaction between human will and social forces—an interaction that surely represents progress, even if it may have been halting and uncertain at various points along the way.

For most of this century, from 1914 to 1970, Dartmouth Medical School administered a two-year program and did not grant the M.D. degree. In 1956, the Association of American Medical Colleges threatened to revoke the School's "Class A" rating, placing the future of even the two-year program in jeopardy. But just 16 short months later, S. Marsh Tenney, a 1944 Dartmouth graduate who had returned to the Medical School and was serving as its director of medical sciences, invited the survey team back to Hanover. They removed the probation, convinced of the importance and vitality of Dartmouth Medical School—a vitality it has continued to exhibit in the years since that time. Meanwhile, the medical world itself was undergoing tremendous change.

Twenty-five years ago, in 1972, Dean Carleton B. Chapman marked the School's 175th anniversary by noting the then-current "uncertainties concerning federal funding, problems with planning for health-care delivery, and numerous strange new currents in medical and health education." How familiar that litany sounds today. The particulars may have changed, but the prevailing sense of tension and of tentativeness about the future of medical education seems to have remained constant.

This symposium, then, rests upon a frank avowal that progress is not without challenge. The purpose of the symposium is to confront our own period of uncertainty with the kind of thoughtful discussion that makes genuine progress possible.

Professor Dudley Herschbach, the Nobel Prize-winning chemist at Harvard, recently summed up, with unsettling irony, the greatest problem that medical education, and the practice of medicine as a whole, now faces: "Our profession has an ancient watchword: 'First, do no harm.' With managed health care, we can do better. Henceforth, let us boldly act on the first law of New Medicine: 'First, do nothing.'" Professor Herschbach's statement suggests two important questions. First, how can we preserve the highest possible standards of health care when physicians and patients may gradually be losing some of their authority to make vital decisions? Second, how should we educate future physicians to function in the new and evolving environment of managed care and health-care reform?

By this point in the development of medicine's changing environment, we are well aware of the economic pressures to increase the number of primary-care physicians and to reduce the number of specialists and subspecialists. We are also aware of the reductions in support for graduate medical education, clinical training, and basic research—changes that have occurred as federal funding authorities have sought to control costs at teaching hospitals.

These developments are profoundly troubling. As Clifton R. Wharton, Jr., former chancellor of the State University of New York and former chairman of TIAA-

CREF, has said, "Experiences that have heretofore been considered part of the teaching mission of traditional hospitals and health-science centers are not seen as integral to the mission of many of the new institutions of health-care delivery. At the same time, established hospitals can compete with the new institutions only by way of the most rigorous cost-containment efforts. Not surprisingly, the most vulnerable targets of cost-cutters are often programs associated with the teaching function."

Once we recognize the growing extent to which economic concerns now encroach upon scientific and educational goals in the practice and teaching of medicine, we begin to appreciate the pertinence that many other disciplines have to medical education. Professor Herschbach's witticism was directed to the economics of managed care, but his statement has a broader reach; it is fundamentally an ethical pronouncement.

As new economics and new technologies reshape the practice and possibilities of medicine, the field of medical ethics necessarily commands a more central role in medical education. And not only ethics, but many other disciplines in the social sciences and humanities—psychology, sociology, history, anthropology—increasingly assert their relevance.

In such circumstances, there must surely be a temptation to avoid the pressure of dealing with so many different disciplines by maintaining, rather than broadening, the current scope of medical education. "Confronted by such problems," President Derek Bok of Harvard wrote in his annual report for 1983, "doctors could easily react by clinging resolutely to their traditional role as applied scientists seeking accurate biomedical explanations for a patient's disease. After all, it is hard enough to cope with the mounting complexity of the biosciences without having to take account of computers, decision trees, health care regulations, ethical constraints, and the vagaries of patient psychology."

But such a narrow definition of the physician's role, even if its stated purpose is to maintain professional autonomy, in the end would clearly compromise that autonomy by ceding authority to bureaucrats and technocrats. Physicians would be consulted principally for their "scientific" opinions, and fundamental decisions concerning patient care and research—often life-and-death decisions—would be left to others: employers, managed-care bureaucrats, benefits administrators, and government officials. If physicians are to be in a position to make their voices appropriately heard, medical education must broaden its conception of the physician's role.

For these reasons, it is essential that medical education, as an academic discipline, conceive of itself as a form of liberal education. The purpose of medical education, whether at a liberal arts college like Dartmouth or at the largest of research universities, is to train men and women in the art of healing and caring. But to heal and to care requires more than scientific expertise, more than technical skill; it requires a rich understanding of human beings, an idealistic engagement with values, and an exposure to the humane lessons of the social sciences and the humanities, not merely as "window dressing," but also as respected parts of the curriculum.

As John Sloan Dickey, the twelfth president of Dartmouth, put it when he spoke at Dartmouth's convocation entitled "Great Issues of Conscience in Modern Medicine" in 1960, "Any man who aspires to minister greatly to any human ill, or need, must be more than merely a skilled professional. Liberal learning is that transcending more, which however it is acquired, gives all callings the possibility of greatness."

At a time when patients are increasingly worried that their best interests may be sacrificed to the imperatives of cost-cutting, the broader perspective that the liberal arts provide becomes especially critical.

The imperative of cost containment is a perfect example of the interaction between social forces and human will, and, as such, reveals the challenges tomorrow's physicians will face. Doctors will need their training in the liberal arts more and more if they are to strike a balance between these two equally compelling forces. It will be incumbent upon physicians to call upon the values of a liberal education in shaping medicine's agenda in the next century, in making their decisions with professional integrity, and in explaining with compassion those decisions to their patients.

Not even the most fervent medical humanist would suggest, of course, that medical schools become liberal arts colleges. But many medical school deans and other members of medical school faculties have urged that the agenda for medical education be shaped by physicians who approach their calling as a liberal art, as an interdisciplinary field of inquiry and practice.

One of Dartmouth College's most accomplished graduates, Dr. Charles E. Odegaard, former president of the University of Washington, has provocatively argued that "medicine is not a science. It is not the function of the physician, *qua* physician, to know; it is his function to acquire a background of knowledge relevant to the problems of patients and then to act in diagnosis, prognosis, and therapy for his particular patient. The physician can gain knowledge from social or behavioral scientists and from humanists relevant to patient care, which may then be used for the potential benefit for the patient."

Medical schools, it should be said, have an important influence on undergraduate education, not least in their admissions policies. In recent years, medical schools have sent gratifying signals that they no longer favor only those applicants who have followed a strict premed course of study, and that they especially welcome applicants who have prepared themselves broadly in the liberal arts.

Medical schools have also sent gratifying signals of their commitment to diversity, reflecting their belief that a diverse student body provides an education in empathy that is essential for establishing compassionate physician-patient relationships. However, African-Americans and members of other minority groups remain underrepresented in the pool of medical school applicants. And that is why medical schools must continue to make known to prospective applicants their strong interest in training a diverse medical profession to provide care for a diverse society.

The successful recruitment of minority medical students will require sustained efforts at all levels of education, as it will also require continued experimentation with intervention programs among high school and college students. These efforts are especially necessary at a time when some seek to dismantle affirmative action programs in this country.

The constitutional amendment prohibiting affirmative action by state agencies in California and the *Hopwood* decision banning affirmative action in academic admissions programs in Texas are discouraging steps backwards on the road to the American ideal of equality. We already know the alarming results at the University of California at San Diego's School of Medicine, where none of the 197 black students who applied for admission this fall [1997] has been accepted; at the law school of the University of California at Berkeley, where only one black student is enrolled in this year's entering class of 270; and at the University of Texas Law School, where only four black students are expected to enroll in an entering class of 468. It would be devastating if other states and other courts were to follow suit.

Justice Harry A. Blackmun in his opinion in the *Bakke* case spoke wisely when he commented that "it would be impossible to arrange an affirmative action program in a racially neutral way and have it successful. To ask that this would be so is to demand the impossible. In order to get beyond racism, we must first take account of race. There is no other way. And in order to treat some persons equally, we must treat them differently."

It would be ironic, indeed, as Justice Blackmun further observed, to interpret the equal-protection clause of the 14th Amendment, which was adopted immediately after the Civil War in order to achieve equality for emancipated Negroes, in a manner that would "perpetuate racial supremacy."

And so it is these interrelated concerns—the threat that managed care poses for graduate medical education and basic research, the relevance of ethics and liberal education to the study of medicine, and the necessity of diversity in medical school student bodies—that present some of the greatest challenges, as well as some of the greatest opportunities for progress, today.

When Dean Chapman concluded his reflections on the first 175 years of Dartmouth Medical School, he took a look forward. "The next 25 years will bring the School to its bicentennial," he wrote. "No doubt some School stalwart, following Phineas Conner's example of 1897, will sum up the record for the two centuries at that time. What those final 25 years of the School's second century will contain no one can say, but it takes no great seer to perceive that they will be the most critical in the School's history; that the School will achieve undisputed greatness, will succumb, or will become something no longer identifiable as Dartmouth Medical School, defined in terms of 1972."

Our celebration belies any fear that Nathan Smith's bold and pioneering "medical school within this college" would succumb to the pressures of the late 20th century. And during the past 25 years, under the leadership of Deans Strickler, McCollum, and Wallace, Dartmouth Medical School has grown, adapted, and prospered without becoming an institution unrecognizable to the preceding generation.

As we contemplate the role of medical education in the American future, I am confident that Dartmouth Medical School will not succumb in the critical years that lie ahead; that it will remain identifiable to us as an integral part of Dartmouth's liberal arts environment; and that as it ventures forth into its third century, guided by the vision and commitment embodied in this symposium, it will prove still again the indisputable truth of progress.

Burgers, Chips, and Genes

JOSEPH L. GOLDSTEIN

Chair, Department of Molecular Genetics, and Paul J. Thomas Professor of Medicine and Genetics, University of Texas Southwestern Medical Center at Dallas, Dallas, Texas 75235-9046, USA

The opportunity to present this opening lecture in celebration of the 200th anniversary of the founding of Dartmouth Medical School caused me to reflect back on my own 35-year career in medicine. I am impressed by one dominant and recurring theme—namely, how a few good ideas and the power of science can radically transform the way we live.

Thirty-five years ago, in September 1962, I began my first day of medical school at UT Southwestern Medical Center in Dallas. During my four years as a medical student, therapeutic medicine was primitive by today's standards. We had no H2 blockers for treating ulcers, no calcium channel blockers or ACE inhibitors for high blood pressure, no statins for high cholesterol, no Prozac for depression, and no vaccines for hepatitis or *Hemophilus influenza*. There were no bone marrow transplants, liver transplants, or heart transplants. Coronary bypass operations and coronary angioplasty did not exist. There were no CAT scans or MRIs. Alzheimer's disease was considered an extremely rare disorder, described briefly in *Harrison's Principles of Internal Medicine* (4th edition, 1962) and not even mentioned in *Cecil-Loeb's Textbook of Medicine* (11th edition, 1963). AIDS did not exist, and sickle cell anemia was the only inherited disease that had been studied at a molecular level. We had no personal computers, and there were only two Xerox machines in our entire medical school in 1962. But most amazing of all—there were no McDonald's restaurants in Dallas. Imagine medical students today without Big Macs!

And this brings me to the theme of this presentation: that the world in general and the world of medicine in particular have been radically changed by three turns of events: burgers, chips, and genes. Let me explain.

BURGERS

First, the hamburger. I ate my first Big Mac in 1968 while I was a resident in medicine at the Massachusetts General Hospital. McDonald's had just opened its first restaurant in Boston. Since the early 1960s, McDonald's has grown from several restaurants in California to 23,000 restaurants in 101 countries throughout the world. Every day, 7% of the U.S. population eats in McDonald's. McDonald's serves 30 million people in the world each day and sells 5 billion hamburgers each year. McDonald's owns more real estate than any other company or person in the world. A new McDonald's opens somewhere in the world every three hours, and each restaurant is in the center of the four-minute universe, which means that in the next few years everyone in the world is going to be no more than a four-minute walk or drive from a McDonald's.[1,2]

If I had bought 100 shares of McDonald's stock after I ate my first hamburger 29 years ago, my investment of $2,000 would be worth about $2,000,000 today. In those days, $2,000 was one-half my annual salary as a medical resident. The genius of Ray Kroc, the founder of McDonald's, was his discovery that people wanted to be served in 60 seconds and his creativity in franchising fast food restaurants.[3] Of all the remarkable things that have happened since I began medical school, McDonald's is the best example of how one good idea by one person can change the way we live. Or, as Woody Allen might say: This is an example of the transmutation of life—by a lowly hamburger.

CHIPS

So much for burgers. Now for the chips, the second McDonald's-like transmutation that has occurred since I entered medical school 35 years ago. Burgers were not invented in Dallas, but chips were, not by Frito-Lay, but by Texas Instruments. I am referring to the silicon chips of the type that led to the revolution in microelectronics and to the birth of the personal computer, the Internet, and the World Wide Web.

In 1959, Jack Kilby, an electronic engineer at Texas Instruments in Dallas, hit on the ingenious idea of integrating all the transistors and other components of an electrical circuit on a single miniature flake of silicon.[4,5] Each silicon chip was only about a quarter-inch square in size, but it did the work of multiple transistors. The idea of the integrated circuit solved the most important engineering problem of this century: It was now possible to create a complex network of electrical circuits without having to wire together multiple transistors.

The first major practical application of the wireless chip came 30 years ago in 1967, when Texas Instruments introduced the first pocket calculator, weighing only 2.5 pounds and having all the electronic transistors squeezed onto a single silicon chip designed by Jack Kilby.[5] At about the same time, Robert Noyce and Gordon Moore founded Intel Corporation in the Palo Alto area with the then-daring idea that they could further miniaturize Kilby's integrated circuit and produce a micropro-grammable computer on a chip that was about the size of the head of a pin—the so-called memory microchip.[6] The rest is history.[4]

Without microchips, there would be no car phones, no cash cards, and no personal computers, not to mention the Internet. The typical American home contains 50 microchips. There are microchips in your microwave, microchips in your doorbell, and microchips in your VCR. In the last five years, the production of microchips and computers accounted for 45% of U.S. industrial growth. By common consent, the Information Revolution created by the microchip industry has been the most life-changing technological revolution since the harnessing of steam power in the 18th century and electricity in the 19th century. Imagine medicine today without CAT scans, PET scans, or MRIs.

GENES

Now let me tell you about the newest McDonald's-like transmutation, one that is changing biomedical science and clinical medicine in ways that will be just as profound as the way McDonald's changed the eating habits of the world and microchips changed the way we devour information.

When I began medical school in 1962, the gene had not yet become a household word. No one had ever isolated a gene or seen a gene. Genes could not be purified or put in a bottle. As medical students, we hardly ever heard about genes or chromosomes. Genetic diseases were believed to be extremely rare, and medical genetics was not considered sufficiently important to be taught as a course in the curriculum. Only three of the 100 medical schools in the U.S. had postdoctoral specialty training in medical genetics.

The year that I graduated from medical school, 1966, was a turning point in the history of genetics. This was the year that the genetic code was completely deciphered. Six years later, in 1972, the technique of recombinant DNA was discovered. By the early 1980s, scientists had perfected the techniques to clone and sequence individual genes and to study their action in living cells of animals and humans. Today, genes can be cloned, sequenced, weighed, counted, visualized, replicated, altered in test tubes, and shuttled from cell to cell in animals and humans. These phenomenal advances could never have arisen without two prior decades of what many considered at the time to be esoteric basic research in pure enzymology. This so-called esoteric research produced the polymerases, ligases, reverse transcriptases, and restriction endonucleases that are the key reagents used by scientists every day to manipulate genes.[7]

Today, manipulating genes is as easy as flipping burgers and surfing the Web. Every week, the front page of every major newspaper reports the discovery of a new disease-producing gene or a potentially new gene-based drug. We may soon live in a world where the Golden Arches yield center stage to the Golden Helices.

Our new power to manipulate genes will allow scientists to obtain the complete DNA sequence of the entire human genome—all 100,000 genes that make up the blueprint of you and me. The ultimate aim of the Human Genome Project is to read each person's genes like a book and discover which genes make Madonna so sexy and Jim Freedman, the president of Dartmouth College, so smart.

Great scientific discoveries in pure basic research virtually always lead to practical applications that benefit society. The birth of the microchip industry in the 1960s was a direct outgrowth of the discovery of the transistor in 1947 by Bardeen, Brattain, and Shockley at Bell Laboratories.[4] For the first few years after its discovery, the Bell Laboratory transistor was considered a laboratory curiosity for amplifying electrical signals and had no practical utility until Kilby hit upon the idea of integrating multiple transistors on a single chip.

Just as basic research on transistors led to the microchip industry, so basic research on genes has led to the creation of the biotechnology industry. The biotechnology industry began only 20 years ago, but even in this short period, its growth and influence, whether measured intellectually or economically, has been extremely impressive. Let me give you one striking example.

In 1975, the Rockefeller University, one of the great biomedical research institutions in the world, received its first payment for patent royalties in the amount of $500. Twenty years later, in 1995, the Rockefeller University received a payment of $20,000,000 from the biotechnology company Amgen for licensing rights to the gene sequence of a hormone called leptin, which is being used to develop a drug for

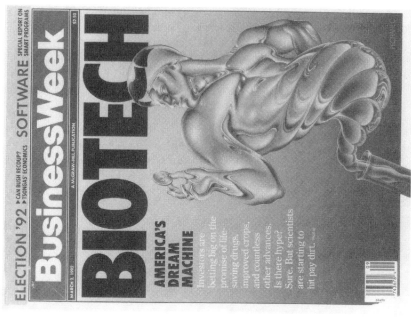

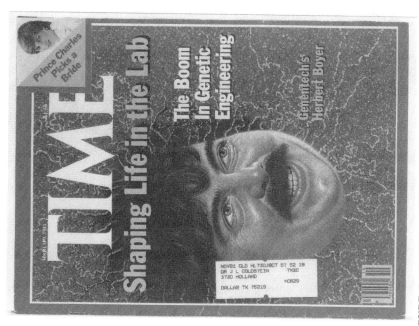

FIGURE 1. (*Left*) Cover of March 9, 1981 issue of *Time* magazine [reprinted by permission. ©1981 by Time-Life]. (*Right*) Cover of March 2, 1992 issue of *Business Week* [reprinted by special permission. ©1992 by McGraw-Hill Companies].

obesity. This phenomenal increase from $500 to $20,000,000 in 20 years is a dramatic example of how the biotechnology industry is changing the style and practice of biomedical research in medical schools and research institutions. (The payment to the Rockefeller University of $500 in 1975 was based on a patent awarded to the Nobel Prize-winning immunologist Gerald Edelman, who is also a participant in this symposium, and who had developed a new method in which antibodies directed against cell surface antigens were attached to nylon fibers for use in isolating intact cells.[8])

BIOTECHNOLOGY AND SURREALISM

In the remainder of my presentation, I will discuss the biotechnology industry, focusing on its dreams and its realities for medicine in the next century. Much of the success of the biotechnology revolution can be attributed to the industry's *style* of operation. Biotechnologists have assumed a style that is reminiscent of an earlier revolution in art called surrealism.[9] Like the surrealist artists of the 1930s and 1940s, today's most creative scientists live and think in a world of fantasy and dreams.

The general public was first introduced to the potential importance of biotechnology on March 9, 1981, when *Time* magazine published a lead story entitled "Shaping Life in the Lab." FIGURE 1 (left) shows the cover of this issue of *Time*, which featured a picture of Herbert Boyer, the scientific cofounder of Genentech, the first major biotechnology company. A notable feature of this *Time* cover is the fact that the engagement of Princess Diana to Prince Charles was apparently deemed less newsworthy than "The Boom in Genetic Engineering" and was thus relegated to the upper right corner of the cover.

In the ensuing decade, many articles on biotechnology were published in all types of magazines read by the lay public. FIGURE 1 (right) shows a cover from the March 2, 1992, issue of *Business Week* that reflects the excitement and hype that the biotechnology revolution had generated in its first decade of existence. In this surrealistic cover picture, the genie in the test tube is delivering the golden egg.

Like journalists, many prominent scientists became seduced by the euphoria of the biotechnology revolution, and they made a number of bold predictions which are listed in TABLE 1. These include:

(1) *Worldwide Shortage of Paper*: Sequencing all 3×10^9 base pairs of DNA that constitute the human genome will produce a severe paper shortage, owing to the in-

TABLE 1. Bold predictions by prominent scientists stimulated by the euphoria of the biotechnology revolution

1. Worldwide shortage of paper

2. Sexual harassment by robots

3. Drugs without side effects

4. Organ replacement with biologically synthesized cells

5. Individual genomes on compact discs (CDs)

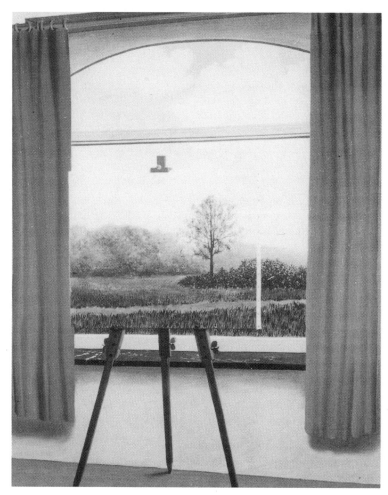

FIGURE 2. René Magritte, 1934. La condition humaine (The Human Condition).
© 1997 C. Herscovici, Brussels/Artists Rights Society (ARS), New York.

crease in computer printouts and proliferation of new journals that will be necessary
to deal with the massive amount of new data.

(2) *Sexual Harassment by Robots*: The actual work of sequencing the human genome is not done by human beings but by thousands of robotic instruments whose
behavior is programmed by humans.

(3) *Drugs without Side Effects*: This development will depend on our being able
to identify genetic differences among individuals and to understand how these genetic differences predispose different people to metabolize the same drug in different
ways. The wonder-drugs of the future will be tailored to the genetic makeup of each
individual and will be without side effects. Today we all take the same penicillin;

TABLE 2. Biotechnology's successes: 17 drugs approved by FDA

1982	Insulin	1991	G-CSF
1985	Growth hormone		GM-CSF
1986	α-Interferon		Glucocerebrosidase
	Anti-OKT3	1991	IL-2
	Hepatitis B vaccine		Factor VIII
1987	tPA	1993	DNAse
1989	Erythropoietin		β-Interferon
1990	γ-Interferon	1994	Anti-IIb/IIIa
		1997	Factor IX

99% of us do not have a problem, but the remaining 1% suffer severe allergic reactions. Doctors today deal in medicines of similarity, while in the future the prediction is that we will have medicines of variation, tailored to our patients' genetic differences.

(4) *Organ Replacement with Biologically Synthesized Cells*: This development will depend on first understanding the basic science of how an organ like the heart is formed in the embryo and on the ability to use that information to persuade the genes that work in the developing embryo to work in a test tube. The goal is to create the new organ, such as a new heart, from the patient's own genes so that there would be no rejection crisis and no need for toxic immunosuppressant drugs. That is a conceivable goal, although I cannot even hazard a guess as to how long it will take to achieve it.

(5) *Individual Genomes on Compact Discs*: Walter Gilbert, an eminent scientist at Harvard University who received the Nobel Prize in Chemistry in 1982 for discovering how to sequence DNA, stated in 1990: "In year 2020–2030 you will be able to go into the drug store, have your DNA sequence read in an hour or so, and given back to you on a compact disc so that you can analyze it."[10] If this turns out to be true, pharmacists are going to play bigger roles in medicine than physicians!

In many of these predictions, the distinction between illusion and reality is blurred, and that is what leads me to suggest that the biotechnology revolution is like the surrealist revolution in art in which the practitioners—artists or scientists—express their creativity by living and thinking in a world of dreams and fantasy. The surrealistic style and spirit of biotechnology is brilliantly captured in many paintings done 50 years ago by the famous surrealist artist René Magritte (1898–1967).

FIGURE 2 shows Magritte's most famous painting, *The Human Condition*, which hangs in the National Gallery of Art in Washington. This is a painting within a painting. It exemplifies the essence of surrealism. The distinction between illusion and reality is called into question. The tree in the painting hides the real tree behind it, outside the house. This is the way biotechnologists and genomic researchers see the world: as a painted dream. Is the tree really outside the room? Will we really have drugs without side effects? Will each of our genomes really be put on a compact disc? Will we really be able to replace organs with cells produced in the test tube? No one can promise with absolute certainty that any or all these dreams will come true, but I can tell (you that a strong start has been made, in large part as a result of the biotechnology industry.

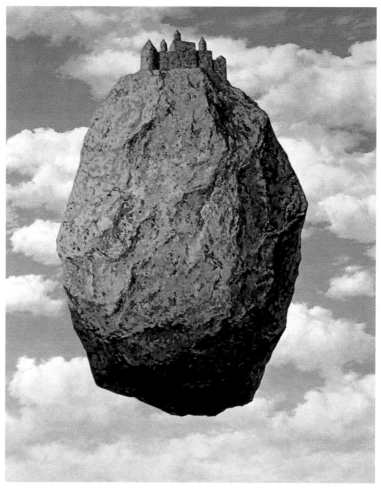

FIGURE 3. René Magritte, 1959. Le château des pyrénées (The Castle in the Sky). © 1997 C. Herscovici, Brussels/Artists Rights Society (ARS), New York.

BIOTECHNOLOGY INDUSTRY IN 1997

At the beginning of 1997, the biotechnology industry consisted of 1,287 companies, of which 23% are publicly owned. It employs 118,000 people; about one-third of them are Ph.D. scientists, and virtually none are patient-oriented researchers. The industry has a market capitalization of $83 billion, product sales of $11 billion, and research and development expenses of $7.9 billion.[11] The biotechnology industry represents the most rapidly growing new industry in our society, but unlike McDonald's and the microchip industry, it has not yet shown profits. The net losses of the industry as a whole were $4.6 billion last year.

TABLE 3. Biotech's "castles in the sky": the second-generation pipeline for drug development

---

New molecules

  Soluble TNF receptors—rheumatoid arthritis and other autoimmune disorders

  Leptin—obesity

  Bone morphogenetic factors—bone fractures

  Glial-derived neurotrophic factor—Parkinson's disease

  Thrombopoietin—platelet disorders

  Inhibitors of angiogenesis and telomerase—cancer

New concepts

  Naked DNA vaccines—AIDS and human papilloma virus

  Universal organ transplants—genetically engineered pig livers

  Protein pills—oral insulin enveloped in coats of polymethacrylic acid

  Intracellular code blockers—antisense DNAs and ribozymes

  Combinatorial chemistry—small-molecule drugs

Gene therapy

  Cancer

  AIDS

  Inherited disorders

Genomics

  Whole-genome sequencing of human beings and their pathogens—
      identification of diagnostic reagents and targets for drugs and vaccines

Proteomics

  Characterization of all human proteins expressed in different cell types in normal vs.
      disease states—identification of diagnostic reagents and targets for drugs

---

Together, the 1,287 companies that constitute the biotechnology industry are the equivalent of one big Merck & Co. Merck employs 100,000 people and has product sales of $11 billion; its market capitalization is $50 billion. The difference is that Merck's annual profit is of the order of $8 billion.[11] One can think of the whole biotechnology industry as one big Merck, without the profits—or even as one Big Mac without the profits!

To date, the biotechnology industry has developed 17 recombinant protein drugs or vaccines that have been approved by the FDA (TABLE 2). The number-one seller is a hormone called erythropoietin, which raises the number of red-blood cells and the hemoglobin concentration in the bloodstream. It is given to patients suffering from chronic kidney diseases, especially those undergoing prolonged dialysis. In 1996, this drug produced more than a billion dollars in sales, and it is the sixth top-selling drug of all pharmaceuticals. The four top-selling biotech drugs—erythropoietin, G-CSF, hepatitis B vaccine, and insulin—are among the 20 best-selling drugs in the pharmaceutical industry as a whole.[11] This is a remarkable achievement for an industry that is so young.

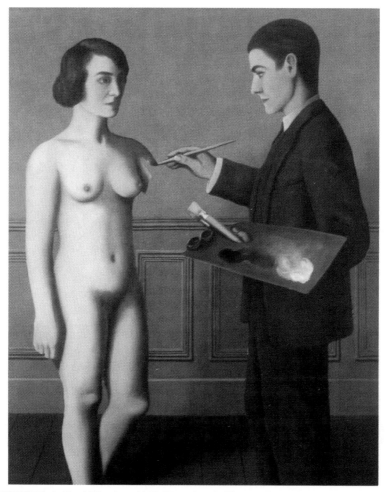

FIGURE 4. René Magritte, 1928. Tentative de l'impossible (Attempting the Impossible). © 1997 C. Herscovici, Brussels/Artists Rights Society (ARS), New York.

The biotechnology industry currently faces a generational crisis in the sense that the "easy targets" that emerged from the first generation of companies (such as insulin, growth hormone, tPA, erythropoietin) have all been identified. Identifying more-complex targets for treating diseases that involve complicated chemical cascades (such as sepsis, degenerative neurologic diseases, skin ulcers) has, to date, totally eluded the ingenuity of the best of biotechnologists.

The successful development of a "second generation" of biotechnology drugs requires creative breakthroughs, and true to their surrealistic spirit, biotechnologists are always cooking up new recipes, which the industry calls "drugs in the pipeline"

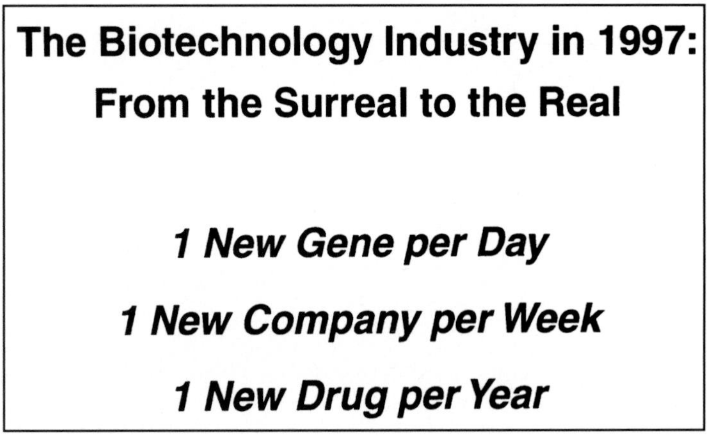

The Biotechnology Industry in 1997:
From the Surreal to the Real

1 New Gene per Day

1 New Company per Week

1 New Drug per Year

FIGURE 5. The Biotechnology Industry in 1997: From the Surreal to the Real.

and which Magritte called *Castles in the Sky* (FIG. 3). A few selected examples of these "castles in the sky" are listed in TABLE 3. Even though most of these ventures are risky and unlikely to produce FDA-approved therapies in the next 10 years, it is only through building "castles in the sky" that new scientific discoveries and *bona fide* therapies will emerge.

Of the five second-generation initiatives in TABLE 3, gene therapy deserves special comment inasmuch as it has received so much attention by the news media. More than 200 clinical trials are currently in progress in the U.S. in which the techniques of gene therapy are being used to treat patients with cancer, AIDS, and inherited diseases. To date, there is no single success story.[12] The Achilles heel of gene therapy is the problem of delivering a gene to the right organ in a patient and having it expressed in a sustained and regulated fashion. This is a formidable challenge and is reminiscent of Magritte's *Attempting the Impossible* (FIG. 4). To be successful, the gene therapist must possess the *superior powers* of the artist who can replace an amputated arm by simply painting it. As shown in FIGURE 4, the artist succeeds through his powers of imagination and his belief in the impossible.

The biotechnology industry has the potential to produce important new medicines as discussed above and as evidenced by the data in TABLE 1. Some would argue that the 20-year-old industry is a big success on the basis of the 17 FDA-approved drugs that are currently being prescribed to patients. On the other hand, the expense and wastage in producing these drugs is enormous, as revealed in FIGURE 5. On average, one new gene is cloned and characterized each day, one new biotechnology company is formed each week, but only one new recombinant drug is approved by the FDA each year. As many as 700 therapeutic products are currently undergoing clinical trials by 167 companies.[11] But 16 of the last 18 drugs failed in Phase 2/3 studies.

If Magritte, the surrealist, were alive today, he might represent the situation shown in FIGURE 6. The top panel shows a reproduction of Magritte's famous painting *The Betrayal of Images*, in which he reminds us that the image of the pipe is not the same as the pipe itself (*Ceci n'est pas une pipe.*). The bottom panel shows a mod-

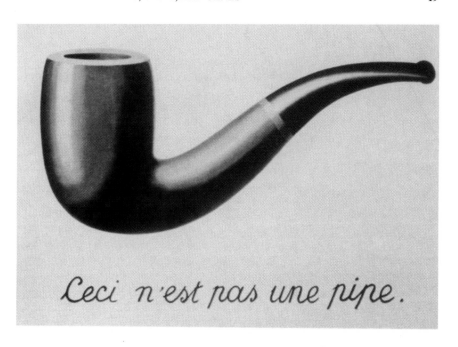

Ceci n'est pas une pipe.

```
CGGGAAAGGA AGCAGGGTCT CTGAAGAAAT ACTTCAGGAG TAGAAAGAGG AAGCTAGAGG
GAGTTAGTAT ATGTCTAGAG GTGTAGTAAA CTAAAACAAG TCTTGAATTG CATACCGCCA
AGGGAAACTG CAACGCCTGT ATTACTAGAT AGCTTTCATC AACAGCTCAA AACCGACAGA
AATTTGGTTT GGATCCCATG CCCATGACCC TGCCAGCTGA CAATTCTAAG CATGCGCAAA
TGGCCCTTTA TGTGAAGTAC CTGGTTTTTC CATTTTCTGT TTTACCATAG GCCTCAGTTC
TCATTCTATT AGATTAAAAA AAAAGAATAC AATGGAAGCC AAGTCATTAA GCTTTCCTTA
AACCGTATTA ACCTACAGAA AATGTCCAGG GAAATGGTCT ATTTCTTATT CTATTTTTGA
TCTCCATCCA CTTCCCTCAG CTTTGGCCTG AAGCTATCTT TAAAGGTACC CTGTACAAGC
TGTTCGATTA GGACACATCT CAGTGGCAGA TAACATGCAA AGTTATTATA TGTATGAACC
GTCTTAAGAC TATAGTAATA TCTTCACTTG AAAAAGCCCT CTATTATTCC TATCTCAGAT
TAATCGCACC TGGCTCTACA AAGCTAGTCT GGACAGACAT TTAAACAATT ATCCTCTAAG
AAAAACCAAA GTGAGCATCC CATCTGTTCC CAGTCAAATG ACCTAGAGCA AAGGACTAGG
CAAATGAATT TGCTTTGTAT ATGAGTGAGA GCAAACACTC TTTATTGTAC AACTTGGGTG
AACGGTTACG TTGGAGTTAA AGGTTAGGAA GAAAACCAAA GGGTAAGAGC TGTTGTTCTG
TGTATATTTT GTAGAAGCAT GTGTGTTGTT GGTTTTTGTG TATGTGTGAG TCTGAAAGAG
TTGACAGATT ATAACTCAGA TGTCTTACTC AGAGCATATG CCTTCCCATT TTCCCCATTA
GCAGACATCT CATACCCCAA ATAGCTAATA TTTTGATAGC TATGATCCTG AACGGCCAAA
TATATTTTAG GCCTTTTCCT TGGCAAGGAT GTTTGGTCAG GGGTTGGCAA AAATAATGCT
CACCAGAAAG TAGTAGAACG CTCCAGGAAG CAAGTCTTTG TCAGGAGTCA GACTAGCTAC
CCTGGCCTAA CTAGCCTACT GAGCTGAGAG ATGTCCAATT TCCCCCCAAT ACACTAACCA
TTCCAATTGC TTAAACAAAT ATGTTCAGTT GTAACTATCA ATACCAGTAT ATAACAGTGT
AGCCAGACAC ATGGTCTTAT GACCGGCGTA CTTACGCAGG GCTTTGCACT GAGACAGGTC
```

Ceci n'est pas un médicament.

FIGURE 6. (*Top*) René Magritte, 1929. La trahison des images (The Betrayal of Images). Text reads "This is not a pipe." © 1997. C. Herscovici, Brussels/Artists Rights Society (ARS), New York. (*Bottom*) A contemporary version of Magritte's painting adapted to the biotechnology industry. Text reads "This is not a drug."

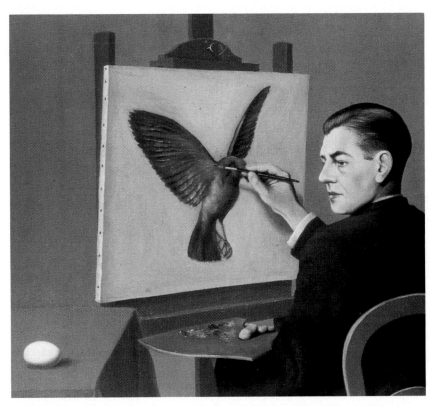

FIGURE 7. René Magritte, 1936. La Clairvoyance (Clairvoyance). © 1997 C. Herscovici, Brussels/Artists Rights Society (ARS), New York.

ern version that reminds us that a gene sequence is not a drug (*Ceci n'est pas un médicament.*).

Cloning a gene is only the first step in producing a drug. The DNA sequence of the cloned gene must be converted into a protein function in order for drug development to occur. Moving from the gene sequence to a drug may take 10 to 15 years if the function of the protein encoded by the gene is known. This process may take 20 to 30 years if nothing is known about the function of the encoded protein.

Fortunately, there is one way to speed the drug discovery process, as illustrated in Magritte's painting *Clairvoyance* (FIG. 7). Here, Magritte teaches us how to create drugs from the DNA sequence. The artist, Magritte himself, is looking at an egg, but he is painting the bird that is implicit in the egg. Such prescience is exactly what scientists of the future will need to learn to do: look at a DNA sequence, deduce the function of the protein, and produce a drug. The scientist of the future must function more and more like an artist, who looks at some amorphous, ill-defined, abstract phenomenon of nature and creates an object of beauty. A major challenge of basic researchers is to learn how to move quickly from the DNA sequence to protein function and ultimately to a drug. An equally important challenge is the need for clinical investigators to acquire the scholarship and the analytical insight that will allow them to point the biotechnology companies in the right direction in selecting the right recombinant molecule for the right disease.[13] In his closing lecture at this bicentennial symposium, Michael Brown will discuss this particular role of the physician-scientist in more detail.[14]

Let us assume that scientists of the future acquire "clairvoyance" á la Magritte and learn how to look at DNA sequences and discover the functions of the 100,000 proteins encoded in the human genome. We will then be in a position to answer, for the first time, the central questions in biology, such as: How does an adult human develop from a simple egg? How do our brains work? How do humans differ from one another? Which specific gene variations and which specific environmental factors predispose different individuals to different diseases?

What will medicine be like in 2097, when Dartmouth Medical School celebrates its 300th anniversary? I will make one prediction that I am absolutely certain will be true: Expect the unexpected. All we need is two or three new McDonald's-like transmutations comparable in impact to the microchip and the gene and, who knows? Perhaps the surreality of the biotechnology industry of today will become the reality of the clinical medicine of tomorrow.

REFERENCES

1. DRUCKER, S. March 10, 1996. Who is the best restaurateur in America? The New York Times Magazine. 45–47.
2. McDonald's Fact Sheet. 1997. McDonald's Corp. Riverside, IL.
3. KROC, R. 1987. Grinding it Out: The Making of McDonald's. 1–218. St. Martin's Paperbacks. Chicago, IL.
4. RIORDAN, M. & L. HUDDESON. 1997. Crystal Fire: The Birth of the Information Age. W.W. Norton & Co. New York.
5. REID, T.R. 1986. Tracing the roots of the microchip. Computerworld 20: 52–65.
6. MOORE, G.E. 1996. Intel—Memories and the microprocessor. In The Power of Boldness: Ten Master Builders of American Industry Tell Their Story. E. Blout, Ed. 77–101. Joseph Henry Press. Washington, DC.
7. KORNBERG, A. 1989. For the Love of Enzymes: The Odyssey of a Biochemist.: 269–296. Harvard University Press. Cambridge, MA.
8. Personal communication from William H. Griesar, Vice President and General Counsel, The Rockefeller University.
9. WILSON, S. 1991. Surrealist Painting. 1–128. Phaidon Press Limited. London.
10. Personal communication from Walter Gilbert, Harvard University.
11. LEE, K.B., JR. & G.S. BURRILL. 1996. Biotech 97 Alignment—The Eleventh Industry Annual Report. 1-78. Ernst and Young LLP. Palo Alto, CA.
12. VERMA, I.M. & N. SONIA. 1997. Gene therapy—promises, problems and prospects. Nature 389: 239–242.
13. GOLDSTEIN, J.L. & M.S. BROWN. 1997. The clinical investigator: bewitched, bothered, and bewildered—but still beloved. J. Clin. Invest. 99: 2803–2812.
14. BROWN, M.S. The making of a physician–scientist: 2000. Ann. N.Y. Acad. Sci. This issue.

Genetics Session: The Human Genome

Prognostications and Predispositions

NANCY WEXLER[a]

*President, Hereditary Disease Foundation, and Higgins Professor of
Neuropsychology, Departments of Neurology and Psychiatry, College of Physicians &
Surgeons of Columbia University, New York, New York 10032, USA*

In reading about the history of the Dartmouth Medical School, I felt a certain affinity
for Nathan Smith's vision, his tenacity, and even for his *name*—my paternal grand-
father was named Nathan Wexler, so maybe they were brothers under the skin.

Here, I would like to talk about the other side of my family—the maternal side—
and an adventure that I've been on ever since I graduated from college. At that time,
I took a trip with my mother to celebrate my graduation, and I noticed that something
was really very amiss with her. She had always been very shy and retiring, even
though she had been a genetics teacher in Harlem. But now she seemed completely
overwhelmed by everything. One vacation we shared a bed, and I noticed that her
feet seemed to be constantly moving and she seemed almost sylphlike and disappearing before my eyes. But I thought, "Well, this is middle age; this is what happens."

Later that year, while my mother was on jury duty in Los Angeles, a policeman
accused her of being drunk at 8:30 in the morning. This really devastated her, for she
knew what it meant. She'd watched her father and three older brothers die of Huntington's disease. She had been told that only men could get it and so had not told
my father when they were married, nor had she mentioned it when both my sister
and I were born. So at the age of 21, I suddenly learned that my mother was dying,
and that my sister (who is three years older) and I each had a one in two chance of
getting Huntington's.

My father, sister, and I got together and started the Hereditary Disease Foundation. We said, "Well, let's just go get it before it gets us. Let's get the gene that causes
Huntington's disease." I feel extremely privileged to have been sent on this voyage,
which is not over yet, not by a long shot. It has made me appreciate many aspects of
what medicine entails today. There is the phenomenal roller coaster of discoveries
and successes that Joseph Goldstein described so eloquently in his opening address.
At the same time, these genetic diseases are wreaking their devastation with mali-
cious disregard. We do not have treatment or even any kind of remediation yet, so
we still have a long way to go.

Let me start with a first principle, namely, that we all have about 50,000 to
100,000 genes, any one of which could potentially go awry. We each carry approximately 10 genes that are sufficiently abnormal to cause serious diseases in ourselves
or our offspring. If you want to find a disease-precipitating gene, you need a family
in which you can see the gene segregating. For reasons that will become apparent, I

---

[a]Present address: 1051 Riverside Drive, PI Annex, Unit 6, New York, NY 10032.

went to Venezuela in search of such a family or families—to Maracaibo, the second largest city in Venezuela, which sits at the neck of a gulf that becomes an enormous lake. Maracaibo did a lot of trading with Europe, and the green eyes and blonde hair of many of its current residents reveal that many of the sailors left their genes behind. There is a phenomenal genetic mix in Maracaibo.

Since 1979, I have been going down to the small fishing villages that rim the shores of Lake Maracaibo. In many of these villages we found the world's largest family with Huntington's disease (HD). It began, as far we can tell, back in the early 1800s, which was just after Dartmouth Medical School was founded. We have now put together a pedigree of more than 16,000 individuals, all of whom are descendants of one woman, who was very aptly named Maria Concepción. Currently, several hundred people in this kindred are living with Huntington's disease, and about 500 have already died of it. Remember—this is a single family, and within this family there's a lot of intermarriage among people who have the HD gene. Almost 3,000 children are gene carriers, and they themselves will develop the disease and die over the next several decades. The HD gene is completely penetrant, meaning that if you carry the gene, you will inevitably fall ill.

The average family size in Maracaibo is 5.6, but it ranges from 1 to 24. The majority of individuals in the kindred are under the age of 40 years. One family that I have studied has 24 kids, all born of the same mother! Another man had over 40 children! For doing a genetic study, it is paradise, especially because the families have been extraordinarily generous in their willingness to be involved.

The families are extremely poor and live in tiny shacks with dirt or concrete floors, tin walls, and tin ceilings. Up to 25 adults and children can live in one tiny shack, which swelters in the equatorial sun, leaks during deluges, and promotes disease. We feel very strongly that if you are doing research you have an obligation to the community where you work and live; those families are now really part of our own families. As part of the research team, we work with a phenomenal person named Dr. Margot deYoung, a Venezuelan physician who is director of research and treatment for our project and provides medical care in the villages year-round. We supply medicines and some food and clothing for these families.

One very special family taught us a great deal about HD as well as about courage and humor in the face of extreme suffering. One member of the family is a little girl who developed Huntington's at the age of six; she died at age 16. Her mother developed the disease at the age of 14 and had four children. The mistake, or mutation, in the little girl's gene, which I will discuss later, was exactly the same as her mother's, and yet there was a big difference in their age of onset of the disease. Most people with the adult-onset type begin to manifest symptoms somewhere between 25 and 50 years of age; rarely, it has been known to show up even as late as age 80. Approximately 20% of all people with HD become symptomatic prior to age 20 years, and another 20% after age 60 years. The children look more like they have Parkinson's disease than Huntington's. They look like little, old, wizened people. They are stiff and very slow-moving. Eating is a major problem for them, and choking is one of the most common forms of death, along with aspiration pneumonia.

Unfortunately, once there is juvenile-onset HD in a family, it seems to be more likely that others in the family who carry the gene will develop the disease while they are young as well. A little boy with juvenile-onset Huntington's had onset of symptoms at age 8 and died at age 17. It is also true that the majority of people who have the juvenile form inherit the disease from their father. This particular little boy's father developed the disease in his 40s. He has families by three different wives, and in his last family, three of his four children have juvenile-onset Huntington's disease, the youngest developing it the most severely and earliest.

Huntington's disease involves a triad of symptoms that are really devastating: loss of motor control—in the adult form, wild, flailing movements of all parts of the body and grimacing; cognitive decline; and psychiatric problems. The last is usually manifested as depression that often ends in suicide, as well as obsessive-compulsive symptoms, mania, and occasionally hallucinations and delusions. The cognitive problems are quite compelling in that people almost always stay oriented as to who and where they are. Although most do not go to school in this Maracaibo population, because even young children in these families must work to bring in a pittance, many are extremely intelligent and do well on our neuropsychological tests.

Perhaps one family above all others pointed our way to the HD gene. In this family of nine siblings, seven children have Huntington's, three with juvenile-onset and the rest with early-onset. Two children became ill at age 12 with the tremor, slowness, and Parkinsonian symptoms typical of children. The youngest child developed HD at age 2—one of the youngest cases in the world—and died at age 9 years. This tiny child had such a severe defect in his HD gene that it helped to identify the correct mutation in the gene. I cannot stress enough how much these illnesses can involve an entire family, all in various stages at any given time and each needing a lot of care.

There is, for example, a woman in her 40s who is tremendously thin. She is absolutely gaunt, even while having a ravenous appetite: both features characterize the disease. Almost all of this woman's many siblings, nieces, nephews, and other relatives have now died of Huntington's disease. Scientific progress to treat or cure this disease is needed desperately, for we are still in the dark ages as far as effective therapy is concerned. We have a long, long way to go.

As I said earlier, our first push on founding the Hereditary Disease Foundation was to try to find the Huntington's disease gene. We knew that it was a gene with an "autosomal dominant" inheritance pattern, which means that the disease occurs equally in both women and men and the gene is not on a sex chromosome. The fact that it is "dominant" means that a person needs to have just one copy of the gene (as opposed to needing two copies as in a "recessive" disorder) to become ill.

Back in 1979, the Hereditary Disease Foundation organized a workshop at the National Institutes of Health (NIH), in which David Botstein and a number of other stellar scientists discussed what might be the best way of finding a disease gene such as the Huntington's gene. There were some heated arguments, considering questions such as: Should we first map the entire human genome and then look for a specific disease gene? Or should we look first for a specific disease? And we concluded that we should try to do both. One needs to concentrate first on the biggest family one can find, because each family might have its own unique mutation. Often the same symptoms in a disease can be caused by different genes, even on different chromosomes. Sometimes there are different mistakes (or mutations) in the same gene in different families. Fortunately, we did not have to deal with that complication; for Huntington's, it turns out, it is the same gene and same mutation worldwide.

Lots of people said that to look for a specific disease gene using DNA markers was a psychotic way to proceed. As David Botstein will tell you, this approach requires so-called "DNA markers," and in 1979 (in contrast to today) we had only one or two DNA markers. Nevertheless, in 1983, much to our astonishment, we did find a DNA marker, which was very tightly linked to the Huntington's disease gene. We saw that every time the Huntington's disease gene was passed down in a family (which you could see by identifying symptoms in a person), a particular variant of this marker got passed down too. This fact told us that the marker must be extremely close to the Huntington's disease gene on the same chromosome. This turned out to be chromosome 4. Our marker was, in genetic parlance, only four million base pairs (or four million rungs on the DNA ladder) below the gene we were seeking.

The marker could be used, then, to predict who in certain families would develop the disease and who would not. However, even though we were close, we still didn't have the Huntington's gene. In just three years we had arrived in its neighborhood, so to speak, and we thought that if we just went knocking door-to-door, behind one of those doors would be the Huntington's gene. Well, it took 10 arduous years of knocking on doors before we succeeded. The task turned out to be a mini-genome project in itself, but we finished it almost before the Human Genome Project even began.

A major advance occurred when Chris Ambrose, a postdoc working in Jim Gusella's lab, sequenced a gene that was found to have a variable number of repeats of just three letters in the four-letter genetic code, namely, CAG (which codes for the amino acid glutamine). This novel gene turned out to be, indeed, the Huntington's gene. Analysis of the Venezuelan child I mentioned earlier, who developed Huntington's at age 2 and died at age 9, revealed well over 100 CAG repeats, whereas normal relatives had only up to about 34. Further analysis showed that all those with Huntington's had 39 or more repeats, and that CAG repeat lengths between 35 and 39 might produce disease or might not. Thus, as few as three repeats (out of approximately three billion base pairs that we all carry in our bodies) could spell the difference between life and death, between having the disease or not having it, between having no symptoms or having terrible symptoms that lead to early death.

These important findings were published by the Huntington's Disease Collaborative Research Group in a paper titled "A Novel Gene Containing a Trinucleotide Repeat That is Expanded and Unstable on Huntington's Disease Chromasomes."[1] The Group consisted of 52 investigators in seven laboratories around the world. Their efforts were really extraordinary; they showed generosity and dedication during a long decade of work, giving each other unpublished materials, working nonstop, and sharing credit. I am very much in their debt, as are all families with HD and related disorders.

We soon learned that the Huntington's disease gene is not the only one to have these long repeats. There are other, mainly neurologic, disorders that involve CAG repeats, and they all show a previously unexpected increase in the number of repeats from one generation to another, resulting, apparently, in worsening of the condition in subsequent generations. It is interesting that all these disorders share approximately the same number of CAGs in a row within the normal range, and that only a subtle increase will take it into the toxic range. And from there the number of repeats relentlessly increases and almost never decreases. It is likely that as we learn more about any one of these conditions, including Huntington's, we will gain valuable insights about the others.

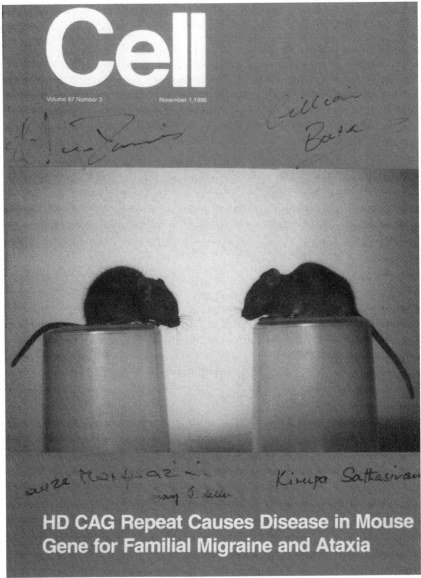

FIGURE 1. Cover of November 1, 1996 *Cell* magazine showing a normal mouse (*right*) and a mouse with Huntington's disease (*left*). The "Huntington's mouse" model has greatly advanced our knowledge about Huntington's disease and similar neurological disorders by demonstrating the lesion in the brain that appears to cause the disease. (Reprinted from *Cell* by permission.)

Remember that most of the children with early-onset Huntington's inherit the gene from their affected fathers. This fact suggested to us that we should try to study sperm, something much easier said than done! Only three or four samples were obtained by investigators at Harvard and Columbia. So in Venezuela, Dr. de Young and I decided to try to collect samples from our large population. At first this was spectacularly daunting. Neither one of us had the right slang vocabulary, and it was culturally rather taboo. But once we endured many embarrassing and often funny moments, we actually did very well. Over the years, we have collected more than 800 sperm samples, from which we learned that some men have really enormous expansions (increases) in the number of CAG repeats in the HD genes in their sperm, while others have rather small expansions. Almost everybody has expansions, unless you begin with a very small abnormal repeat size. The greater the expansion, the more likely it is that there will be further expansion. We also learned that in any one semen sample, almost every single sperm has a different number of repeats, while the size of the HD gene, both in blood and other tissues, is approximately the same. This "stretchiness" of the gene in sperm is primarily responsible for producing new mutations in the gene. The disease can start *de novo*—with no family history—if a person has a repeat size in the intermediate range, which expands into the HD range in subsequent generations. Given the increased vulnerability to expansion found in the HD gene in sperm, the person in whom HD starts *de novo* is more often the child of a man than a woman.

Although all of this progress was fascinating and important, it did not tell us what the protein that is the product of the Huntington's gene does—how that particular protein causes the symptoms of Huntington's. To answer this question, we needed an animal model, such as a mouse, to determine both the normal and abnormal function of the gene and to develop and test new therapeutics. And this leads me to a momentary digression: to emphasize the critical role that animal models play in today's scientific advances. James Freedman outlined many threats to medicine and science today, and I heartily concur with his list. One particular threat is a certain kind of animal activism that stops research in its tracks. Some extremists break into laboratories and animal quarters, releasing animals—experimental models that have been created painstakingly over years of effort—only to have those animals die cruelly outside of the protected laboratory quarters. It is absolutely essential that we continue to fight at all costs, politically and on every front, to maintain the ability to do research with animals.

Let me illustrate the importance of this matter by talking about the mouse model for Huntington's disease, and what important insights we have gained from this model, not only for Huntington's disease, but also for many related disorders.

The little mouse on the left in FIGURE 1 represents a breakthrough that was developed by Gillian Bates and her colleagues at Guy's Hospital in London.[2] Gill Bates was in the collaborating group that had found the HD gene. The gene is enormous, too big to work with easily (more than 3,000 base pairs), so Bates clipped off the first exon of the Huntington's gene, the part that contains the mistake, or mutation. Then, after adding the human gene "promoter," which is like an address system, telling where in the body the HD gene is to express itself or be "turned on," she increased the repeat size to about 150 CAG repeats. (Even though genes are found in the nucleus of every cell, they do not work in every cell. The promoter gives the gene instructions about where to work.) And, lo and behold, it worked: the animals started to shiver and quake, they started getting seizures, and they got very skinny, even

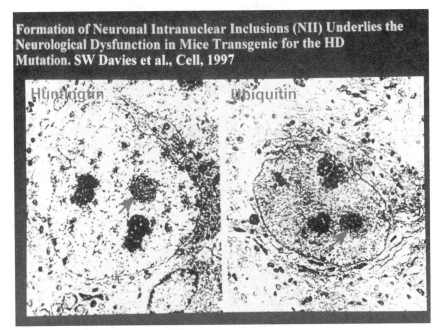

Formation of Neuronal Intranuclear Inclusions (NII) Underlies the
Neurological Dysfunction in Mice Transgenic for the HD
Mutation. SW Davies et al., Cell, 1997

FIGURE 2. Formation of neuronal intranuclear inclusions (NII) underlies the neurological disfunction in mice transgenic for the Huntington's disease mutation. (From S. W. Davies *et al.*, 1997. Reprinted from *Cell* by permission.)

though they were fed chocolate. In short, these new mice are an extraordinarily faithful counterpart of human Huntington's disease.

Nine months after reporting about the mouse model in the journal *Cell*, Gill Bates and Stephen Davies, and their respective groups, had a second cover article in *Cell* devoted to their work.[3] They now reported a shocking new finding about what might be going on with this family of disorders. FIGURE 2 shows a brain cell from one of Bates's mice with the human Huntington's gene fragment, and right in the middle of the cell is a clump called a nuclear inclusion body, which is basically an aggregate of insoluble material formed by the HD protein.

Since 1996 or so, researchers have been saying that the Huntington's disease protein (the product of the Huntington's gene) is located in the cytoplasm, outside the cell nucleus. But Bates and Davies noticed that while the protein starts outside, it then migrates through the nuclear core and forms an insoluble clump within the nucleus. This material reacts with antibodies not only to the Huntington's protein (called "huntingtin") but also to ubiquitin, a protein marker that we associate with targeting a protein for destruction. This suggests that the cell is trying to break down the huntingtin and get rid of it, but apparently it cannot and the clump remains.

What other diseases are also associated with insoluble aggregates? Alzheimer's, Parkinson's, amyloid disorders, amyotrophic lateral sclerosis, and scrapie and other prion disorders, among others. All of a sudden, we have a clue: clumps. This is the last thing that we would have thought was going on in Huntington's. And it required studying the mouse model with fresh eyes to lead us to this critical insight into human diseases.

It is like watching a murder in progress. A tiny fragment of protein wanders into the nucleus, where it doesn't belong. We do not know yet what it is doing there—whether it is interfering with transcription (because the CAG repeats may be masquerading as transcription factors) or "gumming up the works" in some other way. But in the mouse, about a week or so after the protein balls up into a clump in the nucleus of cells, the brain of the mouse starts shrinking, and then the whole animal starts shrinking and getting skinnier. Then, after several weeks, the strange movements start. It is almost like watching cancer begin before you can see the tumor. In the mouse model of Huntington's, you can see the very earliest changes that take place in the brain, very likely causing a tremendous amount of cell compromise, if not cell death, but before the symptoms start.

If you are setting out to find the cure for Huntington's (and for the other similar diseases with expanded CAG repeats), you would logically want to keep the clumps from forming in the first place. And you certainly would like to prevent them from entering the nucleus. Can you put something like a barrier there that would protect the nucleus? Maybe that is the cure. Can you keep the protein clump from rampaging around inside the nucleus, thinking it's a transcription factor or whatever? Is that the cure? The point is that now, with this new mouse model, we have totally new roads to pursue toward a possible specific therapy that we didn't even dream of a month ago. With this sort of new insight, maybe we can prevent the disease before it even starts—which obviously would be the best cure.

Just to keep us humble, I must tell you that back in 1979 some researchers at Columbia University Psychiatric Institute (where I also work) looked at biopsied brain tissue from people with Huntington's disease and said, "Hey, there's stuff in the nucleus of these cells!" But people did not pay enough attention to this finding, and soon everybody forgot about it. In retrospect, we know that the researchers at Columbia saw the clumps partly because they had looked at biopsy tissue (that is, fresh tissue), whereas all other investigators had examined postmortem tissue, where the clumps were harder to visualize. But now, with specific antibodies to the protein, they can be seen quite clearly, especially in children with the disease. The mice awakened us to this critical finding in humans.

So where do we stand now? We have all this incredibly fine research proceeding but, as of yet, no satisfactory treatment. There is commonly an enormous gap (often, many years or even decades) between finding a gene, which allows us to diagnose the disease symptomatically—and, more troublesomely, presymptomatically—and finding satisfactory treatment for that disease. And as long as that gap exists, there is a tremendous risk for insurance discrimination, for stigmatization, for loss of employment, for all kinds of social, ethical, political, and economic problems, and, with them, the potential for devastating human suffering.

As citizens of this society, we are obligated to find solutions to these potential injustices. All of us have some things wrong in our DNA, whether we know it or not. Science must continue so that new treatments can be developed, but we also can and must influence how we deal with the consequences of scientific discoveries, especially, in this instance, of genetic research. Much more will be said here on this important matter, for, after all, the very subtitle for this symposium emphasizes "the ethical and social issues arising out of advances in the biomedical sciences." Let me close, then, by posing some important questions (to which we do not have clear answers) and by relating several dramatic examples of issues people had to face while integrating the knowledge that they carry the gene for Huntington's disease.

Virtually every day, new genes are claimed to have been discovered—genes that supposedly influence such qualities as intelligence, sexiness, sexual orientation, aggression, and emotional disposition. Many persons are concerned that the new genetics is going to wreak unbelievably peculiar changes to the human genome. How much should we tinker with the genome? And how shall we deal responsibly with new genetic information as the human genome is mapped and all genes are found?

One major problem that we must deal with right now concerns genetic testing. What are we doing by offering testing to persons who might or might not have the gene for a serious disease, such as Huntington's? If we could offer effective treatment to those who tested positive, there would be less of a problem. The trouble lies in the gap between our ability to test for the gene and the time when effective treatment becomes available.

There are particular problems that are coming up now in genetic testing, which challenge us as theoretical policies are put into practice. Potentially, there is a special problem in testing identical twins: What if one twin wants to know but the other does not? Should we test either one of them? Who has priority? The guidelines for testing that were developed for Huntington's disease by both families and professionals have recommended that only people 18 or older be tested. This rule is to protect the confidentiality rights of the child. But what if children request testing or parents press to have their children tested? These are guidelines: Who decides?

Currently, we are doing a study at Columbia University with people who have gone through testing so we can learn more about the impact of testing on the lives of those undergoing it. How can we develop better counseling procedures to help people decide whether or not to be tested and to help them cope with test results? Both positive and negative results can be devastating. At a minimum, this is good informed consent. Let me read you some comments from interviews that I conducted in August 1997 with three women who talk about their odyssey in testing:

> I was far more anxious before testing, wondering what my future would bring. The gray area of not knowing was torture for me, because I had big plans, and I really wanted to either feel free to carry them out or alter my course…. That struggle of wondering—if I bumped into a door, if my legs twitched in the middle of the night, or if I forgot my words—that was horror for me. For some reason, knowing that I carry the gene is not that important anymore. I know I'm going to have to deal with it long enough, and there are other things that I want to do.

> You can prepare for testing cognitively…. You can have a support person to talk to for 23 hours out of the 24, and that's the only thing you're thinking about. You think you have all your ducks in a row. And you go to counseling to get prepared for testing, and that can go extremely smoothly. But when you're delivered that information [that you have the gene] you have to remember to breathe again. And then you have to figure out how to go on. And for me, it was extremely difficult to assimilate that information while the world continues to go on, whether you are or not. You know, you have this horrible traumatic experience that you have to internalize. You have to zipper up your trauma and go out and work. I just wasn't good at it.

> My husband and I anticipated I might need a period of time where I wasn't accountable. We played it by ear. We were cognitively prepared for that. What we didn't prepare for, though, was that the weight of that would be so grave. So I went through a period of going through the motions and making sure I had my ducks in a row before I was really able to let my guard down and let this information in. It was a huge struggle.

I had done this testing for myself, but I also wanted to do it for my daughter, who was aged 10, so I could say to her, "Sweetheart, you don't have to worry, we're going to end this right now." I didn't tell her I was being tested. But once I learned I had the gene, I would come home from working all day and try to be a normal, happy mother for my daughter so she wouldn't worry about me. But that really wore me down; it was quite dysfunctional, because we had such an open family.

Finally, my daughter confronted me and said, "Is something wrong? Are you getting divorced? Are you dying? Is Grandma dying? Don't you love me anymore?" So I thought, "Now it's obvious, I'd better tell her," and I did. I really wasn't prepared for the conversation, but it was a relief. At that point I had no choice but to give up my life for six weeks and do nothing. I took off completely, even though we relied on my income. My husband worked three jobs, did laundry, cooked dinner. I walked the dog and went to the beach and cried all day. Then I went to therapy, three times a week, twice individually and once with my husband. It was an accomplishment just to get up and walk the dog. That's all I did for six weeks because that's all I could do. I felt as if part of me had died. I was stuck in my dead body to figure out how to pick up the pieces and go on, because it wasn't over, but a large part of me *was*: my dreams. I thought that after living in a dysfunctional household I had from a sick mother, that I'd pulled myself up by my bootstraps. I was on my road, I was marching in my parade, and then the conductor stopped. I thought that I would be able to give my daughter a better life than what I had had, and here we are challenged by something that was much, much, much more devastating than I could possibly ever imagine.

Finally, here is a quote from someone who had tested positive and then went through prenatal testing:

Many people say, in fact, that to them the uncertainty of finding out they are gene-positive is quite traumatic. Because you can't tell us when the disease will start, only that we have a gene and it will come sometime. All of us have considered suicide, and for many it is not a question of "if," but "when."

I hated the fetal test, and I hated what came after it: having to have an abortion because it was gene-positive—something I've never wanted to have in my life, an abortion .... But here we are, knowledgeable that we have the gene for Huntington's disease and we have a 50/50 chance of passing it on. So we are controlling the destiny of our next generation. In a sense, we have the potential to do that, so we have a sense of responsibility.

Like this woman, I believe that we do have the responsibility for the next generation. But I remain optimistic: I think that with the kind of talent and vision at institutions like Dartmouth Medical School, better times do lie ahead.

REFERENCES

1. THE HUNTINGTON'S DISEASE COLLABORATIVE RESEARCH GROUP. 1993. Cell **72:** 971–983.
2. MANGIARINI, L, K. SATHASIVAM, M. SELLER, B. COZENS, A. HARPER, C. HETHERINGTON, M. LAWTON, Y. TROTTIER, H. LEHRACH, S.W. DAVIES & G.P. BATES. 1996. Exon 1 of the HD gene with an expanded CAG repeat is sufficient to cause a progressive neurological phenotype in transgenic mice. Cell **87:** 493–506.
3. DAVIES, S.W., M. TURMAINE, B.A. COZENS, M. DIFIGLIA, A.H. SHARPE, C.A. ROSS, E. SCHERZINGER, E.E. WANKER, L. MANGIARINI & G.P. BATES. 1997. Formation of neuronal intranuclear inclusions underlies the neurological dysfunction in mice transgenic for the HD mutation. Cell **90:** 537–548.

Of Genes and Genomes

DAVID BOTSTEIN

Chair, Department of Genetics, Stanford University School of Medicine, Stanford, California 94305-5120, USA

Nancy Wexler's presentation gives a clear impression of what motivates researchers to find out what genes do, especially in humans. I'll give you the nuts and bolts of how we learn about genes, how we get and interpret information about our genes, and how the requisite technology led to the Human Genome Project. My view (and I think, now, the general view) is that the Project was the only possible response to the kind of advances in biology that Joseph Goldstein presents in this volume. And I will address my remarks so that they can be appreciated by professors and those that are not—always a difficult task. I will try to boil the subject down to its essence.

FIGURE 1 shows you all that you really need to know about DNA: that it is an information carrier and it makes decisions. DNA contains the instructions for which proteins are to be made and the amino acid sequence of these proteins; in other words, it encodes the information that is required to make the proteins. Proteins do the work in biology; to a first approximation—and everything I say here is a first approximation—proteins do everything.

There is, of course, a genetic code. It was figured out in the 1960s, and it tells how the sequence of letters in the DNA language (the so-called "bases," or "nucleotide bases") is translated into the sequence of amino acids in the proteins. The big insight of our time, arising out of the breaking of the genetic code, is that all living organisms use the same code. This fact makes it possible to express human genes in other

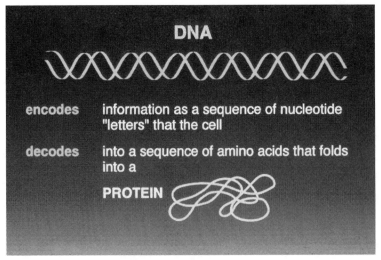

FIGURE 1

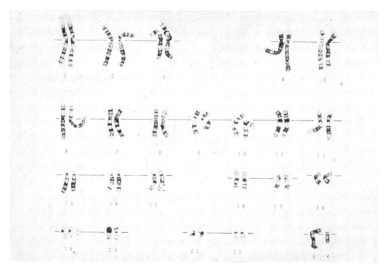

FIGURE 2. Chromosomes of normal human male.

organisms—not just in the mouse but, as we shall see, in truly any living being, plants or animals, even in bacteria and yeast.

FIGURE 2 shows the 23 pairs of chromosomes of a normal human male. All the genetic information about this particular individual is in these chromosomes. Our job as geneticists is to figure out what the information is. Everything that makes one of us different from the other—ignoring, for now, environmental influences—is in the genes that are on our chromosomes.

If humans reproduce in the manner of other organisms, and if our genes follow Mendelian rules (as, indeed, they do), then the following logic can be applied (FIG. 3). If I can distinguish, at any position on a particular chromosome, A1 from A2 by some technical means, I should be able to follow A1 and A2 from a father into his children; and I would find that Mendel's first law applies, namely, that either A1 or A2, but not both, is contributed to an offspring. And which one of the two is passed on to a given child is a purely random event. Likewise, if I can tell A3 from A4 in the mother, I will find that either A3 or A4, but not both, is transmitted to the offspring.

Similarly for B (another locus on another chromosome), Mendel's first law, and therefore the same logic, apply. Also, by looking simultaneously at the results for A and B, I could see that there is no relationship between what happens in A and what happens in B. That is Mendel's second law: of independent assortment.

The point is that if I had yet another locus, C, which happened to be nearby B, then I could show that, whereas A and B are independent and A and C are independent, B and C are not independent—that, in fact, wherever I find B1, I also find C1. The degree to which that last generalization is true has something to do with the distance between A, B, and C; in fact, I can make that relationship a measure of the distance between B and C. And if I do so—and if I limit myself to very short

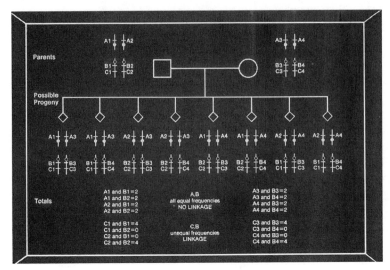

FIGURE 3

distances—I can get a close correlation between B and C (or, in genetic terms, "link-age"). Then, if there is a disease gene that happens to be near B and C (for example, the gene for Huntington's disease), I can follow B and C instead of the Huntington's disease gene (which at that point, I know nothing about) and see that B and C are carried, so to speak, with Huntington's disease. And that's where Nancy Wexler was in 1983.

That was the gist of the workshop that Nancy Wexler referred to in her paper: how we could use linkage to locate and identify genes that cause disease. Unfortunately, the level of genetic education at that time was such that nobody understood the concept of linkage. Nancy's sister, Alice Wexler, has a very amusing description of the workshop in her book, *Mapping Fate*,[1] which is entirely in accord with my recollection. Nobody seemed to understand what we were saying, and we were very frustrated because to us, knowing Mendelism (the principles of genetics), the concept was absolutely elementary.

(The problem, by the way, is one that we should not forget in Dartmouth Medical School's 200th year, namely, that medical education is lousy at dealing with principles. It's great at facts, it's great at practices, it's great at rumors, but it is *not* great with principles. Virtually all medical students shy away from any discussion of principles, especially if it involves a numerical or calculational basis—and genetics, unfortunately, has both. I will say more about this major curricular problem at the end of my this presentation.)

The concept of genetic linkage led to the idea that one wanted to find markers (or pieces of DNA) that fulfill the role of A and B and C, so one could separate A1 from A2, or from A3, or from A4. The short segment of DNA shown in FIGURE 4 was the first useful such marker, isolated by Wyman and White in 1979. The figure shows data from nine randomly selected individuals who happened to give blood at the Uni-

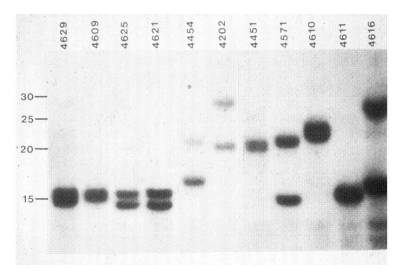

FIGURE 4

versity of Massachusetts in Worcester. (I do not know about informed consent in those days, but fortunately that was not an issue.) The important point is that they were just nine individuals, each different from the others.

It became clear, then, that we wanted to have DNA markers—not just for a single gene in one place (not just, that is, to solve Nancy Wexler's problem of Huntington's disease), but a whole map of markers all over the genome so we could find genes for all diseases. (I need to digress here for just a little bit of vocabulary about markers: a *single copy DNA probe* is a piece of DNA that occurs only once in the genome, which means that we each have two copies of it—one on that specific chromosome from our mom and one on that chromosome from our dad. *RFLP* [restriction fragment length polymorphism] is a technique that allows localization of a gene to a certain chromosome—if you followed the O.J. Simpson trial, you heard this term; and *sequence tag site* [STS] is an even more refined marker than RFLPs, which allows a more precise localization of genes on chromosomes.)

Lots of human disease genes have been mapped by the marker (or linkage) method; I believe the count now is over one thousand. Of course, in 1979 we were told that we were crazy in even proposing to map all of the disease-causing genes. But ultimately, the idea penetrated, thanks in large part to Nancy, and because she found something so quickly. Despite Nancy Wexler's success, however, the concept did not penetrate the establishment to the point where financial support was forthcoming. In fact, the lack of funding forced us to go outside the normal channels and produce a new organization, the Human Genome Project, in order to accomplish what I would have thought the National Institute of General Medical Sciences would have wanted to do as a matter of course. Not at all. They resisted it. To this day, I don't understand why.

In tackling the project, we needed to take into account the size of the human genome. There was the major question of how we would remember the order of things on the map. The 23 chromosomes from our parents contain 3×10^9 base pairs and those from the other parent another 3×10^9 base pairs. There are four bases, so each carries two bits of information; in other words, approximately 12 billion bits of information needed to be stored. In those days, the capacity of a computer was measured in 8-bit units called bytes; but we had need for 750 million bytes (750 megabytes). Joseph Goldstein spoke of the invention of the microchip and the development of compact disks (CDs); today, virtually all medical students have laptop computers with memories that can accommodate the entire human genome.

In addition, of course, we needed lots of polymorphic markers (RFLPs). The original goal, which was regarded as much too ambitious, was one RFLP for every two recombination units (approximately 2 million bases); we now have roughly 20 times that number of markers—approximately one for every 100,000 bases. Thus, it did not turn out to be such a big deal after all. Of course, the sequence in which the bases (strictly speaking, "nucleotide bases") follow one another in any given gene was the ultimate goal; we wanted to know not only the location of the genes on the chromosomes, but also the sequence of the bases (adenine [A], guanine [G], cytosine [C], and thymine [T]—the letters that form the alphabet of the genetic code). We wanted to know the sequence in which these bases are linked, not only in the Huntington's gene and the gene for cystic fibrosis, but, in fact, in all genes.

Eventually, a committee of the National Research Council (NRC), of which I was a member and which was headed by Bruce Alberts, came out with a grand compromise between the people who were for the project and those who were against it. The compromise allotted about a quarter of the total funds towards experiments with model organisms. At that time, I was attacked on this point for feathering my own nest, because I work with such a model organism, yeast. But actually, two things were realized by the committee at this time: one (to which I have already alluded) was the need for a better way of cataloguing the vast amount of information that was to be gained; and the other was the fact that a lot of sequencing in model organisms would have to be a prerequisite for understanding the human genome. Those were scientific insights, and as a direct consequence of the discussion in the committee, the money was made available to realize both of those things.

In regard to the last point, it is worth mentioning that the deliberations of the NRC committee were the only instance that I know of where science policy was made purely on the basis of scientific needs. The credit for this has to go to Bruce Alberts, who emphasized that we needed to take advantage of a major scientific opportunity, and that we should concentrate on what was needed to exploit that opportunity.

In order to give you an idea of the infrastructure that would be required, let me try to illustrate the size of the human genome. FIGURE 5a is a picture of the earth above the Midwest, somewhat comparable to the size of the human genome. As you increase the resolution you see a part of the Midwest, including all of Lake Michigan (FIG. 5b), comparable to the order of resolution of the chromosomes pictured in FIGURE 2. Going further down, you see the Chicago area (FIG. 5c), a specific lakeside marina (FIG. 5d), and finally a person lying on a blanket in a park within the marina (FIG. 5e).

Here is another way of making the analogy: If one compares the human genome (23 pairs of chromosomes) to a map of the United States, one can consider the information on a single chromosome as analogous to the map of a single state. That de-

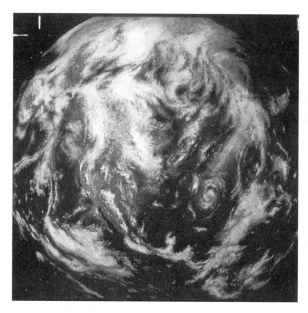

FIGURE 5a. The Earth at 10,000 kilometers above Lake Michigan.

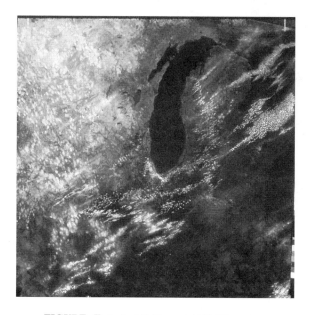

FIGURE 5b. Lake Michigan at 1000 kilometers.

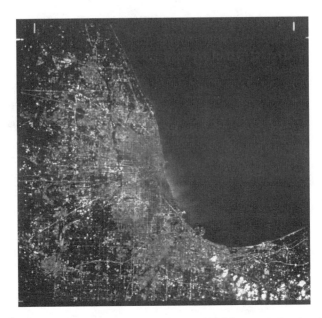

FIGURE 5c. The lower end of Lake Michigan at 100 kilometers showing the Chicago metropolitan area.

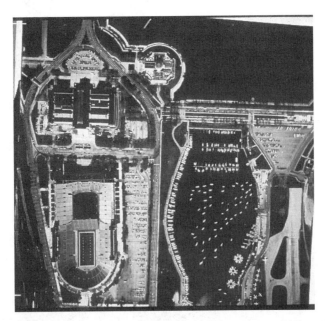

FIGURE 5d. Marina on Lake Shore Drive in Chicago seen at 1 kilometer.

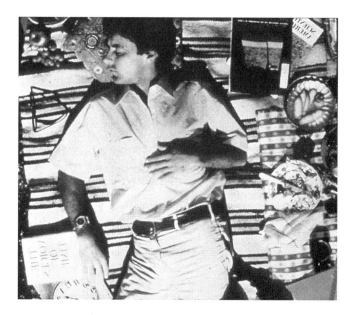

FIGURE 5e. Man on a blanket in park in marina on Lake Shore Drive in Chicago seen at 1 meter. This and FIGURES 5a–d are from *Powers of Ten* by Philip and Phylis Morrison. © 1984, 1992 by the Scientific American Library. Used by permission of W.H. Freeman and Company.

gree of resolution will allow us only to say that a given gene is located on a certain chromosome, like saying we are in Illinois. Obviously, a map of considerably higher resolution is needed in order to determine exactly where on a given chromosome a specific gene is located. That further resolution was provided by finding short sequences of DNA (markers) that are unique to specific locations on a single chromosome, or, to continue the analogy, unique to specific locations in Illinois. The original markers, RFLPs, provided approximate locations on chromosomes, like precincts in Chicago. The resolution was then further improved by STSs (sequence tag sites), allowing us to determine a "street address" for each gene.

And finally, let me put the cost of the Human Genome Project in perspective: Just think how much money must have been expended to get detailed maps of the United States, right down to street addresses. It was a lot. When viewed in that context, the proposed expenditure for the Human Genome Project is really modest.

The invention of the polymerase chain reaction (PCR) eliminated the need to remember probes (the DNA STSs) and store them—a problem of infrastructure that I alluded to earlier. The technique of PCR is completely automatable. It enables one to select a small piece of anybody's DNA and replicate it in such a way that one always gets out exactly the same piece of DNA. With the invention of PCR, all you had to do was to remember a short sequence (say, 50 letters) from the gene in question (e.g., for Huntington's disease, or cystic fibrosis, or neurofibromatosis), and thereafter you could always isolate that particular gene.

Another mapping technique—another form of marker—is to get probes from complementary DNA (cDNA), the subset of DNA that is actually expressed in cells. But that is a further refinement, which is not critical towards understanding the principles that I am trying to explain here.

Now, remember that after you do linkage mapping, you are still at a low level of resolution. Mapping locates the gene only in Illinois, so to speak; it's a U2 spy-plane level of resolution and not a walking-around level of resolution—orders of magnitude too low. To come down on the specific disease-causing gene, you need to have more than linkage mapping; you need a "street map," what is called in genetics a *physical map*. That problem has been solved by David Cox and Rick Myers at Stanford (previously at the University of California in San Francisco), who figured out a way to do physical mapping very efficiently, nearly automatically. Their method is called *radiation hybrid mapping*. I will not describe the details here; suffice it to say that it is an ingenious method that makes it possible to localize—within just a few hours—a given segment of DNA situated somewhere in no less than two million base pairs.

I'm not going to belabor these descriptions of techniques for identifying disease-causing genes. The point I would like to leave you with is that we are now beginning to learn how to use the genomic information in order to look into the future. There is a big opportunity to try to understand what goes on in cancer—because we have reasons to believe that current technology will allow us to discover many genes that have mutated to cause aberrations in growth and differentiation.

In the more general sense, I'd like to leave you with several lessons. One is that principles—for example, the basic principles of how organisms are organized and how one studies these processes—are more valuable than individual facts. Progress is held up if medical students and administrators do not pay enough attention to the basic sciences and to underlying principles as opposed to facts and detailed technologies. The technology that was very important when I was a student is no longer in use today. I spent much of my time as a graduate student aligning a centrifuge that is now a museum piece, if it exists at all. I worked with the same Texas Instruments calculator that Dr. Goldstein spoke of. I learned how to program it and make it go, with its puny memory of 32 bits. The programming stood me in good stead, but the machine is now not even a museum piece; I'm sure it's a metal ingot someplace! So it goes with technology.

However, Mendelism is still with us. The principles of biochemistry are still with us. The rules of inference (of what is a proper control); and statistics (what is the variance, what is the reproducibility, what are the figures of merit)—those things are still with us and will continue to be with us; and those are the things that our students are <u>not</u> learning. That is one issue I'd like to see you concerned about.

My second point is that the conservation, and hence availability, of all the newly-gained information is going to put a great premium on separating the wheat from the chaff. We will have to do very careful and rigorous experiments to figure out what each of these proteins (which are encoded by our roughly 100,000 genes) do in whatever organism can best accomplish the task, be that yeast, or bacteria, or mice. A great unification has been given to us by nature, so that a given gene in yeast may have been preserved in humans and will be responsible for the same function in humans as it has been in yeast (or other micro- or macroorganisms). We had, in fact, no right to such a slow rate of protein evolution; but having seen it, we should take advantage of it. Yeast proteins, for example, can be used to find human genes, and vice versa. Our organism-centric focus must disappear; all these silly barriers—between prokaryotes and lower eukaryotes and higher eukaryotes—all this sort of stuff is going to have to go.

Researchers focus too much on their own work in their own little biological niche. For example, papers in the journal *Cell* make almost no reference to things other than the very narrow area the author is working in. If the author is a good scientist and a little bit of a scholar, the report might go a little further, but anything beyond that, any discussion of principle, is, by and large, not to be found.

So at the end of the day, basic science is important. The explosion of information is going to take all the factoids that you'll remember now, and render them obsolete, if only by swamping them with so many more factoids. We will have to learn how to think about 10,000 facts simultaneously. Remember: rely on much more information technology and much less Tris buffer, and stay close to the basic principles and to the fundamentals.

REFERENCE

1. WEXLER, A. 1995. Mapping Fate. Random House. New York.

The Human Genome Project and the Future of Medicine

FRANCIS S. COLLINS

Director, National Human Genome Research Institute, Bethesda, Maryland 20892, USA

Being in charge of that part of the National Institutes of Health (NIH) that is focused on getting the Human Genome Project done involves funding the right people and holding them accountable—not only to complete work on time but also to accomplish it on an economy of scale one expects with a project of this size. By and large, things have worked out well. The Genome Project has benefited greatly from some excellent advisers, including the chair of this session, David Botstein.

You have already heard a very eloquent description of the principles of Mendelian genetics and the mapping and sequencing of genes—not only the genes that cause disease, but also the other 98% of the genome. My task is to look at the medical consequences of this project. As I do so, I will talk a little about the past and present, but mostly about the future, because this is a symposium that is looking forward. I will argue, as have the preceding two presenters, that we are embarked upon a genuine revolution in genetics that is going to find its way into every nook and cranny of the practice of medicine: diagnostics, prognostics, therapeutics, and the rest. Our current training of physicians does not prepare them well for this new science, and I will harp on that theme as well (though perhaps slightly more gently than Dr. Botstein did —more gently only because that's my nature, not because I feel less passionately about the problem).

My basic premise—and I challenge you to disagree with me—is that every disease (except some, but not all, cases of trauma) has a genetic component. This premise conflicts with the more classic view of medical genetics as a specialty devoted to the study of rare Mendelian disorders or unique chromosomal abnormalities that are unlikely to be encountered by most physicians in their daily practice. This premise is not new, because it's been known all along that virtually every disease has a tendency to track in families. What has changed is that, whereas until recently we thought we could do little about such disorders, we are now beginning to see possible therapeutic approaches based on gene discoveries that will change the way medicine is practiced.

The degree to which a particular disease is determined by a specific DNA sequence depends a lot on the disease. Genes are involved in everything from cystic fibrosis, where, if you have inherited two misspelled copies of a particular gene on chromosome 7, you're going to get the disease (provided they're misspelled in a certain way), to something like AIDS, which is, after all, an infectious disease. Why is AIDS included? In the last year a subset of the population has been characterized that can be exposed repeatedly to the HIV virus and yet individuals in it do not develop the syndrome of AIDS—or develop it very slowly—because they possess certain genetic factors that give them protection from the virus. But most diseases are like diabetes, hypertension, coronary artery disease, or the common mental illnesses, for example, where we know they tend to run in families but they don't follow Mendelian rules. Those diseases are harder to understand, but in the aggregate they are vastly more important in their impact on the health of our population, because they are such common disorders.

The goal of the Genome Project from a physician's point of view is to try to understand the genetic underpinnings not just of the rare, single-gene disorders, but of virtually all diseases.

There are two ways to find a gene that contributes to a disease: You can carry out solid physiologic and biochemical studies, figure out exactly what is functionally wrong in the given disorder, and then use that information to find the gene; or if that approach is not available, you first locate the gene on a map and then trudge around in a complex area of DNA, looking at all the genes in the region until you find the right one. How do you know when you've found the right gene? It must show a difference in its sequence in the affected individuals as compared to the unaffected ones; otherwise, it's just a gene in the neighborhood and not the one for which you are looking.

The latter approach, called *positional cloning* is a relatively new activity, which succeeded for the first time only 11 years ago. This approach was described by Nancy Wexler for Huntington's disease and by David Botstein for the Genome Project in general. *Functional cloning*, on the other hand, where you examine the physiology and biochemistry first and can identify the functional abnormalities, has been around a lot longer. But unfortunately we cannot utilize this approach for the more common disorders, such as diabetes, because we still know too little about the underlying biochemical processes and which genes might regulate them.

Let's quickly review positional cloning for a simple, classical Mendelian disorder. Cystic fibrosis (CF) is a recessive disease, which means that in order for a child to have CF, both parents must carry one abnormal copy of the CF gene and they must both pass the abnormal copy on to the same child. On a statistical average, one in every four of their children may get CF; it is possible, however, that none would get it or that more than one out of four would, since we are talking about a statistical probability. Many of you in this room are carriers of CF because one in 25 Caucasians carries one abnormal copy of the gene, so the probability of a Caucasian couple having a child with CF is one in 2,500 — $25 \times 25 \times 4$.

We knew a lot about the physical problems in cystic fibrosis back in the '70s and early '80s, but not enough about how the gene might function. So the way the gene for CF was identified was to take advantage of positional cloning using what was then a rather rudimentary set of genetic markers that David Botstein described, and testing those markers on families with cystic fibrosis. After a great deal of labor, Lap-Chee Tsui's group[1] and mine identified a marker on chromosome 7 that tended to predict which child in a family got cystic fibrosis and which didn't. By the rules that David Botstein went over, that could be the case only if the specific marker was physically close to the gene. The next step was to place many other markers on that particular chromosome and check them out for their proximity to the CF gene, narrowing the region down as much as possible (much as you saw, in the analogy David borrowed from the Morrisons, coming in from outer space towards Chicago). It meant, ultimately, having to trudge through a DNA region of about one-and-a-half million base pairs looking for the right gene.

I agree with David that it's not worth stuffing your head full of facts, but it might be useful to bear in mind just a few numbers. The human egg and sperm combine to form a cell with three billion base pairs. These three billion base pairs contain approximately 100,000 genes, which means there is a gene about every 30,000 base pairs. If you're searching in a stretch of a million-and-a-half base pairs—a typical situation for a simple genetic disease like cystic fibrosis—you have about 50 genes to consider as candidates. Only one of them will be the one for which you are looking; the other 49 may be interesting to somebody else. The motto of the positional cloner, at least as I've perceived it, is best exemplified in a quote from Winston Churchill: "Success is nothing more than going from failure to failure with undiminished enthusiasm." You know you're going to fail repeatedly before you finally find the right gene.

This process led to the detection[2] in 1989 of what looked like a pretty bland change in the gene of most individuals with cystic fibrosis, namely, the deletion of just three base pairs: a CTT, which is present in the sequence of the normal gene but missing in the cystic fibrosis gene. Remember that each set of three base pairs codes for a specific amino acid. So if you drop out three, you don't scramble everything downstream from that point; in fact, the effect of the deletion in CF is to drop out a single amino acid, a phenylalanine. Although that change doesn't look very impressive, it is, nevertheless, the most common cause of cystic fibrosis.

This deletion of just one amino acid should cause us to stop for a minute and notice the enormous capability of a subtle change in sequence: just three missing bases out of three billion, and it creates a disease with enormous complexity and one that causes much human suffering. Though the genome is large, subtle changes can have big effects if they happen to lie in vulnerable positions.

This effort to find the CF gene took about 10 years, occupied most of the 1980s, and cost roughly $50 million. We can't use this approach for the thousands of genes that afflict us, especially because most of them are even more complicated than the CF gene. Some technical advances introduced since then would make the task somewhat less expensive now, but not nearly enough so. So a major reason for the Genome Project is to make this kind of process much more efficient. When we were searching for the CF gene we had to use approaches that hadn't been tried before; every time we landed in a region of DNA, it was uncharted territory where nobody had been before. The goal of the Genome Project is to decipher the whole thing once and for all, so that whatever gene you're looking for, somebody has been there ahead of you and laid out all of the map information and, ultimately, the sequence. That work is already saving us many years and millions of dollars.

By the way, there's an assumption in this whole symposium that all these gene discoveries are going to change medicine for the better and benefit patients. One little girl who has CF certainly made that assumption when she wrote the following in her diary on the day the CF gene was cloned, August 25, 1989: "Today is the most best day ever in my life. They found a jean [sic] for cystic fibrosis," she wrote. But let's look carefully at what underlies that assumption. Was the little girl right to have that kind of optimism? Here we are in 1997, eight years later, and the management of her disease has not changed in any significant way by finding the gene (although, fortunately, she's doing pretty well). But I will predict that in the course of the next 10 years, management of CF will change. Already several new ideas are emerging about how to treat the disease, ideas that are based on our understanding of how the gene works. The healthy form of the gene itself may even be used in so-called gene therapy.

More than thirty thousand genes have been mapped in the last 15 years; many genes have been cloned and the defects in them (the mutations) have been defined. As Nancy Wexler described for Huntington's disease, the immediate consequences of finding a particular gene are often diagnostic, enabling us to predict those who are at risk even before they develop the illness, or those whose children might be at risk even before those children are conceived. But I would argue that the place we really wish to get to is further on, where we use the information about the gene in order to understand the disease well enough to come up with new treatments. As Joseph Goldstein told you, that effort is a long, drawn-out process. Understanding the basic biological defect is indeed often assisted critically by cloning the gene, but that understanding does not just happen overnight. Thus, for many genetic diseases, we will be living for awhile in an interval where diagnostics are improving while therapeutics are still around the corner. We are in an intermediate state where we have valuable new information, but not yet the kind that we would most like to have, that is, how do you cure this darned thing? When we get to that point many of the dilemmas will melt away.

The Human Genome Project was designed largely according to the plans of the NRC (National Research Council) committee, which was chaired by Bruce Alberts. The plan organized the work to be performed and, importantly, included work on model organisms, which would facilitate our understanding of the functional significance of the data on humans. For human DNA there were three major goals: (a) to build genetic maps, constructed by classical Mendelian studies of families or populations; (b) to build physical maps, constructed by analysis of the anatomic location of genes along the chromosomes; and (c) ultimately, to determine the DNA sequences of the genes.

The genetic maps were achieved almost two years ahead of schedule. The physical maps, which David showed you as computer representations, are 98% complete. We are now beginning to sequence the human genes. Having practiced successfully on viruses, bacteria, yeast, and the roundworm, and to some degree the fruit fly, we were able to ramp up the human sequencing in earnest, beginning in 1996. About a dozen centers around the U.S., and an additional four or five internationally, are involved in this effort. The total completed human genomic sequence at the present time is about 70 million base pairs of DNA. That sounds like a lot—and it is a whale of a lot compared to what we had even two years ago— but that's still only slightly more than 2% of the total. So we're very much on the rising part of an exponential curve, or a curve that one *hopes* will be exponential; it's always a little hard to make that prediction so early in a project.

Will we get there? The next couple of years are going to be absolutely critical toward answering that question, but at present the signs are all quite encouraging. It is now possible to sequence human DNA in large amounts, and to do so accurately— something upon which we have insisted at the Genome Institute because there's no point in doing it in a sloppy fashion and requiring everybody to go back and clean up a lot of mistakes later on. The sequence in the public database, to which everybody will have access, must be accurate to no more than one mistake in every 10,000 base pairs. Also, we demand that our genome centers release new sequences into a public database on a nightly basis so that there will be no hoarding of information.

What about the cost? At the present time [September, 1997], and at the best centers, the cost for sequencing stands at approximately 40 to 50 cents per base pair. At that rate, the budget available for this project will not allow the work to be completed by the year 2005, so the cost must be reduced. It has already come down 20-fold over the last six or seven years. There's good reason to believe that if we can reduce it to just 20 cents a base pair, we can complete the entire Human Genome Project by 2005; and if we can get it down to 10 cents a base pair, it can be completed even sooner. And then perhaps we can throw the mouse genome sequence in for free. That would be great! (I, for one, will be glad to go on record as saying the Genome Project will be a disappointment if we can't also sequence the mouse genome.) So the Project is going well, but only the next two years will tell whether we are indeed on an exponential curve.

By the way, people often ask me, "Whose DNA is being sequenced?" Many comments have been made that it ought to be Walter Gilbert's, or James Watson's, or perhaps that of the person who is willing to contribute the most money. Until a couple of years ago, most of us would have said this is a non-question, but then a change in the technology caused the sequencing centers to lurch in the direction of one particular library, made from one particular individual. It began to look as if a large fraction of the human sequence might be derived from a single postdoctoral fellow who was working in a laboratory somewhere on the West Coast!

Would that be good for that person's well-being? Well, maybe not, for he or she might be exposed to some risk of people poring through the database, looking for glitches, which inevitably will be present; we all have "glitches" in our genomes. In fact, the estimates are that we have between five and perhaps as many as 50 mutated genes that could have serious consequences, depending on the circumstances. There are no perfect human specimens that we can just pluck out and sequence. So the issue of protecting that individual against potential discrimination loomed large, and we produced new libraries from individuals who were volunteers, and whose identity shall remain unknown forevermore. The human genome sequence that will be produced over the next seven or eight years will come from between five and ten anonymous donors. In any case, that really doesn't make a lot of difference, because the point of the project is to look at a so-called reference sequence; the first pass through the human genome will not focus on human variation. That comes next, or maybe in parallel, as I'll explain later.

Inasmuch as all our sequences are 99.9% identical, it doesn't make much difference whose sequence we are describing. The remaining 0.1% is very interesting because it accounts for all the variability in our species. But from the point of view of the Human Genome Project, at least in this first phase, variation is not the part we're trying to figure out. It's the 99.9% of identity in our approximately 100,000 genes that we're after, for that is the part that carries the instruction book for human biology.

I would like to turn now to considering some of the dilemmas that arise increasingly as we locate and describe new disease genes. Let me do so by talking about one particular example, one that has been very much on the public's mind and is in many ways paradigmatic of the problems we are facing as we begin to apply gene discoveries to clinical medicine. That example is breast cancer. It has been known for decades that breast cancer has a tendency to run in families. If you have a first-degree relative with breast cancer, and you're a woman, your risk of getting breast cancer goes up, particularly if your affected relative got the disease at an early age, had bilateral disease, or also had ovarian cancer (or some other relative did). The estimates now are that about 5% of breast cancer arises in individuals who have inherited a very strongly acting mutation in one of perhaps three or four genes, two of which have been found: BRCA1 and BRCA2. If you are a woman who has inherited a BRCA1 mutation, your risk of getting breast cancer is about 55% (we used to say 85% but that number has been revised downward based on more recent studies). Your risk of getting ovarian cancer is about 16%, which is dramatically higher than that of the general population. If you are a man with a BRCA1 mutation, your risk of cancer is not so dramatic, but you probably are at increased risk for prostate cancer. Carriers of a BRCA2 mutation have similar cancer risks.

The first important question is, would you want to know whether or not you have the BRCA1 or BRCA2 gene? If breast cancer runs in your family and a test were made available, would you sign up? If I set out a booth in the lobby during lunch, and said, "Free genetic testing here for BRCA1," how many people would walk up and stick out their arm for blood sampling and say, "Sure, I want to know that, let me know." That's not an easy question to answer. How would this information help you? How would it change what you're currently doing?

Here is one immediate problem: If I were going to set up that booth, it would have to contain very high-tech equipment, because there are more than 200 mutations in BRCA1 and BRCA2 scattered all over the genes. This is not like sickle cell disease, where you look at one single base pair in one location in one gene, and it's always the same base pair, which has mutated from an A to a T to cause sickle cell disease. Nor is it like cystic fibrosis, where a three-base-pair deletion accounts for the majority of the disease. Nor like Huntington's disease, where every affected person has an easily recognizable expanded triplet repeat. Rather, with BRCA1 and BRCA2 there are mutations scattered throughout these very large genes; if you're going to set up a clinical test, you have to be able to find any of them. You can't just look in one part of the gene, you've got to look at the whole thing. There are exceptions, however. You may have heard, for example, that in the Ashkenazi Jewish population there are only a couple of mutations in BRCA1, and another one in BRCA2, which appear to be rather common and which are easier to test for because you don't have to study the whole gene. But in most other, more outbred groups, you have to look all the way across the entire gene if your test is to have any clinical usefulness.

So the first challenge is a technical one. How can we solve it?

Joseph Goldstein spoke about hamburgers, chips, and genes. The last two items have now been combined into a single entity called a "gene chip," a high-density array to look at gene expression. David Botstein, in his talk, showed you an example, and our version—which for the sake of time, I will not describe—applies the same principles. Most of us are pretty optimistic that this new technology will soon revolutionize our ability to look for subtle sequence changes in almost any gene at a reasonable cost. Once the chips have been designed, they can be mass-produced, and DNA can be analyzed within two or three hours and at an estimated cost of something like $10 to $20 per test. So this technological development opens up the possibility in the future of testing for sequence changes in any one of us, for almost any gene, at a fairly modest cost. We are probably two to three years from making this technology a reality. So if I did set up that booth out there and I had a chip machine, I might be able to tell you by the end of this symposium whether you have a mutation in BRCA1 or BRCA2. Again, would you want to know?

Let's look at a specific family. I will confess right off that I will show you a "best case" for the usefulness of this technology. Then I'll tell you that it may not be representative of the most common problems, and why. FIGURE 1 gives the pedigree of a family I know pretty well. I first met them seven years ago, at the University of Michigan, when they came in for counseling because so many women in the family were dying of breast and ovarian cancer. A 35-year old woman, in particular, was desperately concerned because she had watched both of her sisters develop breast cancer (one of them twice), her mother had breast cancer, and her aunt had died of ovarian cancer after surviving breast cancer in her mid-forties. Of course, the woman herself was sure that she had to be next. After all, she had no unaffected first-degree relatives. And while we counseled her in 1990—not knowing very much about the genetics of this disorder—that her risk was probably close to 50%, we really didn't know if this number was correct. We were pretty sure it wasn't 100%, which was her assumption, but that's about all we could say.

Subsequently, the BRCA1 gene was mapped by Mary-Claire King,[3] and then cloned by Mark Skolnick and others.[4] With those developments, it became possible to determine that this family has a four-base-pair deletion in BRCA1, which is fairly easy to find once you know exactly where to look. That information allowed us to inform members of the family whether they were at risk. Before we did so, however,

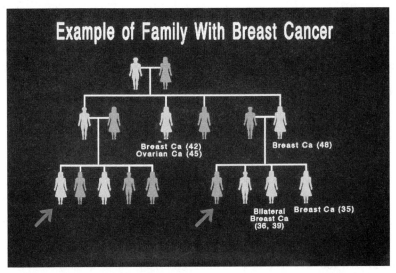

FIGURE 1. Pedigree of a family with breast and ovarian cancer. A 35-year-old woman, designated by the *arrow at right,* sought medical advice because her mother and two sisters had breast cancer, and an aunt had died of ovarian cancer after surviving breast cancer in her mid-forties. The family requested genetic testing; lighter figures tested positive for a BRCA1 mutation. Just three days before surgery to perform prophylactic mastectomy, the 35-year-old woman discovered she was not a carrier of a mutation in the BRCA1 gene, and therefore was not at increased risk of breast cancer. A female cousin designated by the *arrow at left,* who thought she did not carry an increased risk of cancer, discovered she had inherited a BRCA1 mutation from her father. Immediate testing revealed she already had cancer, though early diagnosis and treatment have increased her chance of cure.

we asked them, "Do you want to know?" In this family, they desperately wanted to know because they were already living with such a high level of anxiety, especially the woman who had come to consult me. In fact, she had decided on the basis of what she perceived to be an unacceptably high risk to go ahead with prophylactic bilateral mastectomy. Only three days before that surgery was to be done we learned, through testing, that she does not carry the mutation that her two sisters and her mother carry.

This particular woman was spared needless surgery. She had lived with this anxiety for at least 10 years, and her fears about her daughter (who is not shown in the diagram in FIGURE 1) were also greatly reduced, because the daughter can't carry the mutation if the mother doesn't carry it. (Of course, this mother and daughter can still get breast cancer just like anybody else, but their risk is now at the baseline of the general population, not the exorbitant number that it had seemed to be before.) I will tell you, however, that my patient had a great deal of trouble adjusting to the good news after the initial exhilaration wore off, because she felt profoundly guilty about the outcome. Just like survivors of the Holocaust who are described as having "survivor guilt," she found it very difficult to deal with the fact that the other women in her family had suffered and died from this terrible disease, while she had been spared. This burden had been something they had shared; it was part of their family bond. Now she was in a different category. She was let off the hook as a consequence of the test.

Thus, this story illustrates the power of genetic information and how critical it is that we support people going through this experience, even when they get good news. We must make sure that these people have adjusted to their new view of themselves, a goal that can be accomplished through excellent genetic counseling. As testing becomes generally available, we will need counseling for large numbers of people, and we currently have only a thousand genetic counselors in the country. I will return to this problem at the end of my talk.

Another interesting (and disturbing) result occurred in another part of the family —cousins of the people I have just described. They participated in our research study and decided they wanted to know their results—partly, perhaps, because none of the women in this part of the family had an affected first-degree relative, so they assumed they were not at any increased risk of cancer. As FIGURE 1 shows, however, their father had the mutation. Although he was O.K., he had passed the mutated gene to two of his daughters, who had no clue they were at high risk. When these daughters came in to learn the results of their tests, they were, understandably, deeply shaken to realize they were in the same situation as their cousins, who already had cancer at that age. The older daughter was forty at the time. After learning of her high risk, she decided to be examined right away, because she'd never had a mammogram and had not practiced self-examinations. On physical examination, there were no palpable lumps in her breasts. But the mammogram, done the same day she got the results of the genetics test, unfortunately showed an alarming-looking, though small, lesion in the right breast. It was biopsied the next day and turned out to be cancer.

This woman was put through an enormously wrenching experience. In 24 hours she went from thinking she was at low risk, to finding out she was at high risk, to discovering she already had cancer and having to face choices about what she could do. Furthermore, she also learned that she might get cancer in the opposite breast, which is common in this high-risk situation; and she might even get ovarian cancer as well.

This woman decided to proceed with bilateral mastectomy. Her chances of being cured of the cancer are extremely high, because of its small size and because all the lymph nodes were unaffected. She believed for her the right thing to do was also to remove the opposite breast, in order to minimize the risk of having another breast cancer. But we had to tell her that we don't yet know how much this procedure reduces her risk; some women have developed breast cancer in the small amount of epithelial tissue that remains after surgery, even years after prophylactic mastectomy. Finally, after another year of thinking about it and deciding she didn't want to have any more children, she had her ovaries removed as well.

These are tough choices. These are drastic options. We all wish we had something better to offer women in these circumstances. There are other options, but we don't yet have the data to predict their outcomes. Instead of removing the left breast, this woman could have chosen to have mammograms at regular intervals, just like the one that picked up the cancer in her right breast. Could she count on that regimen picking up the next cancer quickly? In this high-risk situation, we simply don't know the answer to that important question. And there is no truly effective screening for the associated risk of ovarian cancer. So you can appreciate the complexities of the situation: Pandora's box is potentially opened when we offer testing to someone. We cannot easily answer the patient's question, "How would this information help me?"

The introduction of BRCA1 testing to the general public presents barriers and is an area of enormous controversy. Searching for a possible mutation through a large gene is technically complex and therefore expensive. A commercial test costs approximately $2,400, and is currently not reimbursed by many third-party payers. It is unclear how best to medically manage somebody found to have a mutation. Genetic counseling on a large scale will surely be required once an inexpensive screening test becomes available. Researchers do not yet know whether some mutations are worse than others. Should we be quoting everybody the same cancer risk, or do some mutations carry a higher risk or a lower risk, or perhaps even no risk? And finally, I am sorry to say, this information could be used against individuals who have mutations.

Another, very recent, finding carries presymptomatic testing one step further. It concerns the Ashkenazi Jewish population, on which much genetic research has focused in the last 20 years, because this population went through a fairly narrow genetic bottleneck. It had a limited number of "founders," meaning the population is derived from a small number of ancestors and thus has a narrow range of genetic variation. When you search for a specific alteration in a gene, you may find it at higher frequency in a narrow population than in an outbred one, such as the population of the entire United States. Bert Vogelstein's group published an article in *Nature Genetics*, in which they reported a sequence change in the so-called APC (adenomatous polyposis coli) gene.[5] If this gene is completely inactivated, a relatively rare condition ensues called familial adenomatous polyposis. Individuals with this disease will get colon cancer 100% of the time if their colons are not removed by the age of about 30, because they have hundreds or even thousands of polyps, and eventually one of those polyps will degenerate into a cancer. But the individuals studied by Vogelstein's group did not have that kind of syndrome; they had only a few polyps, maybe 4 or 5, and yet their risk of cancer was still about twice that of the general population.

The subtle mutation that the Vogelstein group identified involves a change in just a single nucleotide, from a T to an A, which changes one amino acid to another, an isoleucine to a lysine. While sometimes a change in a single amino acid can be deleterious, in this instance the change doesn't affect the function of the encoded protein. This finding therefore suggests a brand new mechanism, and Vogelstein and his coworkers present evidence that, while in itself the sequence change is probably benign, it creates a potential for further mutation in the DNA. There are now 8 "A"s (adenines) in a row in the mutant sequence, which makes it difficult for the cell to copy the gene and to make the protein product. And so the cell sometimes makes a mistake—not frequently, but a lot more frequently than if it were copying the normal gene. Consequently, there is an occasional polyp that may progress to cancer, much less frequently than in the full-blown disease of familial adenomatous polyposis, but still at a greater frequency than in the normal population.

The greatest impact of this new finding on medical practice may be that this particular alteration is very common. It is found in about 6% of Ashkenazi Jews. In Jews with colon cancer, it is found in 10%; in those with colon cancer at an early age, 16%; and in those with colon cancer and a positive family history, 28%. It is a smoking gun, which says that this particular sequence change in the DNA confers an increased risk of familial adenomatous polyposis. Statistically, the risk goes up about twofold for those having the mutation.

Researchers have hotly debated how to use this information. The discoverer, Bert Vogelstein, argues that every Jewish individual with a family history of colon cancer should be tested for this new type of mutation, and if it is found, he or she should undergo a program of regular colonoscopy beginning at age 35 and repeated every two years for the rest of their lives. After all, he argues, we know that colon cancer of this type begins as a benign polyp and only after many years may develop into an invasive carcinoma. One would predict, therefore, that such a program of regular colonoscopy applied to these high-risk individuals would save lives. While that prediction is indeed plausible, I think we should insist on examining more data before we rush into the new preventive regimen proposed by Dr. Vogelstein, for it would entail major inconvenience and expense for a very large number of people, perhaps hundreds of thousands. With luck, we will have the data very soon. As in so many other instances, one has to worry about the people who have tested positive for the genetic alteration and who might need the colonoscopy. Will they discover their health insurance has been canceled, so they will be deprived not only of the colonoscopies but also of all other health care? This is not an idle question.

Let us now consider the influence of inheritance on much more common diseases. The leading causes of death in the United States in 1995 were heart disease, cancer, cerebral vascular disease, emphysema, bronchitis, accidents, pneumonia, influenza, diabetes, AIDS, suicide, and liver disease. In my opinion, genetics is involved in all of these diseases except accidents; and even there inherited predisposition may play a role. We should therefore want to uncover the genetic roots of all of these causes of death, particularly those for which medical surveillance or lifestyle changes would reduce risk.

A new kind of future might be only ten years hence. At the age of 18 individuals might go to their physician, undergo tests that will accurately predict risk for a considerable list of conditions for which effective interventions will be available, and then follow a program of medical surveillance, diet, and lifestyle that would reduce the risks. Such a program would be true preventive medicine, practiced on a genotype-specific basis as opposed to our current one-size-fits-all recommendations. Of course, people need to be reassured, before they sign up, that the information derived from genetic testing will benefit them; I'll come to that aspect in a minute. The point is we could undoubtedly make a dent in some of the leading causes of death if we could identify those at highest risk.

How will we get there? Not by continuing the current strategy, because most of the successes we've achieved so far in identifying genetic contributions to common diseases have been for those with low-frequency but high-penetrance mutations. I've talked about BRCA1 and BRCA2 as examples, but they account for only 5% of breast cancer cases. What about the other 95%? Many of those seem to have hereditary influences, but much weaker ones. Genes for diabetes, called MODY-1, -2, and -3, have been found in the last three years, but they account for only about 5% of adult-onset diabetes. What about the other 95%? Research in Parkinson's disease was electrified recently [mid-1997] by the discovery of a mutation in a gene on chromosome 4, which codes for a protein called alpha-synuclein. But so far this mutation has been identified in only about five families, and most people with Parkinson's disease do not have that alteration. And yet, there does seem to be a hereditary component in Parkinson's disease.

How, then, can we make progress with the more common disorders, those due to high-frequency, low-penetrance mutations? I have already talked about the I1307K mutation that causes colon cancer in the Jewish population. Perhaps the best example right now is the apoE mutation in Alzheimer's disease. There are three common kinds of apoE: apoE2, apoE3, and apoE4 (I don't know what happened to apoE1). ApoE4 predisposes to Alzheimer's disease, so if you have one copy of it, your risk goes up substantially, and if you have two copies, you're probably going to have Alzheimer's disease by age 75 or 80. Yet, apoE confers a relatively weak genetic influence so one can't use it right now clinically, particularly because as yet we have nothing therapeutic to offer the persons at high risk. This relatively weak predisposition is probably the way genetics will work for most common diseases: more like the apoE example than the BRCA1 example.

Perhaps we could come up with a strategy to understand the common diseases more quickly. Like many others in the genetics community, I am spending a lot of my time thinking about a new approach, which might very well need to be taken on as an additional goal of the Genome Project. That approach might identify the functional variations in the human genome that actually contribute to common diseases. There may not be all that many. You recall that 99.9% of our sequences are identical, which means that approximately 0.1% of them, or about 3 million, are variations that may contribute to common diseases. Moreover, most of those 3 million are in regions that ostensibly do nothing; they constitute the so-called "junk" (actually, this is most of our DNA), which neither codes for protein nor regulates gene expression. If, say, 1% of the 3 million variations are in genes, then we would have approximately 30,000 variations that might be involved in common diseases. That estimate is a very squishy number that might be off by a factor of 2 or 3; but it is in the ballpark of the total number of common functional variations in our genome that distinguish us from one another. Maybe we should try to catalogue those relatively few variants because many of them will, in fact, turn out to play a role in health and disease.

If you had those variants catalogued, and you had classified people into those who have a given disease and those who do not, you could screen the affected and the unaffected for association with one or more of the approximately 30,000 variants, using microchip technology. That's called an "association" study, which is easier to do than a pedigree study because you do not have to find families with many affected individuals. You have to be careful, however, that the affecteds and the unaffecteds are not different in some other genetic way, such as coming from a different ethnic population, because you could then get spurious correlations. But if you take that precaution, this strategy has greater power to detect a gene involved in disease than does the pedigree approach, and it is also easier to implement because you don't have to find those rare pedigrees with multiple affected individuals.

Of course, to use this approach at the present time, one has to make a guess about which gene to study, and typically that guess is wrong. We ought to find the variations in all our genes, all 80,000 to 100,000 of them. Of these, approximately one-half to one-third will have common functional variants, and once we have those variants, we would perform a whole genome association study with the common diseases. That approach would be radical—something we've never even thought of doing. Completion of the entire Genome Project is not a prerequisite for getting started on such a project soon.

We probably already have a pretty good idea about what kinds of genes are contributing to the common diseases. Joseph Goldstein and Michael Brown work on cardiovascular disease and cholesterol metabolism. Thanks mainly to their work, we already know a lot about the pathway that regulates cholesterol. If we wanted to figure out why one person's cholesterol is higher or lower than another person's, we could identify a list of 20 or 30 candidate genes likely to set the level of blood cholesterol. By characterizing their common functional variants, we could identify the source of that human variability in a particular population. The same is true for hypertension. We already know a lot about which genes contribute to the regulation of blood pressure, but nobody has made a list, characterized common variants, and carried out a big experiment on a population. That experiment ought to be done. We have the requisite technology, and the power of an association analysis is going to be substantially greater than that of a family-based analysis.

However, the cost of finding those variants is a very important issue. It will be expensive and time-consuming to study a single gene in a small lab and try to characterize its variation. I'm going to argue that we should—right now [1997] and with public funds—set out to characterize the common functional variants in as many genes as we can get our hands on, and keep on going until we have them all.

There is another, scary reason why this project ought to be done very soon. You may not realize it, but a functional variation in a human gene is patentable. If you pluck a gene out of nowhere, test a hundred people to determine the sequence of that gene, and then find variations in the sequence, you can, believe it or not, patent each variation. It is not unimaginable, and is perhaps even probable, that if the project is not done with public funds within the next three or four years, someone in the private sector will assemble databases for the common functional variants of the human genome, and patent those databases. If we allow that to happen, investigators who wish to study a disease might have to work out licensing agreements with 10 or 20 different companies before they can even start to perform one experiment. That outcome would be very unfortunate. I think, therefore, that the NIH ought to step forward and carry out the project as quickly as possible. Preferably, the NIH would do it in partnership with some of the large pharmaceutical companies, who share our view that our genes are a research tool and not a property, and that, therefore, the databases ought to be available to anybody who wants them.

Let me end by emphasizing some of the major ethical and social issues being raised by the Human Genome Project, a topic that is, after all, the major theme of this entire bicentennial symposium. I have already alluded to some of these issues as I reviewed specific examples. Clearly, as we move forward with the science of the Genome Project—and we *should* move forward as aggressively as we can—we also have to take responsibility for how this information will be used. That is our obligation as scientists, as citizens, and as human beings. James Watson, the first director of the Human Genome Project, saw this need from the very beginning, when he and Nancy Wexler started the ELSI (Ethical, Legal, and Social Implications) Program, a program that has been very successful in producing quality research into the ethical and legal issues associated with the Genome Project. The Program is now furnishing us with policy recommendations that are being adopted by leaders in the administration and in Congress.

The ELSI Program identified four major priorities deserving of close attention: (1) health insurance for those known to be at genetic risk; (2) employability for those known to be at risk; (3) privacy of health records; and (4) education of health professionals. I will take up each of these, in turn.

Perhaps the major worry for most people is the possibility that they will be denied health insurance because they are found to be at genetic risk for illness, even though they are currently healthy. The Kassebaum–Kennedy bill made substantial progress with this problem last year [1996], but some loopholes remain. On July 14, 1997, the President of the United States put his support behind plugging those loopholes. Discrimination in health insurance is both unjust (because we don't choose our DNA) and unworkable (because we are all at genetic risk for some illnesses). Ultimately, nobody will be insurable if genetic predisposition to illness is the reason for exclusion. In fact, insurance companies themselves are not opposed to eliminating the discrimination. We need to come to grips with this problem, and we must do so at the federal level in order to avoid a lot of variation among states. Rights to employment by those at risk pose an analogous issue.

The problems of insurability and employability also involve the need for privacy of health records. Legislative efforts to avoid discrimination will be successful only if health records are kept confidential. Not only should information about a person's health not be generally available, but it should also be forbidden to even ask people about their health—just as it is already prohibited, in certain settings, to inquire about race; otherwise, mischief will ensue. A national debate on privacy of medical records is already under way, and genetics are going to be an important part of that debate.

The fourth major issue is one that I am personally deeply concerned about, and it is highly relevant to the future of medical practice. Are our health care professionals ready for the genetic revolution? Surveys have shown repeatedly that, by and large, physicians are unprepared to deal with genetic information. A recent report in *The New England Journal of Medicine*[6] showed that fully one-third of physicians who informed their patients about the results of a genetic test for colon cancer failed to understand what the test meant. Understanding that test does not require filling one's head with factoids—a practice which I, like David Botstein, decry. Rather, it requires the mastery of *principles*, of basic Mendelian inheritance and penetrance and probabilities of risk. Beyond that, physicians and other professionals who perform genetic counseling will need a humane approach to patients, and they will need to learn how to be nondirective in situations where the correct course of action may be ambiguous. Currently, we physicians are poor at these skills, and yet most medical schools still do not teach genetics in a way that will rectify this shortcoming.

Some groups are working on this problem, however. The American Medical Association and the American Nurses Association have formed a coalition with the NHGRI to assemble an electronic database that will allow busy physicians and nurses, as well as patients, to find out what they need to know when dealing with complex genetic situations.

Sir William Osler's words are singularly appropriate, both for what we have been trying to accomplish for the last 200 years, and certainly for what we should accomplish for the next century. Medicine is all about this:

> To wrest from nature the secrets which have perplexed philosophers in all ages; to track to their sources the causes of disease; to correlate the vast stores of knowledge that they may be quickly available for the prevention and cure of disease. These are our ambitions.

These principles drive the Genome Project, and are, I think, what's driving every medical school. Wayne Gretsky put it even more succinctly: "Skate where the puck is going to be."

REFERENCES

1. 1985. Science **230:** 1054–1057.
2. 1989. Science **245:** 1059–1065.
3. 1990. Science **250:** 1684–1689.
4. 1994. Science **266:** 66–71.
5. 1997. Nature Genetics **17:** 79–83.
6. 1997. N. Engl. J. Med. **336:** 823–827.

Commentary on the Genetics Session

CHARLES N. COLE

*Professor of Biochemistry, Dartmouth Medical School, Hanover,
New Hampshire 03755, USA*

Dartmouth College was 100 years old, and Dartmouth Medical School about 70, when the principles of genetics were first deduced by Gregor Mendel. Although Mendel's experiments marked the beginning of the scientific study of heredity, genetics actually had played a central role in the development of our civilization over thousands of years prior to Mendel. Our major food crops and the domestication of animals resulted from the practice of genetics, beginning at the end of the last ice age and continuing into the present time. Early people examined their crop plants and domesticated their animals, and they selected those with the most desirable traits for further breeding and propagation. They thus were aware that desirable traits could be passed along to the progeny, even though these advances took place with little or no understanding of the principles underlying genetics. Our ancestors probably noticed that children bore a physical resemblance to their parents, and most likely they were also aware that some diseases occurred within families. Yet many more centuries were required before genetics would become a central foundation of the biological sciences.

It is worthwhile to briefly review the experiments of Mendel—ingenious, conclusive, profound, yet simple—which he performed in the 1860s. He crossed pea plants having different properties (phenotypes) with one another and observed the patterns by which the properties of the parents were inherited by the offspring (the first generation offspring are the F1 generation; crossing F1 offspring with one another yields the F2 generation, and so forth). Mendel crossed pea plants that differed from one another in a single property (e.g., short versus tall plants, yellow versus green seeds, wrinkled versus smooth seeds, and so forth). In some cases, all offspring resembled one of the parent plants, but not the other, in respect to a particular trait—a phenomenon that we recognize today as genetic dominance. When these apparently identical F1 plants were bred with each other, Mendel observed that the parental trait that was not detectable in the F1 progeny reappeared in the F2 progeny. He interpreted this result to mean that traits were specified by particulate factors, transmitted intact from parent to offspring, and that the phenotype does not necessarily reveal the genotype.

The particulate factors are now known as genes. Alleles are different varieties of the same gene, able to produce or contribute to different phenotypes. Mendel noticed that sometimes, even when the progeny resembled neither parent in respect to a particular trait, the parental phenotypes reappeared when these F1 plants were crossed. For example, crossing a plant having white flowers with one having red flowers could yield an F1 generation of pink plants; but crossing the pink plants to one another led to an F2 generation with white, red, *and* pink plants—always in the same ratio. This finding indicated that plants contained genes with genetic information from each parent and that these different forms of the same gene (alleles) were distributed independently to the offspring through gametes (eggs and sperm in animals). The principle of segregation of alleles during the formation of gametes is now known as Mendel's First Law.

Mendel also carried out crosses between plants that differed in two traits (e.g., smooth yellow seeds versus wrinkled green seeds). He observed that in each cross, the different traits were inherited independently. Progeny were obtained that had smooth green seeds, wrinkled green seeds, smooth yellow seeds, and wrinkled yellow seeds—again, in highly reproducible and predictable proportions for each phenotype. This result indicated to Mendel that seed color was inherited separately from smoothness, leading to Mendel's Second Law, the principle of independent assortment. Today we understand that independent assortment means that different genes are located on different chromosomes. Gametes are haploid, meaning that only a single copy of each gene, or a single copy of each chromosome, is found in the gametes. All other cells are diploid, containing two copies of each chromosome and each gene. Mendel's Second Law indicates that gametes containing DNA from both parents gave rise to the gamete-producing organism.

Although Mendel's work was published in the 1860s, it attracted little attention at that time. His principles were rediscovered at about the time that Dartmouth Medical School celebrated its first centenary, namely, in the late 1800s. The past 100 years have seen an accelerating interest in and understanding of genetics. Determining the chemical nature of the genetic material (genes) was the focus of many years of investigation; it culminated in Avery's discovery, in 1944, that DNA was the carrier of genetic information.[1] He and his coworkers were able to transfer the properties of one strain of bacteria to another by adding the DNA from the first to cells of the second. And this important work was followed, in 1953, by another pivotal milestone, the elucidation of the structure of DNA by Watson and Crick.[2] It was the seminal contribution by Watson and Crick that ushered in the era of molecular genetics —a revolution (in the words of several speakers at the symposium) that has brought us today to a sophisticated understanding of what genes and chromosomes are, how the information in DNA is expressed as protein via an RNA intermediate, how genes are regulated, and how complex genetic programs operate during development and differentiation.

As Dartmouth Medical School celebrates its 200th anniversary, we can look back over a century of progress in genetics, and we can look forward to the central role that this scientific discipline will play in the next century. It is conceivable, in fact, that the next century will someday be looked back on as "The Genetic Century." Given the central role that the discipline is playing in the biological and biomedical sciences today, it is perhaps not surprising that this symposium opened with a session on this topic.

Nancy Wexler, cofounder with her father and sister of the Hereditary Disease Foundation, and currently its president, described her long odyssey toward finding the gene responsible for Huntington's disease. It is a fascinating and dramatic story, not least because the Huntington's gene, which is inherited in an autosomal manner, is carried in Wexler's family. As she recounts it so poignantly in her presentation, Nancy Wexler was 21 years old when she learned that her mother was dying of this incurable disease and that she and her sister each had a 50% probability of having inherited the defective Huntington's gene. Her contribution toward isolating the gene by going to Lake Maracaibo in Venezuela, where Huntington's disease runs rampant in an extended family with more than 16,000 individuals, is legendary. That work also led to the painful awareness that the disease becomes more severe and has an earlier age of onset in subsequent generations.

In the early 1980s the problem of finding the Huntington's gene amidst 100,000 other human genes was daunting. As Nancy Wexler and David Botstein make clear in their presentations, the task was accomplished through a marvelous, concerted, and cooperative effort by a number of laboratories in the United States and England. They credit Bruce Alberts, now president of the National Academy of Sciences, with having had the vision and leadership to guide the project in the right directions.

One seminal contribution that greatly aided the effort was a landmark paper published in 1980 by David Botstein, Ray White, Mark Skolnick, and Ron Davis.[3] They proposed a novel method for identifying disease genes and other genes of interest, through the use of a "marker" called restriction fragment length polymorphisms (RFLPs). These markers were key toward the ultimate success of finding an allele that differed dramatically from normal and was present in all people who had developed Huntington's disease,[4] as well as in many younger individuals who had not yet come down with the symptoms of Huntington's disease. We now know that the mutated form of this gene is the causative agent of Huntington's disease. This mutant allele acts dominantly and with 100% penetrance so that all individuals who inherit one copy of the mutant allele eventually succumb to Huntington's disease. The successful culmination of the project represented an important breakthrough, since it permitted the development of a test that today allows prenatal determination of whether or not a fetus has the Huntington's gene.

However, as Nancy Wexler related at the end of her talk, and as Francis Collins also described for other diseases, such testing brings with it major psychological and ethical problems. A prenatal test is useful if the presence of the mutation causes the disease 100% of the time. If other factors (e.g., other mutations or environmental factors) are also required, then simply finding a mutant allele is insufficient for predicting whether or not the disease will appear later. This makes it difficult to decide whether or not to terminate a pregnancy.

The difficulties related to testing after birth would be in large measure alleviated if effective therapy for the diseases being tested were at hand. Often, however, there is a lag of many years—even decades—between the time when a test to detect a mutant gene becomes available and when effective treatments can be applied. Although we now know where on chromosome 4 the Huntington's disease gene is located, what the sequence of amino acids in the encoded protein is, and how this protein is altered in people who carry the mutated gene, we have little understanding of how this particular genetic defect produces the profound and ultimately fatal neurological and behavioral abnormalities of Huntington's disease. Animal models of human diseases frequently play crucial roles in understanding a disease and developing effective treatments. And so it appears to have been with the recent development of a mouse model for Huntington's disease, which, as Wexler relates, may soon result in our understanding of how the mutant gene causes Huntington's disease and how, therefore, we might be able to treat and prevent it.

David Botstein, professor and chair of Genetics at Stanford University, discussed the basic principles of genetics, especially in relation to the various kinds of markers that are used for mapping genes. There are two types of maps: a genetic map and a physical map. A genetic map—likened so clearly by Dr. Botstein to a map of the United States divided into just states—tells us the relative order of genes on a chromosome. This is often called linkage analysis and is conducted by determining the frequency with which two different genetic markers are inherited together. A physical map—compared by Dr. Botstein to a detailed street map of Chicago—gives precise "street addresses" for each gene on a given chromosome. It tells us physically the order of different segments of DNA. This permits us to identify and clone genes, including those responsible for causing diseases. The development of many, ever more refined markers, and of new and more efficient approaches to mapping, has enabled geneticists to construct increasingly detailed physical maps of the entire human genome. As maps improve, we can find the physical location of specific genes with increasing precision. The ultimate physical map of the human genome is the complete sequence of every human chromosome, and it is essential for finding every human gene.

Botstein also stressed the importance of working with model organisms. In fact, when the decision was made to sequence the human genome, it was decided to sequence the genomes of several model organisms as well. Models in wide use today include the common intestinal bacterium of humans, *E. coli*; baker's yeast (*Saccharomyces cerevisiae*); the fruit fly (*Drosophila melanogaster*); the nematode worm (*Caenorhabditis elegans*); and the mouse (*Mus musculus*). A small plant that is a member of the mustard family, *Arabadopsis thaliana*, has become the model of choice for studies of plant biology.

Many factors enter into choosing model organisms. These include ease of growth under laboratory conditions, the ability to obtain large numbers of organisms, and the ability to visualize cytologically processes within the cells of these organisms. One of the most important properties for most model organisms in use today is that they are highly amenable to genetic analyses. This means that mutants can be readily isolated and crossed, both to determine whether two genes are linked, and to generate organisms carrying both mutant genes.

The great utility of model organisms is a reflection of the remarkable unity of molecular and biologic processes within living systems. This unity derives from the general rule that biologically useful functions tend to be preserved during evolution. By and large, even very complex biological processes occur by identical or nearly identical mechanisms, using closely related proteins, in all organisms that use a given process. Thus if a certain process occurs in yeast cells (e.g., secretion, transcription, and signal transduction) and also in multicellular organisms (even including humans), then yeast cells are usually an ideal model system for understanding that process. This rule generally holds so true that in some cases the human homologue of a yeast protein can function as well in yeast as can the yeast's own protein. It is for these reasons that yeast is a favored model organism for studying basic cellular processes. Some processes, however—for example, development and cellular differentiation—are far more complex in metazoan (multicellular) organisms than in the one-celled yeast. Therefore, the fruit fly, the worm, the mouse, and the frog *(Xenopus laevis)* serve as models for studying these processes.

These days, as soon as a human disease gene is identified and sequenced, computer analyses are conducted to determine whether a homologous gene exists in yeast or has been identified in metazoan models. And if such homologues exist, an investigator immediately turns to one of the model organisms to determine the function and mechanism of action of the affected gene and its protein product, and to identify other proteins that are involved. Obviously, one can search for homologues in model organisms only if their genome has been sequenced, and that is why geneticists advocate the completion of the genome projects not only for humans but also for the other models—a point emphasized for the mouse, for example, by Francis Collins in his presentation. The sequencing of the genomes of baker's yeast and the worm has been completed,[5,6] and finishing the sequencing of the genomes of all the other important model organisms is in progress. Model organisms can also be of great utility in designing and testing drugs that can be used to block the action of specific mutant gene products. Botstein emphasized that basic research, including studies of model organisms, is absolutely essential for progress in the treatment of human genetic disorders—as, indeed, it is for progress in the treatment of all diseases.

Francis Collins, director of the National Human Genome Research Institute, spoke next. He has been responsible for putting in place the complex infrastructure needed for sequencing the human genome. His talk focused on the medical consequences of the Human Genome Project, a theme touched on by both Wexler and Botstein. Collins reemphasized that we are in the midst of a revolution in genetics that will have profound effects on all aspects of medicine. He underscored the emerging view that all diseases—even many cases of trauma—have a genetic component.

Over the past few decades, we have gone from thinking of human genetics as a subspecialty of pediatrics, focused on developmental disorders and rare diseases with relatively simple Mendelian inheritance, to the current view that genetics is of great importance and relevance for all branches of medicine. Genetic mechanisms underlie both normal and pathologic aspects of human health—the ways in which humans develop and the diseases we acquire as we age. Human genetics is now as important in a department of medicine or a section of endocrinology as it used to be (and continues to be) in departments of pediatrics. Most medical schools in the United States have established distinct departments of genetics or of human genetics.

The importance of genetics for human medicine is likely to increase dramatically in the next decade, when it will become possible to know the makeup of each person's genome. This capability can lead to development of strategies for lifelong medical care designed specifically for that person and based on his or her genotype. Thus genetic advances will permit development of entirely new approaches to the treatment and prevention of disease.

The revolution in genetics has several aspects. One is that the discipline is now taking up a new challenge: to define the influence of each of multiple genes in the causation of our most common diseases. For disorders inherited in a Mendelian pattern, and therefore caused by mutation at a single locus, isolating the affected gene is now routine. But most medical conditions are far more complex, and reflect the interplay of many genes and their protein products. Dozens of genes are involved in diseases such as cancer, diabetes, heart disease, stroke, and mental illness, to mention a few. Determining how each member of a diverse set of genes contributes to such diseases or to specific biological processes is one of the formidable tasks that lies ahead.

A second aspect of the revolution is our ability to handle and analyze the ever-increasing volume of information, a point also emphasized by David Botstein. Collins discussed the emerging technology of DNA chips, where DNA probes specific for thousands of genes can be attached to a conventional microscope slide, and then used to analyze the patterns of gene expression in different cells and tissues, and in healthy versus diseased conditions. These gene chips are likely to be adapted to measure genetic diversity within the human population. The mere numbers are staggering: The genome of the chimpanzee is 99% identical with ours, yet the differences between humans and chimps are profound. Each human shares 99.9% of its DNA with any other human, which means, nevertheless, that there are approximately three million differences in the complete DNA sequence between any two people. Although most of these differences are not expressed as altered protein products and therefore do not influence function or health, still, two humans will produce different proteins from several thousand genes. In many cases, change in a single amino acid caused by a difference of a single DNA sequence, yields a protein that remains fully functional in spite of the amino acid difference. But in other cases, a change in a single DNA sequence can eliminate a protein, destroy its activity, or empower it with new activities so that it causes disease. Once the human genome has been sequenced, it will prove possible to determine precisely how much variability exists within the human population at each genetic locus. And by comparing the genomes of two advanced primates, the chimpanzee and the human, we should gain new insights into human evolution.

In a series of poignant examples—relating to cystic fibrosis, breast cancer, and colon cancer—Collins highlighted the ethical, legal, and social implications of the accelerating revolution in genetics. As had Nancy Wexler, so Collins pointed out that decades of additional work may be required before effective treatments are developed to prevent, control, or cure various inherited diseases that we can currently predict and diagnose. Clearly, there will be an increasing number of situations where identifying disease genes will lead to effective treatments. At that point, identifying carriers of a defective allele will permit treatment that prevents a disease from occurring or ameliorates its symptoms and effects.

In the meantime, clinical medicine must confront questions such as these: Should genetic tests be generally available? Would most people wish to know at an early age —or would they rather not know—that they are highly likely (or certain) to develop a serious disease? For example, should some women undergo preventive bilateral mastectomy if they carry a defective gene that can result in breast cancer? Not all people with these mutations develop breast cancer, and even radical surgery may not prevent the appearance of cancer at other sites in these individuals. Should certain Ashkenazi Jews undergo frequent colonoscopies for the rest of their lives because they carry a gene that predisposes them to colon cancer? Effective treatments exist for colon cancer if it is detected at an early stage. How do we prevent misuse of genetic information, which might lead to discriminatory employment practices or refusal of health and life insurance? All of us must be prepared to participate in the resolution of these profound questions.

Collins concluded by emphasizing a point made earlier by Botstein: that we must revise medical curricula so that new physicians are knowledgeable about and comfortable with modern genetics. If they and other health professionals are to counsel patients competently, it is essential that they know the principles of genetics, beginning with Mendel, including how genes function and are regulated. In an era when information about human health and disease is expanding at an accelerating rate, physicians will need to rely on fundamental principles of basic science in order to make their way through the forest of medical information.

The final presentation in the genetics session was delivered by Richard Axel,[a] an investigator of the Howard Hughes Medical Institute and a professor of biochemistry and of pathology at Columbia University. At an early point in his education, Axel decided to devote his energy to basic research. His work represents a superb example of how modern approaches, including those of genetics, can be used to understand fundamental aspects of neurobiological function.

A major focus of Dr. Axel's studies has been to understand the biology of perception, specifically the molecular basis of smell.[7–9] He pointed out that smell is the most primitive of our senses, probably because it is linked to the ability of organisms to find food and mates and to avoid predators, that is, to survive and propagate. A sense of smell enables organisms to detect various chemicals in the air, to transmit the information to the brain, and to evaluate this information so that a representation within the brain will reflect the smell of the outside world. This information can then be the basis for action. The brain, said Axel, is an assembly of highly organized, specialized cells adapted for perception, cognition, and memory—and these cellular functions are encoded in our genes. The importance of the sense of smell in evolution is reflected in the fact that 1 to 2% of the entire complement of genes—the largest gene family known—is devoted to odor perception, from the worm *C. elegans* to mammals.

One major problem of olfaction is to understand how our brains are able to distinguish among thousands or tens of thousands of different odors. Two very similar chemical substances can have very different odors, and the brain has little trouble distinguishing between them. In addition, smells are often linked to deep emotions and distant memories—as with Marcel Proust's madeleines. How do we recognize this diversity of odors and couple the information with memory and feeling? Axel's research is beginning to provide answers to these questions.

Humans and most other mammals have two olfactory systems: the general system that detects odors, and the vomeronasal system, which subserves mating. The detection of odors begins with the olfactory epithelium, located at the rear of the nose. One type of cell located there, a bipolar neuron, extends specialized dendritic processes to the epithelium, where they connect to an array of cilia that are thought to interact with the odorant through specific proteins called "receptors." The energy of binding of special chemicals to the cilia of these detectors on the surface of these neurons is relayed electrically to a portion of the brain called the olfactory bulb. The region then projects into the neocortex and somehow facilitates connection of odors to memories and emotions.

The vomeronasal organ, or the "erotic nose," is more primitive, bypassing the cognitive brain. It recognizes pheromones, chemical compounds that influence the behavior of members of the same species and are involved in detecting mates and

---

[a]Regrettably, it was not possible to publish as a part of these proceedings the presentation made by Dr. Axel entitled "Towards a Molecular Biology of Perception." However, the main points he made are summarized here. ED.

avoiding competitors. Axel and his associates have been able to isolate the genes that encode the odorant receptors of both the main olfactory system and the vomeronasal organ.

Since mammals have about 100,000 genes, and 1 to 2% of those genes are devoted to the sense of smell, that means a remarkable 1,500 genes or more encode for olfactory receptors. Most likely, though, we can detect many more than 1,500 odors because these genes act in a combinatorial manner, as is the case with genes that encode antibodies.

So how does the brain know what the nose is smelling? Do different receptors sensing different odors activate different spatial regions within the brain? Put another way, how does the brain know which of the numerous receptors has been activated? There may be an analogy here with the immune system: Although organisms can produce thousands of different antibodies, any given lymphocyte produces only a single type of antibody. The ability to recognize an enormous array of foreign substances (e.g., proteins, viruses, bacteria) derives from the fact that antibodies are composed of two types of proteins, a heavy and a light chain, and that the genes encoding antibodies undergo mutation to generate better antibodies as the immune response develops. Is it possible, therefore, that each bipolar neuron is able to transmit messages from only one of thousands of receptors—that receptor being specific for a single odor—and that all neurons expressing the same receptor project to a fixed site within the brain? That would mean that different odors would interact with different receptors, activating different regions of the brain.

To test this model, Axel's lab turned to the mouse, the most commonly used mammalian model organism. Techniques have been developed over the past 20 years that permit individual genes within the mouse genome to be deleted or altered, or new genes to be inserted. These so-called "transgenic" or "gene knockout" approaches were developed primarily in the laboratories of Oliver Smithies[10,11] and Mario Capecchi.[12]

Axel's laboratory modified the gene encoding one odorant receptor so that the protein produced was a fusion between the beta-galactosidase gene (called the "reporter gene") and a specific odorant receptor. This reporter gene codes for an enzyme that metabolizes certain substrates to produce a blue color. Therefore, a blue color will be produced in any cell that expresses the odorant receptor of interest, and the color will track the neuron(s) from the specific receptor to the specific area of the brain to which the neuron projects. This experiment yielded the remarkable result that all neurons expressing a specific receptor projected to a singular fixed point in the brain. Thus there is a map that relates where a bipolar olfactory neuron projects and what odors it can sense. Put another way, our olfactory bulb contains a two-dimensional map of receptor activation. Different odors activate different receptors, leading to different but reproducible patterns of electrical activity within the olfactory bulb of the brain.

In the final part of his talk, Axel turned to the more difficult questions of how the map is formed and how the map is read. One of the simpler models to explain how the map is formed is that the receptor could be located not only on the epithelial surface where it interacts with odors, but also on the axon that extends from the olfactory neuron to the olfactory bulb in the brain. Such an arrangement might allow individual receptors to find their way to the proper locus in the brain, because an axon expressing an individual receptor could have unique interactions with other cells that could guide it to the proper location. To test this idea, Axel and his colleagues produced another transgenic mouse where the odorant receptor had been inactivated, so it could not detect odors, but where the beta-galactosidase portion of the fusion protein remained functional. How would the map be affected by producing a nonfunctional receptor? The answer was clear-cut: The axons expressing this receptor did not converge on a single site in the brain, but instead wandered randomly. In this way, the receptor plays critical roles both in recognizing the odorant and in forming the map within the brain. Next comes the challenging task of determining how experience and memory can be linked to this two-dimensional map.

Axel's discoveries demonstrate the power of molecular genetics and model organisms to reveal the mechanisms of perception and neural function. It is likely that the next century will see the application of similar approaches to an enormous range of medical and biological processes.

Many unsolved problems remain in the biological and biomedical sciences. Understanding consciousness, learning, and memory—which were the topics of the next session in the symposium—represent major frontiers intimately connected to who we are. What is the biological and genetic basis for personality and emotion? How are facts and feelings encoded, stored, and retrieved? Why do some older people remember in exquisite detail experiences from their youth, yet have difficulty remembering what happened yesterday? Why do some students learn so well from lectures while others learn best from visual demonstrations? These questions lie at the interface between genetics and neuroscience. Clearly, dysfunction of the nervous system is related to mental health, but we still have only a limited understanding of the mechanisms at work and of how they are specified by genes.

Perhaps a symposium will be held 100 years from now when Dartmouth Medical School celebrates its third centenary. By that time, the genomes of all organisms of scientific, medical, or agricultural interest will have been determined, and as we compare our genomes with those of other animals we will gain important insights into the origin and evolution of the life on earth. We will understand how much genetic diversity there is among humans. We will understand how genetics contributes to virtually all diseases, even when a large number of different genes interact to produce the pathology. We will understand how the genetic program underlying development operates. We will have developed chemicals that can modify genetic programs. And we will likely have gained profound insights into the biological basis of mind, emotion, and personality.

Obtaining the answers to these important questions will require not only a continuation of the genetic revolution now occurring, but also the development of close collaborations between geneticists and both other basic science and clinical investigators—the kind of mature and unselfish collaboration that Nancy Wexler referred to when she related how the Huntington's gene was found. Francis Collins saw the need for this kind of collaboration clearly when, a couple of years ago, he joined forces with the then-president of the American Physiological Society, Allen Cowley, to advocate the discipline of "functional genomics." This development led, in 1999, to the publication of a new journal, *Physiological Genomics*, by the American Physiological Society. In addition to fostering such collaborations, we must make a commitment to train future generations of medical and graduate students so that they can understand and use genetic information and the knowledge that flows from its application. And we must equip all people with the knowledge and understanding that society will need to make decisions based on genetic information.

REFERENCES

1. AVERY, O.T., C.M. MACLEOD & M. MCCARTY. 1944. Induction of transformation by a deoxyribonucleic acid fraction isolated from pneumococcus type III. J. Exp. Med. **79:** 137–158.
2. WATSON, J.D. & F.H.C. CRICK. 1953. Molecular structure of nucleic acids: a structure for deoxyribose nucleic acid. Nature **171:** 737–738.
3. BOTSTEIN, D., R.L. WHITE, M. SKOLNICK & R.W. DAVIS. 1980. Construction of a genetic linkage map in man using restriction fragment length polymorphisms. Am. J. Hum. Genet. **32:** 314–331.
4. GUSELLA, J.F. & M.E. MACDONALD. 1995. Huntington's disease. Sem. Cell Biol. **6:** 21–28.
5. GOFFEAU, A. *et al.* 1997. The yeast genome directory. Nature **387** (Suppl. 6632): 1–105.
6. THE *C. elegans* SEQUENCING CONSORTIUM. 1998. Genome sequence of the nematode *C. elegans*: a platform for investigating biology. Science **282:** 2012–2018.
7. DULAC, C. & R. AXEL. 1998. Expression of candidate pheromone receptor genes in vomeronasal neurons. Chem. Senses **23:** 467–475.
8. MOMBAERTS, P., F. WANG, C. DULAC, R. VASSAR, S.K. CHAO, A. NEMES, M. MENDELSOHN, J. EDMONDSON & R. AXEL. 1996. The molecular biology of olfactory perception. Cold Spring Harbor Symp. Quant. Biol. **61:** 135–145.
9. AXEL, R. 1995. The molecular logic of smell. Sci. Amer. **273:**154–159.
10. BRONSON, S.K. & O. SMITHIES. 1994. Altering mice by homologous recombination using embryonic stem cells. J. Biol. Chem. **269:** 27155–27158.
11. SMITHIES, O. 1993. Animal models of human genetic diseases. Trends Genet. **9:** 112–116.
12. CAPECCHI, M.R. 1994. Targeted gene replacement. Sci. Amer. **270:** 52–59.

Neuroscience Session: Intelligence—
The Origin and Substrate of Thinking

Introduction to the Session

PASKO T. RAKIC

Chair of Neurobiology, Yale University School of Medicine, New Haven, Connecticut 06520-8001, USA

It is my pleasure and privilege to introduce this session on neuroscience. Earlier we heard about exciting developments in molecular biology and genetics as they pertain to many different organs. This session is devoted to a single organ, the brain. There are many reasons why the brain might deserve such special attention. Most beds in our hospitals are filled with patients suffering from diseases that are related to the brain—and unlike cancer, heart disease, and many other diseases, those of the brain, by and large, do not interfere with longevity. Our prisons are crowded, due in part to problems with the brain. And I am sure that each of you knows someone who has a brain disorder but is neither hospitalized nor incarcerated. Thus, diseases of the brain engender enormous expenses for society and incalculable suffering for individuals and families.

Furthermore, the quality of our lives depends on the brain. No matter who you are, at some point in your life you will have to cope with some problem related to the function of your brain, be it sensory, motor, or a dysfunction caused by aging—loss of memory being one that we all fear as we get older.

But there is an even more compelling reason why we devote ourselves to studying the brain: Study of the brain is a study of ourselves. The brain is the organ that sets us apart from any other species. It is not the strength of our muscles or of our bones that makes us different, it is our brain. The brain holds the key to our mental capacity, to our creativity. Our civilization is a product of the brain. So we should be interested in how we came to be what we are on this planet, what makes the human species unique from any other. Religion, art, and philosophy have perhaps provided some of the answers, but certainly not all of them. Many people believe that the ultimate answer will come from study of the brain.

Neuroscience is a separate discipline that was created about three decades ago. Some say that in these three decades we have learned more about the brain than was learned during all of the rest of history. If indeed that is true, the reason is not that we are smarter than those who preceded us, but rather that we were given the tools with which to study the brain—those truly marvelous new techniques of molecular biology, of neuroanatomy, of neurophysiology. Numerous major problems remain to be solved, and, judging by the bright young people interested in neuroscience today, we can be optimistic that they will be solved.

Some day, those who follow us may look back on the 21st century as the "Century of the Brain." Last year, when I served as president of the Society of Neurosciences, we held our annual meeting in Washington, D.C., with 25,000 participants—the largest gathering of neuroscientists in the world. Twenty-five years earlier, that meeting drew only 500 people. The Society has grown so fast that, someone has calculated, by the year 2200 all people in the United States will be neuroscientists! Francis Collins just talked to me about this calculation; he said, "How about geneticists?" "Well," I said, "by that time the human genome will have been mapped and geneticists will work as postdocs in neuroscience laboratories."

For this session, we have selected just a few subjects that fall under the broad field of neuroscience. Dr. Gerald Edelman will talk about the evolution of the brain, I will speak about its development, and Drs. Marcus Raichle and Steven Pinker will discuss the function of the cerebral cortex—that part of the brain which has reached its highest development in mammals, especially in humans.

Building a Picture of the Brain[a]

GERALD M. EDELMAN

Chair of Neurobiology, Scripps Research Institute, LaJolla, California 92037, USA

The brain is among the most complicated material objects in the known universe. Even before the advent of modern neuroscience, it was a commonplace that the brain is necessary for perception, feelings, and thoughts; today this is considered a truism.[1] What is the connection? Can we build a picture of the structure and dynamics of this extraordinary object that can account for the origin of the mind? This is in fact the main goal of modern neuroscience, and, when reached, it will have large consequences for humankind.

In this essay, I want to touch upon some features of the brain that make it special, features that challenge the picture of the brain as a machine. In doing so, I shall suggest alternative views to such a picture and shall range over various levels of organization of the brain, from its most microscopic structural aspects to its most abstract functions. My position shall be that the human brain is special both as an object and as a system—its connectivity, dynamics, mode of functioning, and relation to the body and the world is like nothing else science has yet encountered. This, of course, makes building a picture of the brain an extraordinary challenge. Although we are far from a complete view of that picture, a partial view is better than none at all. Before attempting a synopsis, an examination of some key features and properties of the brain is required.

THE PRIMACY OF NEUROANATOMY

If someone held a gun to my head and threatened oblivion if I did not identify the single word most significant for understanding the brain, I would say "neuroanatomy." Indeed, perhaps the most important general observation that can be made about the brain is that its anatomy is the most important thing about it.[2]

The brain of an adult human is about three pounds in weight. It contains about 30 billion nerve cells, or neurons. The most recently evolved outer corrugated mantle of the human brain, the cerebral cortex, contains about 10 billion neurons and one million billion connections, or synapses. Counting one synapse per second, we would just finish counting 32 million years from now. If we consider the number of ways in which circuits or loops of connections could be excited, we would be dealing with hyperastronomical numbers: 10 followed by at least a million zeros. (There are 10 followed by 79 zeros, give or take a few, particles in the known universe.)

---

[a]The following article is reprinted here in lieu of Gerald Edelman's remarks at the symposium; it covers virtually all the material that he presented in his address, which was titled "Darwinian Competition Among Neurons." The article is reprinted by permission of *Daedalus, Journal of the Academy of Arts and Sciences,* from the issue entitled "The Brain," Spring 1998, Vol. 127, No. 2. ED.

Neurons have a great variety of shapes but in general they have tree-like projections called dendrites, which receive connections. Neurons also have a single longer projection called an axon, which makes synaptic connections at the dendrites or cell bodies of other neurons. No one has made an exact count of different neuronal types in the brain, but a crude estimate of 50 would not be excessive. The lengths and branching patterns of dendrites and axons from a given type of neuron fall within certain ranges of variation, but even in a given type, no two cells are alike.

How the brain is connected provides the major ground for understanding its general function. We know that the brain is interconnected in a fashion no man-made device yet equals. First of all, proceeding from the finest ramifications of its cells up to its major pathways, its connections are all three-dimensional, or 3D. (A computer chip can be connected to others in 3D, but it is inscribed in 2D.) Second, a brain's connections are not *exact*. If we ask whether the connections are identical in any two brains of the same size, as they would be in computers of the same make, the answer is no. At the finest scale, no two brains are identical, not even those of identical twins. Furthermore, at any two moments, connections in the same brain are not likely to remain exactly the same. Some cells will have retracted their processes, others will have extended new ones, and certain other cells will have died. This observation applies to patterns at the finest scale, consisting of individual neurons and their synapses. Thus, although the *overall* pattern of connections of a given brain area is describable in general terms, at the level of its synapses the patterns are extraordinarily complex and variable.

As an example, consider a so-called pyramidal cell in a particular layer of the six-layered cerebral cortex. It typically has as many as 10,000 synapses connecting it with distant or neighboring cells. If one moved over to the next pyramidal cell of the same type, the number of synapses could vary widely and the pattern of their contacts could be quite different. Yet in a given area of the cortex (say, that for vision), these two cells will resemble each other more than one of them would resemble a cell from another area of the cortex, for example, that for controlling movement. One conclusion we can draw from such observations is that, while there are close similarities in certain regions, there are no absolutely specific point-to-point connections in the brain. The microscopic variability of the brain at the finest ramifications of its neurons is enormous, making each brain unique. These observations provide a fundamental challenge to models of the brain based on instruction or computation. As I shall discuss, the data provide strong grounds for so-called selectional theories of the brain—theories that actually depend upon variation to explain brain function.[3]

Two key characteristics of neuronal patterns at the microscopic level are their density and their spread. The body of a single neuron measures up to about 50 microns in diameter, although its axon can range from microns to meters in length. In a tissue like the cortex, neurons are packed together at an extraordinary density; if all of them were stained with silver in the so-called Golgi stain, the section would be pitch black. (Actually, the usefulness of this stain rests on the fact that it affects only a very small fraction of cells in a given area.) Interspersed among the neurons are non-neuronal cells, called glia, that have developmental and physiological functions supporting neuroanatomy and neural activity. In some places, glia even outnumber neurons.

In the dense networks of the brain, it is the spread of neuronal arbors—of dendritic trees and axonal projections—that is perhaps the most striking feature. In some places, the spatial spread of an axon forming an arbor can be more than a cubic millimeter. Overlapping that arbor with all its intricate branchings can be arbors from countless other neurons. The overlap can be as great as 70 percent in three-dimensional space. (No self-respecting forest, made of trees and root structures, would permit such a large overlap.) Moreover, as the axonal arbors overlap, they can form an enormous variety of synapses with cells in the paths of their branches, resulting in a pattern that is unique for each brain volume. To this day, while we can trace the full arborization of a single nerve cell, we have no clear picture of the microanatomy of the interspersed arbors of the many neighboring cells at the scale of their synapses. In summary, the main microstructural features that arrest attention are the density, the overlap, the individual branching, and the uniqueness of neuronal structures, even in the face of the quite specific higher-level patterns that characterize the neuroanatomy of a given brain region.

These larger-scale patterns and the overall functioning of the brain depend on how neurons function and exchange signals.[4] The general cellular functions of neurons—such as respiration, genetic inheritance, and protein synthesis—are like those of other cells in the body. The special features related to neural function mainly concern synapses. Neurons come in two flavors, excitatory and inhibitory, and the fine structure of their synapses varies accordingly. But for each the basic principles are similar and they involve both electrical and chemical signaling. While in certain species some synapses can be completely electrical, the vast majority of the synapses we are concerned with in human brains are chemical. In most cases, the presynaptic and postsynaptic neurons are separated by a cleft forming a single synapse. Neurons are polarized in electrical potential between the inside and outside of their cell membrane. As a result of the flow of ions across a particular portion of the cell membrane, the cell is locally depolarized. A wave of depolarization called an action potential spreads down an axon and, when it reaches the region of the synapse, causes the release of neurotransmitters from a series of vesicles in the presynaptic neuron. If the neuron is excitatory, neurotransmitters will then cross the cleft, bind to specific receptors on the postsynaptic neuron, and cause the postsynaptic neuron to depolarize. These processes occur over time periods of tens to hundreds of milliseconds. If the postsynaptic neuron depolarizes sufficiently after several such events, it will fire (i.e., generate an action potential of its own), relaying the signal in turn to other neurons to which it is connected.

A key point is that the statistics of the release of these neurotransmitters, their distribution at the microscopic level, and their binding to receptors all govern the thresholds of the response of neurons in an extraordinarily intricate and variable manner. As a result of transmitter release, electrical signaling not only takes place but also leads to changes in the biochemistry and even in the gene expression of target neurons. This molecular intricacy and the resulting dynamics superimpose several more layers of variability on that of the neuroanatomical picture, contributing to what may be called the historical uniqueness of each brain.

Despite the microanatomical variability of the brain, at its higher levels of anatomical organization it falls nicely into areas, regions, and specialized parts that, in general, are functionally segregated or specialized. In examining such regions, it is tempting to assign necessary and sufficient functions to each area. As I shall discuss below, this has historically led to paradoxes that place the local and global aspects of brain function in sharp contrast to each other. In the case of vision, for example, there are as many as three dozen (and probably more) different areas in the monkey brain, each contributing to a different function—such as the detection of line orientation, the movement of objects, or the construction of color. These areas are widely distributed over different regions of the brain, and yet there is no one master area coordinating all their functions to yield a coherent visual image or pattern. Nevertheless, coherent perceptual patterns of this kind are in fact generated by the brain.

This distributed property of different, segregated functions raises extraordinary difficulties for attempts to understand how brain anatomy relates to brain physiology. One feature found in monkey brains that affords a helpful basis for resolving these difficulties is as follows: Of the more than 305 connection paths (some with millions of axonal fibers) between members of the set of functionally segregated visual areas, more than 80 percent have fibers running in both directions. In other words, the different functionally segregated areas are for the most part reciprocally connected. These reciprocal pathways are among the main means that enable the integration of distributed brain functions. They provide a major structural basis for reentrant signaling, a process that, as I shall describe later, offers the key to resolving the problem of integrating the functionally segregated properties of brain areas despite the lack of a central or superordinate area.[5]

In this abbreviated account I have not mentioned the variety of other important brain structures—such as the cerebellum, which appears to be concerned with coordination and synchrony of motion; the basal ganglia, which consist of nuclei connected to the cortex that are involved in the execution of complex motor acts; and the hippocampus, which runs along a skirt near the temporal cortex of the brain and which has a major function in consolidating short-term memory into long-term memory in the cerebral cortex. The specific ways in which these different structures interact with the cortex are of central importance, but the principles and problems connected with analyzing their functions remain similar to those I have already mentioned.

One of the main organizing principles of the picture we are trying to build is that each brain has uniquely marked in it the consequences of a developmental history and an experiential history. The individual variability that ensues is not just noise or error. As we shall see, it is an essential element governing the ability of the brain to match unforeseeable patterns that might arise in the future of a behaving animal. No machine we are familiar with incorporates such individual diversity as a central feature of its design. The day will certainly come, however, when we can build devices that incorporate some of the formative patterns and connection rules that we see in brains. One can safely foresee that a quite different kind of memory and learning will be exhibited by such constructions than those we currently attribute to computers.

THE SPECIALNESS OF THE BRAIN

Our quick review of neuroanatomy and neural dynamics indicates that the brain has special features of connectivity that do not seem consistent with those operating in computers. If we compare the signals a brain receives with those of such machines, we see a number of other features that are particular to brains. In the first place, the world cannot function as the unambiguous input device that a piece of computer tape is. Nonetheless, the brain can sense the environment, categorize patterns out of a multiplicity of signals, initiate movement, mediate learning and memory, and regulate a host of bodily functions.

The ability of the nervous system to carry out the perceptual categorization of various signals for sight, sound, and other sensory inputs, dividing them into coherent classes without a prearranged code, is certainly special. We do not presently understand fully how this is done, but, as I shall discuss later, I believe it arises from a special set of mapped interactions between the brain, the rest of the body, and various rearrangements of signal configurations originating in the environment.

Another distinguishing feature of the brain is how its various activities are dependent on constraints of value. I define value systems as those parts of the organism (including special portions of the nervous system) that provide a constraining basis for categorization and action within a species. I say "within a species" because it is through different value systems that evolutionary selection has provided a framework of constraints for those somatic selective events within the brain of each individual of a particular species that lead to adaptive behavior. Value systems can include many different bodily structures and functions (the so-called phenotype); perhaps the most remarkable examples in the brain are the noradrenergic, cholinergic, serotonergic, histaminergic, and dopaminergic ascending systems. During brain action, these systems are concerned with determining the salience of signals, setting thresholds, and regulating waking and sleeping states. Inasmuch as synaptic selection itself can provide no specific goal or purpose for an individual, the absence of inherited value systems would simply result in dithering, incoherent, or nonadaptive responses. Value constraints on neural dynamics are required for meaningful behavior and for learning.

If we consider neural dynamics, the most striking special feature of the higher vertebrate brain is the occurrence of the process I have called "reentry."[6] Reentry depends on the possibility of cycles in the massively parallel graphs of the brain, such as are seen in their most elementary form in reciprocally connected brain maps. It is the ongoing recursive dynamic interchange of signals occurring in parallel between maps that continually interrelates these maps to each other in space and time. If I were asked to go beyond what is merely special and name the *unique* feature of higher brains, I would say it is reentry. There is no other object in the known universe so completely distinguished by reentrant circuitry as the human brain. While a brain has similarities to a large ecological entity like a jungle, no jungle shows anything remotely like reentry, nor do human communication systems; reentrant systems in the brain are massively parallel to a degree unheard of in our communication nets, which, in any event, deal with coded signals.

All of these special features of the brain—the connectivity, the categorizing ability, the dependence on value, the reentrant dynamics—operate in a very heterogeneous fashion to yield coordinated behavior. As I hinted above, the nonlinear aspects of the interaction between the brain, the body, and various parallel signals from the environment must be considered together if we are to understand categorization, movement, and memory.

Finally, there is also something quite special about the brain when considered from an evolutionary point of view. While the human brain can be viewed in terms of the immense anatomic, biochemical, and dynamic complexity that is built up during individual development and behavior (a complexity that includes an enormous variety of different events), its actual evolution can only be explained by a relatively small number of selectional events or transcendences.[7]

Understanding the specialness I have touched upon here sets a good part of the research agenda for modern neuroscientists, who are attempting to build a picture of the brain and thus understand its functions. This understanding and its research agenda require a robust theory—one that provides insights into the biological origins of pattern formation, the nature of complexity, and the correlation of brain activity with psychological functions. I turn now to a brief description of one such theory.

NEURAL DARWINISM

The diversity and individuality of the multilayered structures and dynamics of each brain pose major challenges to the formation of any theory proposed to account for global brain function. Machine analogies simply will not do. I believe that these challenges can be met by turning to population thinking. Charles Darwin invented population thinking, the idea that variation in individuals of a species provides the basis for the natural selection that eventually leads to the origin of other species. Darwin's description of the combined processes of variation and selection in populations has since been shown to be the most fundamental of biological principles. This population principle not only provides the basis for the origin of species but also governs processes of somatic selection occurring in individual lifetimes. An example is the immune system, in which the basis for molecular recognition of foreign molecules is somatic variation in antibody genes, leading to a vast repertoire of antibodies with different binding sites. Exposure to a foreign molecule is followed by the selection and growth of cells bearing just those antibodies that fit a given foreign structure sufficiently well, even one that has never occurred before in the history of the earth. The mechanisms and the timing differ in evolution and immunity but the principles are the same—the Darwinian processes of variation and selection.

Almost two decades ago, I began to think about how the mind could arise in evolution and development.[8] It seemed to me then, as it does now, that the mind must have arisen as a result of two processes of selection: natural selection and somatic selection. The first is hardly doubted except perhaps by some philosophers and theologians. Thinking about the second led to the proposal of a theory concerned with the evolution, development, structure, and function of the brain.

This theory of neuronal group selection (TNGS), or neural Darwinism,[9] has three main tenets: (1) *Developmental selection:* During the development of a species, the formation of the initial anatomy of the brain is constrained by genes and inheritance, but connectivity at the level of synapses is established by somatic selection during an individual's ongoing development. This generates extensive variability of neural circuitry in that individual and creates groups made up of different types of neurons. Neurons in a group are more closely connected to each other than to neurons in other groups. (2) *Experiential selection:* Overlapping this early period and extending throughout life, a process of synaptic selection occurs within the diverse repertoires of neuronal groups. In this process, certain synapses within and between groups of neurons (locally coupled neurons) are strengthened and others are weakened. This selectional process is constrained by value signals that arise as a result of the activity of ascending systems in the brain, an activity that is continually modified by successful output. (3) *Reentry*: Spatiotemporal correlation of selective events in the various maps of the brain is mediated through the dynamic process of reentry. This occurs via the ongoing activity of massively parallel reciprocal connections, and it correlates events of synaptic selection across disjunct brain maps, binding them into circuits capable of coherent output. Reentry is in fact a form of ongoing higher-order selection, a form that appears to be unique to animal brains.

Because of the dynamic and parallel nature of reentry and because it is a process of higher-order selection, it is not easy to provide a metaphor that captures all of its properties. But as an example, imagine a string quartet in which each player responds through improvisation to ideas and cues of his own as well as to sensory cues of all kinds in the environment. Since there is no score, each player decides what notes to play and so is not coordinated with the other players. Now imagine that the players are connected to each other by myriad threads so that their actions and movements are very rapidly conveyed by back-and-forth signals. Signals that instantaneously connect all four players would lead to the correlation of their sounds, and thus a new, more cohesive, and integrated sound would emerge out of the independent efforts of each player. This correlative process would alter the next action of each player and the process would be repeated but with new emergent and more correlated melody lines. Although no conductor would instruct or coordinate the group, the players' productions would tend to be more integrated and more coordinated, leading to a kind of music that each one alone could not produce.

One of the striking consequences of the process of reentry is the emergence, as with the players in our example, of widespread interactions among different groups of active neurons distributed across many different and functionally specialized brain areas. The resultant spatiotemporal correlation of the activity of widely dispersed neurons is the basis for the integration of perceptual and motor processes, which is characterized by the global coherency and unified character of such processes. Indeed, if reentrant paths connecting cortical areas are disconnected, these integrative processes are disrupted. Reentry allows for a unity of perception and behavior that would otherwise be impossible given the absence in the brain of a unique central processor with detailed instructions or algorithmic calculations for coordinating functionally segregated areas.

Following a brief account of this theory in 1976, I published a trilogy between 1987 and 1989 describing its various aspects ranging from neuroanatomical development to consciousness.[10] In addition, along with my colleagues, I published a series of papers that analyzed various aspects of the theory, describing a number of simulations and models that tested its self-consistency.[11] Since that time considerable evidence to support the theory has accumulated, and no disconfirming evidence has emerged.[12] Nevertheless, it has become obvious that much remains to be clarified and explained in greater depth. One of the most important issues concerns analyzing and understanding the complexity of the brain that underlies its integrative capacities.

COMPLEXITY AND DISCONTENTS

The ideal of science is to provide the simplest account possible of the facts of the world. As Einstein put it, a theory must be as simple as possible but no simpler. The fact is that the world of biology and particularly that of the brain, not to speak of the world of human experiences, leaves us almost stupefied with complex chains of events and at the same time hardly satisfied with naive attempts at simple reduction. I began this essay with the statement that the brain is among the most complicated natural objects in the known universe. This is both a challenge and a source of discontent; it does not appear that the brain will yield itself to simple mathematical reduction. What one would like to have, nevertheless, is a measurable characterization of the brain's complexity that clarifies the relations between its functions and its structure. This requires the creation of a yardstick or measure of complexity that captures the essential elements of the brain's connectivity and dynamic interactions.

What is complexity? Ideas of heterogeneous mixtures, of multiple levels and scales, of intricate connectivities, and of nonlinear dynamics spring to mind.[13] One approach to relate these matters is in terms of the degree of independence and mutual dependence of the functions of the brain's multiple elements. This provides a means to define a complexity measure for the brain: It turns out that, using such an approach, we can apply the concepts of statistical entropy and mutual information that have been successfully applied to the analysis of multivariate processes. I will attempt here only to give a qualitative feeling for the quantitative approach that my colleagues have applied to derive various measures of complexity.[14]

If the components of a system are independent, entropy (which is a measure of disorder) is maximal and the mutual information between the system's parts is zero. If the system has any constraints resulting from interactions among its parts, however, they will deviate from statistical independence; mutual information will in general increase, and entropy is reduced. To provide an intuitive feel for a complexity measure based on entropy and mutual information, consider that it would have a low value for an ideal gas, which has statistically independent components (high entropy), as well as for a perfect crystal that has totally integrated units (low entropy but no local segregation or functional segregation) and in which all regions resemble all others.[15] This is certainly not generally true of brains—brains are functionally segregated into a diversity of different units and regions essential for different tasks. The derivation of complexity measures rests on reconciling this diversity with the global exchange and overall integration of different segregated areas.[16]

A word about functional segregation in the brain is in order. During development and behavior, neuronal groups are formed that consist of local collectives of strongly interconnected neurons that share inputs, outputs, and response properties. Each group is connected to only certain subsets of other groups and possibly to particular sensory afferents or motor efferents. In a given brain area, different combinations of groups are activated preferentially by different input signals. In the visual cortex, for example, at the level of brain maps there is a functional segregation into areas, each responding to different stimulus attributes such as color, motion, or form. Functional segregation is clearly revealed by the appearance of specific perceptual and motor deficits that result from lesions to particular cortical areas.

A sharp contrast to this kind of specialization is provided by equally strong evidence for global integration. This occurs across many levels, ranging from interactions among neurons to interactions among areas to concerted outputs that lead to particular behaviors. Integration results jointly from the patterns of connectivity among neurons and their dynamic interactions. Any two neurons in the brain are separated from each other by a relatively small number of synaptic steps. Moreover, the pathways linking the functionally segregated neuronal groups are often reciprocal.

This reciprocity provides the necessary substrate for reentry, which I have already described as a central integrative process of ongoing recursive signaling occurring along multiple, massively parallel paths. Simultaneous activity in subsets of these paths allows for selection and correlated activity among neuronal groups in the same and different areas and even between distant mapped areas.

Although much evidence exists both for localization of function and for global processes, conflicts in interpreting this evidence have given rise to long-standing controversies in brain science. To explain brain function, "localizationists" favor specificity of local brain modules whereas "holists" stress global integration, mass action, and Gestalt phenomena. As is often the case, when viewed from the proper vantage point, these controversies turn out to be misguided. This vantage point is provided by formulating a framework for an analysis of brain complexity that suggests that effective brain function arises both from the combined action of local segregated parts having different functions and from the global integration of these parts mediated by the process of reentry.

A brain organized in this fashion is not just a complex system, it is a complex selectional system. It consists of a series of repertoires—variants of neural circuits that are selected by interactions with inputs and that engage in signaling to outputs. Various signals from the environment provide sensory input to such repertoires, and the selection of appropriate neural circuits results in a matching or a fit to that input. The complexity of repertoires is in fact an essential property in the success of this process. After repeated episodes of selection, a complex neural system can generally come to match the overall statistical structure of signals from the environment by changing which paths are favored.

At any one time, an individual input or stimulus inevitably contains only a very small subset of the regularities that are potential in this statistical structure. Nonetheless, after selection, a given stimulus that is consistent with the overall statistical structure of previous inputs will tend dynamically to enhance the set of intrinsic correlations already present in the neural system. Thus, the functional connectivity of the brain and the presence of memory, which I shall discuss below, provide an intrinsic context that by necessity dominates the brain's dynamic response to any single stimulus. This is perhaps not surprising given the fact that, in mammalian brains, most neurons receive signals from other neurons, rather than directly from sensory inputs. The reentrant recursive signaling among multiple sets of neuronal groups across massively parallel reciprocal connectivity assures that such an intrinsic context is made available in a rapid fashion in very short time periods. A set of examples of this process may be seen in a series of functioning computer models of the cerebral cortex.[17]

By such means, a complex brain that has undergone neuronal group selection and reentrant interactions can go beyond the information given—it can generalize, fill in ambiguous signals, and generate various sensory constancies. The synaptic changes that are essential to these processes are connected to the emergence of memory, one of the most fundamental properties of neural systems.

NONREPRESENTATIONAL MEMORY: A SYSTEM PROPERTY

To say, as is commonplace, that memory involves storage raises the question: What is stored? Is it a coded message? When it is "read out" or recovered, is it unchanged? These questions point to the widespread assumption that what is stored is some kind of representation. This in turn implies that the brain is supposed to be concerned with representations, at least in its cognitive functions. In perception, for example, even before memory occurs, alterations in the brain are supposed to stand for, symbolize, or portray what is experienced. In this view, memory is the more or less permanent laying down of changes that, when appropriately addressed, can recapture a representation—and, if necessary, act on it. In this view, learned acts are themselves the consequences of representations that store definite procedures or codes.

The idea that representational memory occurs in the brain carries with it a huge burden. While it allows an easy analogy to human informational transactions embedded in computers, that analogy poses more problems than it solves. In the case of humans working with computers, semantic operations occurring in the brain, not in the computer, are necessary to make sense of the coded syntactical strings that are stored physically in the computer either in a particular location or in a distributed form. Coherency must be maintained in the code (or error correction is required) and the capacity of the system is quite naturally expressed in terms of storage limits. Above all, the input to a computer must itself be coded in an unambiguous fashion: it must be syntactically ordered information.

The problem for the brain is that signals from the world do not in general represent a coded input. Instead, they are potentially ambiguous, are context-dependent, are subject to construction, and are not necessarily adorned by prior judgments as to their significance. An animal must categorize these signals for adaptive purposes, whether in perception or in memory, and somehow it must associate this categorization with subsequent experiences of the same kinds of signals. To do this with a coded or replicative storage system would require endless error correction, and a precision at least comparable to and possibly greater than that of computers. There is no evidence, however, that the structure of the brain could support such capabilities directly; neurons do not do floating-point arithmetic. It seems more likely that such mathematical capabilities have arisen in human culture as a consequence of symbolic exchange, linguistic interactions, and the application of logic.

Representation implies symbolic activity. This activity is at the center of our semantic and syntactical skills. It is no wonder that, in thinking about how the brain can repeat a performance, we are tempted to say the brain represents. The flaws with such an assertion, however, are obvious: there is no precoded message in the signal, no structures capable of high-precision storage of a code, no judge in nature to provide decisions on alternative patterns, and no homunculus in the head to read a message. For these reasons, memory in the brain cannot be representational in the same way as it is in our devices.

What is it, then, and how can one conceive of a nonrepresentational memory?[18] In a complex brain, memory results from the selective matching that occurs between ongoing neural activity and signals from the world, the body, and the brain itself. The synaptic alterations that ensue affect the future responses of the brain to similar or different signals. These changes are reflected in the ability to repeat a mental or physical act in time and in a changing context. It is important here to indicate that by the word "act," I mean any ordered sequence of brain activities in a domain of perception, action, consciousness, speech, or even in the domain of meaning that in time leads to neural output. I stress time in my definition because it is the ability to recreate an act separated by a certain duration from the original signal set that is characteristic of memory. And in mentioning a changing context, I pay heed to a key property of memory in the brain: that it is, in some sense, a form of *recategorization* during ongoing experience rather than a precise replication of a previous sequence of events.[19]

What characteristics must the brain possess to show memory without coded representation? Just those characteristics, I believe, that one would find in a selectional system. These are a set of mappings making up a diverse repertoire, a means of changing the population characteristics of the repertoire with varying input signals, and a set of value constraints acting to enhance adaptation by repeating an output. Signals from the world or from other brain parts will act to select particular circuits from the enormously various combinatorial possibilities available in a given brain area. Selection occurs at the level of synapses through alteration of their efficacy. Which particular synapses are altered depends on previous experience as well as upon the variously combined activities of ascending value systems such as the locus coeruleus, raphé nucleus, and cholinergic nuclei.

The triggering of *any* such set of circuits resulting in a set of output signals that are sufficiently similar to those that were previously adaptive provides the basis for a repeated mental act or physical performance. In this view, a memory is dynamically generated from the activity of certain selected subsets of circuits. These subsets are degenerate in the sense that comparison would indicate that different ones contain circuit topologies or patterns that are nonisomorphic; nevertheless, any one of them can yield a repetition of some particular output. Under these conditions, a given memory cannot be identified uniquely with any single specific set of synaptic changes. This is so because the particular set of changed synapses that leads to a given output, and eventually to a performance at a given time, is itself continually changing. So it must be the adequate *pattern* underlying a performance, not its detail, that is repeated.

We conclude that synaptic change is essential to memory but is not identical to it. There is no code, only a changing set of circuit correspondences to a given output. The equivalent members of that set can have widely varying structures. It is this property of degeneracy that allows for changes in particular memories as new experiences and changes in context occur. Memory in a degenerate selectional system is recategorical, not strictly replicative. There is no prior set of determinant codes governing the categories, only the previous population structure of the network, the state of the value systems (which interact combinatorially according to context), and the physical acts carried out at a given moment. The dynamic changes linking one set of circuits to another within the enormous graph set of neuroanatomy allows the brain to create a memory. By these means, structurally different circuits within the degenerate repertoires are each able to produce a particular output leading to repetition or variation of a given mental or physical act. This property underlies the well-known associative properties of memory systems in the brain, for each member of the degenerate set of circuits has different network connections.

In this view, there are many hundreds, if not thousands, of separate memory systems in the brain. They range from all of the perceptual systems in different modalities to those systems governing intended or actual movement to those of the language system and speech sound. This gives recognition to the various types of memory tested by experimentalists in the field—procedural, semantic, episodic, and so on—but it does not restrict itself only to these types, which are defined mainly operationally and to some degree biochemically.

While individual memory systems differ, the key general conclusion is that memory itself is a system property. It cannot be equated solely to circuitry, synaptic changes, biochemistry, value constraints, or behavioral dynamics. Instead, it is the dynamic result of the interactions of *all* of these factors within a given system acting to select an output that repeats a performance. The overall characteristics of a particular performance may be similar to a previous performance within some threshold criterion, but the structures underlying any two similar performances can be quite different.

Besides guaranteeing association, the property of degeneracy also gives rise to the robustness or stability of memorial performance. There are large numbers of ways of assuring a given output. As long as a sufficient population of subsets remains to give an output, neither cell death, nor intervening variables competitively removing a particular circuit or two, nor switches in contextual aspects of input signals will, in general, be sufficient to extirpate a memory.

It might be argued that, even in a selectional system, the entire set of all the responses that give a repeated performance can be considered to be a representation. To accept this, however, would tend to weaken the notion of selection, which is a dynamic one. Selection is *ex post facto;* no code or symbol stands for a given memory, and very different structures and dynamics can give rise to the same memory. Above all, the structures underlying memory change continually over time. It seems senseless to conflate such dynamic properties with those that we know are characteristic of the coded representational systems, which we have consciously constructed under a code for human communication and cultural purposes.

It may be illuminating to try to envision the operation of a nonrepresentational memory by using an analogy. The geological example I use here is somewhat trivial and in only four dimensions, but I believe it can be generalized to higher dimensions. Consider a mountain, with a small glacier at its top, under changing climatic conditions or contexts leading to melting and refreezing. Under one set of warming conditions, a certain set of rivulets will merge downhill to a stream that feeds a pond in the valley below. Let that be the output leading to a repeated performance, i.e., the thawing of ice and its flow into the pond has occurred before. Now change the sequence of weather conditions, freezing some rivulets then warming them, leading to a merger with some other rivulets and the creation of new ones. Even though the structure at the heights is now changed, the same output stream may be fed exactly as before. But given even a small further change in the temperature, wind, or rain, a new stream may result, feeding or creating another pond, which may be considered to be associated with the first. With further changes, the two systems may merge rivulets and simultaneously feed both ponds. These may in turn become connected in the valley.

Consider the value constraints figuratively to be gravity and the overall valley terrain, the input signals to be the changes induced by contextual alterations of weather, the synaptic change to involve freezing and melting, the detailed rocky pattern down the hill to be the neuroanatomy, and you have a way of repeating a performance dynamically without a code. Now switch and imagine the vast set of graphs constituted by the actual neuroanatomy of the brain and consider that their connections define an *n*-dimensional space. By extension of the dimensionality of the process I have described, one can at least figuratively see how a dynamic nonrepresentational memory might work.

Such a memory has properties that allow perception to alter recall, and recall to alter perception. It has no fixed capacity limit since it actually generates "information" by construction. It is possible to envision how it could generate semantic capabilities prior to syntactic ones. It is robust, dynamic, associative, and adaptive. If such a view is correct, every act of perception is to some degree an act of creation and every act of memory is to some degree an act of imagination. Biological memory is creative and not strictly replicative.

A final word on the general significance of biological memory. Elsewhere, I have suggested that the ability to repeat a performance with variation under changing contexts first appeared with self-replicating systems under natural selection.[20] The action of natural selection then gave rise to various systems for which memory is critical, each having different structures within a given animal species—structures that range from the immune system to reflexes and even to consciousness. In this view, there are as many memory systems as there are systems capable of autocorrelation over time, whether constituted by DNA itself or by the phenotype that it constrains. Morphology underlies the particular properties of a given memory system. In turn, memory is a system property, allowing the binding in time of selected characteristics having adaptive value. If symmetry is a great binding principle of the physical universe, memory in selectional systems may be seen as a great binding principle in the biological domain.

CONSCIOUSNESS: THE REMEMBERED PRESENT

The greatest challenge to modern neuroscience is to provide an adequate explanatory basis for consciousness.[21] My purpose here is not to review the various attempts to provide such a basis. Instead I want to consider a proposal for the neural origin of consciousness consistent with selectional brain theories. It is important to point out some limits on such an enterprise. The first has to do with evolution. Consciousness depends on a certain morphology. Insofar as that morphology is the product of evolutionary selection, consciousness is also such a product. At the outset of any sensible scientific consideration of consciousness, we must confront the peculiarities and limitations that arise from these conclusions.

The only morphology providing a secure functional basis for scientific assertions about consciousness is that of our own species. There are two reason for this. First, each of us knows what it is like to be conscious as human beings but not directly what it is like to be conscious as some other animal might be; and second, we can use linguistic exchanges together with objective scientific examinations to confirm causes or correlations related to consciousness in a way that other animals cannot. The first reason recognizes that, as a process, consciousness occurs in individuals (and in the human case, in selves or persons). This reflects the fact that, in its fullest expression, consciousness is epistemically subjective: all exhaustive and historical accounts of an individual's consciousness can be provided only by that individual and cannot be directly shared or experienced by any other. The second reason recognizes that even the most parsimonious scientific (i.e., epistemically objective) account of consciousness can only be useful if our measurements and models are accompanied by correlation with reportable subjective states.

Having said that our best bet is in investigating consciousness first in human beings, we must still consider the criteria by which other animals may be investigated. Here, though, there will inevitably be additional methodological limits, and certain familiar cautions against conflating analogy and homology are bound to arise. At the anatomical level, we are on reasonably sound ground—it is known, although perhaps not exhaustively, which structures in the human brain are necessary and sufficient for consciousness. The presence of such structures in a nonhuman animal that demonstrates behavior indicative of the exchange of signs or of symbolic reference provides at least some justification for the working hypothesis that that animal is conscious. The *absence* of such structures will not allow us to say dogmatically that a particular organism is *not* conscious, but on evolutionary and functional grounds we may surmise that whatever phenomenal experience that organism has, it will not resemble ours. Given the other methodological limitations, the matter must be left at that.

Consciousness is a subjective state of sentience, unique in each subject but with properties shared by different subjects. It is implicitly felt by us as much by the recall of its absence (in deep sleep, in drugged or anesthetic states, or post-traumatically) as it is by its presence in various degrees of awareness. William James stressed that it is a process that is personal, continuous but ever-changing, selective in time, dealing mainly but not exclusively with objects independent of the self, and not exhaustive of the objects with which it deals. A predominant property of consciousness, involving referral to objects, has been termed "intentionality" by Brentano. But note that intentionality is not always present—one can be aware of a mood without any reference to objects.

There is in most states of consciousness some kind of location in time and space that is not necessarily coherent, as dreams attest. There is usually the experience of mood, and above all of so-called qualia—the subjective experiencing of the sensory modalities of sight, hearing, touch, olfaction, and taste, proprioception, and kinesthesia. And, of course, there are what might be called the "super qualia"—the philosopher's exemplary companions, pleasure and pain.

A biological theory of consciousness must describe how such properties arise in terms both of ongoing neural structure and function and of evolutionary events. In formulating such a description, it is useful to distinguish primary consciousness and higher-order consciousness. Primary consciousness is seen in animals with brain structures similar to ours (such as dogs) that appear able to construct a mental scene but seem to have very limited semantic or symbolic capabilities and no true language. Higher-order consciousness (which presumes the coexistence of primary consciousness) is accompanied by a sense of self and the ability to construct past and future scenes in the waking state. Higher-order consciousness requires, at the minimum, a semantic capability and, in its most developed form, a linguistic capability.

What structures and mechanisms must be described to account for the consciousness that we ascribe to dogs and to ourselves when, in certain of our subjective states, we are least in bondage to language? Here we must face four complex processes and their interactions. The first is a property shared by all animals—perceptual categorization, the ability to carve up the world of signals into categories useful for a given phenotype in an environment that has physical constraints but which itself contains no such categories. Along with the control of movement, perceptual categorization is the most fundamental process of the vertebrate nervous system. I have suggested that it occurs in higher vertebrates as a result of reentrant signaling among mapped and unmapped brain areas.[22] It occurs, usually simultaneously, in a number of modalities (sight, hearing, proprioception, et cetera) and in a variety of submodalities (color, orientation, and forms of motion, for example).

The second process required for the understanding of primary consciousness concerns the development of concepts that provide the ability to combine different perceptual categorizations related to a scene or an object, and thus to construct a "universal" reflecting the abstraction of some common feature across a variety of precepts. I have proposed that concepts arise from the mappings of the activities of the brain's various areas and regions by the brain itself.[23]

The third and fourth processes contributing to the emergence of primary consciousness are those related to memory and value. According to the theory of neuronal group selection, memory is the capacity specifically to recategorize, or to repeat or suppress, a mental or physical act. That capacity arises from combinations of synaptic alterations in reentrant circuits. As a result of categorical selection biased by value systems to yield such synaptic change, the entire sensorimotor system is *constrained* to give a particular range of outputs for a particular combination of inputs.

Inasmuch as a sectional nervous system is not preprogrammed, it requires such value constraints to develop categorical responses that are adaptive within a species. Certain value systems are specifically adapted to signal salience, as can be seen in the workings of the diffuse ascending systems of the brain. Such systems—the locus coeruleus, raphé nucleus, cholinergic nuclei, histaminergic systems in the posterior hypothalamus, and various dopaminergic systems—may interact combinatorially to signal salience after receiving some particular signal sequence or after instituting an action.

Value systems of these kinds are richly connected to the concept-forming regions of the brain, notably the frontal and temporal cortex but also the parietal regions and hippocampus. These regions affect the dynamics of memories that, in turn, are established or not, depending upon positive or negative value responses. The synaptic alterations that combine to develop such a "value-category memory" are essential to a model of primary consciousness.

With the notions of perceptual categorization, concept formation, and value-category memory in hand, we can formulate a model of primary consciousness.[24] The model assumes that, during evolution, the cortical systems leading to perceptual categorization were already in place before the connections that led to primary consciousness appeared. With further development of secondary cortical areas, conceptual memory systems appeared. At a point in evolutionary time corresponding roughly to the transition between reptiles branching to birds and to mammals, a new anatomical connectivity appeared. Massively reentrant connectivity arose between the multimodal cortical areas carrying our perceptual categorization and areas responsible for value-category memory. The key candidate structures for this connectivity responsible for the emergence of consciousness are the specific thalamic nuclei, modulated by the reticular nucleus in their reentrant connectivity to cortex, the intralaminar nuclei of the thalamus, and the grand systems of corticocortical fibers.

The dynamic reentrant interactions mediated by these connections occur within time periods ranging from hundreds of milliseconds to seconds—the "specious present" of William James. What emerges from these interactions is an ability to construct a scene. Through corticothalamic reentry, the ongoing parallel input of signals from different sensory modalities in a moving animal results in a grouping of perceptual categories related to objects and events. Their salience is governed in that particular animal by the activity of value systems. This activity is influenced by that animal's history of rewards and punishment accumulated during its past behavior. The ability of an animal to connect events and signals in the world (whether they are causally related or merely contemporaneous), and thereby to construct a scene that is related *to its own* value-category memory system, is essential for the emergence of primary consciousness.

The ability to construct such a scene is the ability to construct, within a time window of fractions of seconds up to several seconds, a remembered present. An animal without such a system could still behave and respond to particular stimuli, and, within limits, even survive. But it could not link events or signals into a complex scene, constructing relationships based on its own unique history of value-dependent responses. It could not imagine scenes and evade complex dangers. It is this ability to imagine that underlies the evolutionarily selective advantage of primary consciousness.

How can such a picture be reconciled with our empirical program of starting with the human experience of consciousness? To confront this issue, we must consider the later evolutionary appearance of brain structures leading to higher-order consciousness. An animal having primary consciousness alone can generate a "mental image" or a scene. This is based in part on immediate multimodal perceptual categorization in real time, and is determined by the succession of real events in the environment. Such an animal has biological individuality but no concept of self and, while it has a "remembered present," it has no concept of the past or future. These are characteristics that emerged in evolution when semantic capabilities appeared, perhaps earliest in the precursors of hominids. When linguistic capability appeared in the precursor of *Homo sapiens,* higher-order consciousness flowered. Syntactical and semantic systems provided a new means for symbolic construction and memory. As in the case of primary consciousness, a key step in evolution was again the development of the neural substrate that permits the brain to construct another novel reentrant connectivity, this time between the symbol-based sensorimotor memory systems for language and the rest of the brain.

The emergence of speech and of these new connections allowed reference to objects or events between two or more early humans or protohumans under the auspices of a symbol. The development of a lexicon of such symbols, probably initially based on the nurturing and emotive relationships between mother and child, led to the discrimination of individual consciousness and the emergence of a self. And with narrative capabilities linked to linguistic and conceptual memory, the emergent higher-order consciousness could foster the development of concepts of the past and future related to that self and to others. At that point, the individual self is freed to some extent from bondage to the remembered present. If primary consciousness marries the individual to real time, higher-order consciousness allows for a kind of occasioned divorce made possible through the creation of concepts of time—concepts of the past and the future. A whole new world of intentionality and awareness, of categorization and discrimination can be experienced and remembered by these means. Extraordinary powers are rendered by these evolutionary developments; as a result, concepts and thinking can both flourish.

The building up of a system of higher-order consciousness capable of rehearsal and planning based on value-laden memory and linguistic capabilities is accompanied by phenomenal experience and feeling. The neural processes underlying that feeling can have far-reaching causal consequences—as we know by witnessing the concomitants of pain or pleasure. Feelings or sensations are the identifiers to a conscious individual of particular sets of neural states. The discussion so far has not addressed the origins and basis for feelings themselves. The issue of qualia is considered by some to be the sticking point and major obstacle to any theory that attempts to explain consciousness as a causal consequence of neural events. I have pointed out, however, that a scientific theory of consciousness, like any other scientific theory, implies intersubjective communication between at least two human beings. For that communication to be scientifically successful, we must already assume that the prior transactions of each of the two communicants must allow both to experience qualities: warm, green, rough, and so on. These are aspects of qualia, and thus it may seem we are in a circular situation: to explain qualia scientifically, we must assume their existence. Our theory proposes, however, that embodiment is a source of meaning and that experiences leading to meaning certainly involve qualia —to be conscious is to experience qualia. There is no qualia-free human observer; actual scientific observers must have sensations as well as perceptions. There is thus no God's-eye view of consciousness that would succeed in conveying or explaining what "warm" is to a hypothetical, qualia-free observer. Description, scientific or otherwise, must not be confused with embodiment: being is not describing. Despite this limitation, we can account scientifically for the discriminability of qualia and for their refinement as species of higher-order categorizations that are carried out by complex reentrantly connected brains.[25]

If indeed there is one central organizing principle underlying the appearance of consciousness it is the emergence of a few specific but very critical reentrant systems in evolution. These served to relate new forms of memory to perceptual and conceptual activities in the brain under the constraint of values. Following the emergence of primary consciousness, the development of linguistic capabilities through new reentrant connections of the language areas of the brain to various distributed areas mediating concept formation led to higher-order consciousness, which flowered in humans. Unraveling the complex of neural connections (mainly in the thalamocortical system) that gave rise to these extraordinary processes remains as a central challenge for modern neuroscience.

THE PICTURE OF THE BRAIN: TWO EXCLUSIVE VIEWS

In considering how we may build a picture of the brain I have deliberately emphasized one view, in full recognition of the fact that it is not the most widespread or the received view. Indeed, at least by contrast, it might be called a radical view.[26]

It may be useful to highlight the contrast between the received and the radical views to indicate how differently our factual picture of the brain is presently interpreted. In the received view, the brain is an information machine with precise circuit functions and mechanisms to react to and store signals in a more or less orderly and coded fashion. In this view, anatomy involves precise connectivity with high specificity. If variation exists, it is error, or else it is ignored in the focus on precise circuit functions. Physiology, according to the received view, consists of highly defined circuit functions governed by a form of intensity or amplitude coding in which synaptic change mediates the storage of information in order to call up coded specific circuits later for specific functions. The brain is considered to carry out computations and, indeed, is felt by many to be a special kind of computer. It is implicit in this view that input to the brain from the world is somehow syntactically parsed, as in a computer.[27]

In the received view, the world presents *information* to the brain in the sense that the ordering of input signals follows certain objective categories of grouping that go beyond mere energy differences between neighboring sources of signals. Memory involves the storage of this information, presumably via a variety of codes at synapses. Recall involves calling up patterns of such stored codes. The purpose of memory and learning is to yield coordinated output according to appropriately coded routines. The various functions of perception, sensation, movement, attention, sleep, and consciousness are integrated in much the same manner as they would be if they were programmed in a computer. While, like all summaries, this one is to a degree overdrawn, I believe its flavor is right.

What about the radical view, one version of which I have emphasized in this essay? According to this view, the brain is a dynamic system that emerges from a selectional interaction with the world. The selection is constrained by evolved value, not by instructions or codes, and is actually determined by sensorimotor encounters with a world of signals. This world does not contain unambiguously parsed cues but acts with the brain to permit construction of adaptively valuable behavior. If one could look inside an appropriately selected set of brain repertoires and could read the translation to and from the phenotype, one would see an enhanced capacity for certain complex dynamics but no code. Thus one would not see uniquely mapped representations.

In the radical view, anatomy is a composite made up of patterns with underlying variability at the finest ramifications of neural connectivity. This variability and local diversity is looked upon not as noise, potentially leading to error in a code, but rather as an essential substrate for selection—what is called the primary repertoire, made up of highly diverse circuits in a given brain area.[28] A key element of neuroanatomy is the existence of massive reciprocal connectivity, which provides the structural basis for reentry. A major emphasis is placed on degeneracy, the existence of many nonisomorphic pathways that can nonetheless lead to similar functional outcomes.

At the level of gross physiology, circuits are functionally segregated parts that have significance only in the context of the action of very large correlative networks. Synaptic change within these networks is a reflection of selectional events. While the amplitude of neural impulses is important, the temporal correlation of neuronal firing across these large networks is also considered to be critical. The most prominent dynamic principle underlying such correlation is reentry. Reentry is the large-scale recursive interaction of ongoing neural activity, both locally and in different areas across massively parallel reciprocal connections. It is most clearly seen within and between neural maps. The concepts of functional segregation, temporal correlation, and reentry are consistent with the units of selection existing at a much higher spatial scale than that of the functional components (such as the individual neurons) that play a major role in the received view. Indeed, in the radical view, the unit of selection necessary for perceptual categorization is considered to be a global mapping, a large-scale circuit made up both of cortical maps and subcortical structures whose operation is capable of yielding output that results in behavior.

In the radical view, the selectional system in the brain is capable of dynamic reconstruction of outputs under the constraints of value, selecting from a large number of degenerate possibilities. As such, this view rejects codes, representations, and explicit coded storage. Memory is nonrepresentational and is considered to reflect a dynamic capacity to recreate an act (or specifically to suppress one) under such constraints. The brain is not a computer, nor is the world an unambiguous piece of tape defining an effective procedure and constituting "symbolic information." Such a selectional brain system is endlessly more responsive and plastic than a coded system. In it the homunculus disappears, its role ceded to a self-organizing and necessarily complex biological system.

It is my belief that the radical view will become the received one within the next decade. Predictions are precarious, however, and we must remain open to the possibility that as a result of continuing discovery in neuroscience, an entirely new view of the brain will emerge.[29] One prediction nevertheless stands out as more secure than practically any other: the results of neuroscientific discovery will have enormous implications for our view of our position in nature. Establishing the proper picture of the brain will remain at the center of human concern.

NOTES AND REFERENCES

1. By the time of the French Revolution a picture was emerging of what was in the head, although almost a century would have to pass for the emergence of what we would accept as scientific data. An amusing indication of an earlier view can be found in *Le Rêve de d'Alembert* by Denis Diderot, in which d'Alembert's mistress, Mademoiselle de l'Espinasse, queries the physician, Dr. Bordeu, about the causes of d'Alembert's disturbed dreams:

   BORDEU: Because it is a very different thing to have something wrong with the nerve-center from having it just in one of the nerves. The head can command the feet, but not the feet the head. The center can command one of the threads, but not the thread the center.

   MADEMOISELLE DE L'ESPINASSE: And what is the difference, please? Why don't I think everywhere? It's a question I should have thought of earlier.

   BORDEU: Because there is only one center of consciousness.

   MADEMOISELLE DE L'ESPINASSE: That's very easy to say.

   BORDEU: It can only be at one place, at the common center of all the sensations, where memory resides and comparisons are made. Each individual thread is only capable of registering a certain number of impressions, that is to say sensations one after the other, isolated and not remembered. But the center is sensitive to all of them; it is the register, it keeps them in mind or holds a sustained impression, and any animal is bound, from its embryonic stage, to relate itself to this center, attach its whole life to it, exist in it.

MADEMOISELLE DE L'ESPINASSE: Supposing my finger could remember.

BORDEU: Then your finger would be capable of thought.

MADEMOISELLE DE L'ESPINASSE: Well, what exactly is memory?

BORDEU: The property of the center, the specific sense of the center of the network, as sight is the property of the eye, and it is no more surprising that memory is not in the eye than that sight is not in the ear.

MADEMOISELLE DE L'ESPINASSE: Doctor, you are dodging my questions instead of answering them.

BORDEU: No, I'm not dodging anything. I'm telling you what I know, and I would be able to tell you more about it if I knew as much about the organization of the center of the network as I do about the threads, and if I had found it as easy to observe. But if I am not very strong on specific details I am good on general manifestations.

MADEMOISELLE DE L'ESPINASSE: And what might these be?

BORDEU: Reason, judgment, imagination, madness, imbecility, ferocity, instinct ....

BORDEU: And then there is force of habit which can get the better of people, such as the old man who still runs after women, or Voltaire still turning out tragedies.

[Here the doctor fell into a reverie, and MADEMOISELLE DE L'ESPINASSE said:] Doctor, you are dreaming.

BORDEU: Yes I was.

MADEMOISELLE DE L'ESPINASSE: What about?

BORDEU: Voltaire.

MADEMOISELLE DE L'ESPINASSE: What about him?

BORDEU: I was thinking of the way great men are made.

2. Two reasonably elementary books for a lay reader are Gordon M. Shepard, *Neurobiology* (New York: Oxford University Press, 1983) and Gordon M. Shepard, *The Synaptic Organization of the Brain* (New York: Oxford University Press, 1990).
3. Gerald M. Edelman and Vernon Mountcastle, *The Mindful Brain: Cortical Organization and the Group-Selective Theory of Higher Brain Function* (Cambridge, Mass.: MIT Press, 1978); Gerald M. Edelman, *Neural Darwinism: The Theory of Neuronal Group Selection* (New York: Basic Books, 1987); Jean-Pierre Changeux and Antoine Danchin, "Selective Stabilization of Developing Synapses as a Mechanism for the Specification of Neuronal Networks," *Nature* **264** (December 1976): 705–712.
4. Shepard, *Neurobiology* and Shepard, *The Synaptic Organization of the Brain*; Eric Kandel, James H. Schwartz, and Thomas M. Jessell, Eds., *Principles of Neural Science* (New York: Elsevier, 1991).
5. Giulio Tononi, Olaf Sporns, and Gerald M. Edelman, "Reentry and the Problem of Integrating Multiple Cortical Areas: Simulation of Dynamic Integration in the Visual System," *Cerebral Cortex* **2** (July/August 1992): 310–335.
6. Edelman, *Neural Darwinism;* Tononi, Sporns, and Edelman, "Reentry and the Problem of Integrating Multiple Cortical Areas"; Gerald M. Edelman, *The Remembered Present: A Biological Theory of Consciousness* (New York: Basic Books, 1989).
7. Edelman, *Neural Darwinism*.
8. Edelman and Mountcastle, *The Mindful Brain*.
9. Ibid.; Gerald M. Edelman, "Through a Computer Darkly: Group Selection and Higher Brain Function," *Bulletin of the Academy of Arts and Sciences* **36** (October 1982): 20–49; Gerald M. Edelman, "Neural Darwinism: Selection and Reentrant Signaling in Higher Brain Function," *Neuron* **10** (February 1993): 115–125.
10. Edelman and Mountcastle, *The Mindful Brain;* Edelman, *Neural Darwinism;* Edelman, *The Remembered Present;* Gerald M. Edelman, *Topobiology: An Introduction*

to Molecular Embryology (New York: Basic Books, 1988).

11. Tononi, Sporns, and Edelman, "Reentry and the Problem of Integrating Multiple Cortical Areas"; Olaf Sporns, Giulio Tononi, and Gerald M. Edelman, "Modeling Perceptual Grouping and Figure-Ground Segregation by Means of Active Reentrant Connections," *Proceedings of the National Academy of Science* **88** (January 1991): 129–133; Geroge N. Reeke, Jr., Olaf Sporns, and Gerald M. Edelman, "Synthetic Neural Modeling: The 'Darwin' Series of Recognition Automata," *Proceedings of the Institute of Electrical and Electronics Engineers* 78 (September 1990); 1498-1530; Karl Friston *et al.*, "Value-Dependent Selection in the Brain: Simulation in a Synthetic Neural Model," *Neuroscience* 59 (March 1994): 229–243.

12. Charles M. Gray and Wolf Singer, "Stimulus-Specific Neuronal Oscillations in Orientation Columns of Cat Visual Cortex," *Proceedings of the National Academy of Science* 86 (March 1989): 1698-1702 and Michael M. Merzenich *et al.*, "Topographic Reorganization of Somatosensory Cortical Areas 3b and 1 in Adult Monkeys Following Restricted Deafferentation," *Neuroscience* **8** (January 1983): 33–55.

13. Two nontechnical books are M. Mitchell Waldrop, *Complexity: The Emerging Science at the Edge of Order and Chaos* (New York: Simon & Schuster, 1992) and Roger Lewin, *Complexity: Life at the Edge of Chaos* (New York: Macmillan, 1992).

14. Giulio Tononi, Olaf Sporns, and Gerald M. Edelman, "A Measure for Brain Complexity: Relating Functional Segregation and Integration in the Nervous System," *Proceedings of the National Academy of Science* **91** (May 1994): 5033–5037 and Giulio Tononi, Olaf Sporns, and Gerald M. Edelman, "A Complexity Measure for Selective Matching of Signals in the Brain," *Proceedings of the National Academy of Science* **93** (April 1996): 3422–3427.

15. Tononi, Sporns, and Edelman, "A Measure for Brain Complexity."

16. Tononi, Sporns, and Edelman, "A Complexity Measure for Selective Matching of Signals in the Brain."

17. Tononi, Sporns, and Edelman, "Reentry and the Problem of Integrating Multiple Cortical Areas"; and "Sporns, Tononi, and Edelman, Modeling Perceptual Grouping and Figure-Ground Segregation."

18. Daniel L. Schacter, *Searching for Memory: The Brain, the Mind, and the Past* (New York: Basic Books, 1996).

19. Gerald M. Edelman, *Bright Air, Brilliant Fire: On the Matter of the Mind* (New York: Basic Books, 1992).

20. Ibid.

21. Edelman, *The Remembered Present.*

22. Tononi, Sporns, and Edelman, "Reentry and the Problem of Integrating Multiple Cortical Areas"; Sporns, Tononi, and Edelman, "Modeling Perceptual Grouping and Figure-Ground Segregation."

23. Edelman, *The Remembered Present.*

24. Ibid.

25. John R. Searle, *The Mystery of Consciousness* (London: Granta, 1997).

26. In making this distinction, I am aware of the fact that certain scientists in neurobiology proper would agree, more or less, with the radical view. The fact remains, however, that many neurobiologists talk of the brain's carrying out of computations utilizing codes. In doing so, they do not account for the brain's enormous structural and dynamic variability. Moreover, cognitive psychologists, workers in artificial intelligence, and a good number of linguists all hew to the notions I have bundled together as the received view. Naturally there are as many variants in each position as there are individual scientists but the two positions are, I believe, usefully contraposed.

27. George N. Reeke, Jr., and Gerald M. Edelman, "Real Brains and Artificial Intelligence," *Daedalus* **117** (1) (Winter 1988): 143–173.

28. Edelman, *Neural Darwinism.*

29. It is not possible to predict precisely what we will learn about the brain in the future. Consistent with my position here, I will put forth the conjecture that in carrying out a function such as speech, the interaction of the parts of the brain will not resemble those of an orderly machine but will more resemble a crazy quilt, the parts of which are connected in no uniformly systematic fashion. Evolution tinkers, it does not plan, and natural selection acts on functional outcomes of the individual organism, not on design drawings. I will also hazard a guess: as has been the case in other domains of science, once we know the facts and principles of brain function and structure more securely we will be able to imitate nature to a limited extent. At such a time, we will construct a conscious artifact. If we can give it the basis for language, we will be able to ask whether it categorizes or "carves nature at the joints" the way we do. The answer will perhaps provide as exciting or terrifying a prospect as hearing from intelligent life somewhere else in the galaxy. The ethical implications are obvious, if not easily resolvable. A more modest prediction is that we will build devices that incorporate what we have learned about brain functions and structures into new kinds of artifacts, mixing what we already know about computers with components capable of perceptual functions. This is already on its way.

The Importance of Being Well Placed and Having the Right Connections

PASKO T. RAKIC

Chair of Neurobiology, Yale University School of Medicine, New Haven, Connecticut 06520-8001, USA

It is probably safe to state that deciphering the mechanisms by which our brain develops and functions is the most challenging scientific goal for the next millennium. After all, ultimately the solution to most problems facing humanity depends on this remarkable organ. Research on the brain has been aided greatly by the remarkable new tools of molecular and cellular biology. These tools have brought with them, however, enormous possibilities for manipulating the development and function of the brain by tampering with genes, and this fact has introduced new and equally challenging ethical, moral, social, and philosophical problems.

For this talk, I chose the title "The Importance of Being Well Placed and Having the Right Connections" not because I had in mind the possible advantages of attending a prestigious educational institution such as Dartmouth, but rather to emphasize the two properties of the brain that make it uniquely different from all other organs of our body. One can argue, of course, that in most biological aspects the brain is similar to all other tissues in that it is composed of individual cells that have a nucleus with the same genetic code, as well as the usual complement of cytoplasmic organelles enclosed in a common membrane bilayer. Likewise, brain cells abide by the same laws of physics, chemistry, and biology as do cells in all other tissues. But if I had to give a single answer to the question "What is so special about the brain that makes it different from any other organ?" I would say that it is a structure in which the *position* of the cells within the brain and their *connections* with other brain cells play an absolutely critical role in determining their function. Nerve cells (called neurons) can be seemingly identical in their shape and chemical makeup, and yet perform totally different functions, depending on their location and connections. It is probably for this reason that the loss of as little as 0.001% of neurons in a particular position within the brain may result in 100% loss of the function usually represented in that area of the brain—which stands in sharp contrast to the fact that an individual can lose one-third of the liver, or an entire kidney, and yet continue to function normally. The cells of our brain are organized as functional units—as maps of our bodies on which are superimposed maps of the outside world as perceived through our senses, and then maps of our experience over time, our memories. These interconnecting cortical maps hold the secrets not only to success but also to the limits of our species.

In order to understand how the brain works, we must understand how these maps are formed—how brain cells attain their positions and become stereotypically interconnected in order to perform complex functions. In the past we could not even think scientifically about such problems; the consideration of higher brain functions that are performed by the cerebral cortex—perception, reasoning, emotion, esthetic preferences, planning, decision-making—was relegated to theology and philosophy. Actually, as Steven Pinker will show later in this session, those are valid approaches that have brought advances in our understanding of the brain. However, it is only during the past 25 years or so that scientists have been able to delineate how genes, molecules, and cells construct the interconnected maps that form the basis of our intelligence, our creativity, and our uniqueness. The development and function of our brain can be formulated as a set of concrete scientific problems that will be amenable to experimental testing and that, therefore, may be solved during the next century. You may have noticed that I said "a set of problems," because I doubt that full understanding of the brain can be achieved by a single quantum leap or discovery, similar to the deciphering of the double helix structure of DNA. Much more likely, I think, we will sequentially identify a variety of mechanisms, occurring in precise combinations and temporal sequences, that build a functioning adult brain. Today, I will outline briefly our state of knowledge, as well as prospects for future advances, in the development and evolution of the cerebral cortex—a topic that is central to most theories of human intelligence and creativity.

FIGURE 1 shows a map of the human cerebral cortex as created at the turn of the 20th century by the German neurologist Korbinian Brodmann. He suggested that segregation of nerve cells into definable fields localized the function of those particular nerve cells to certain areas of the brain. Seeing Brodmann's map was actually the very reason that I decided to devote myself to research on brain development. After completing medical school in Belgrade, I started training in neurosurgery, and I quickly learned that after opening the skull, the neurosurgeon has to be careful not to cut certain areas of the cerebral cortex. If the surgeon cuts the wrong area, the patient loses sensation, or movement of part of the body, or capability in some aspects of speech—depending on the location of the erroneous cut. To avoid such dire consequences, neurosurgeons were guided mainly by Brodmann's map.

So, with my interest aroused, I asked my professor, whom I had assisted in one of the operations, "If this map is so constant from individual to individual, how was the map constructed in the first place?" He looked at me and asked, "Do you read German?" He then referred me to Brodmann's book, which was published in 1905. Well, I thought to myself, I'm training at a backward institution. So in the mid-1960s, I went to Harvard Medical School, to the Massachusetts General Hospital (MGH), which was at that time the mecca for neurologic scientists. And I very quickly learned that the neursurgeon at the MGH opened the skull in the same way as was done in Belgrade, and he voiced the same caution about avoiding damage to the functionally critical areas. So I asked him the same question: "How was this map of the cortex created?" And he looked at me and said, "Do you read German?" And he referred me to Brodmann's book.

I have related this little anecdote to illustate the modest level of understanding about human brain development at the turn of the century, and the minimal progress in such understanding that was made during the ensuing 60 years. It wasn't that Brodmann and his contemporaries were incapable of asking the critical questions, only that the techniques required to provide the answers to those questions were not available to them. In contrast, our generation has been lucky to have access to truly remarkable new methods that have allowed us to gain new insights into the principles and mechanisms of brain development. It is often stated that we learned more about our brain in the last three decades than during the entire history of mankind, and this statement certainly is true for the cerebral cortex.

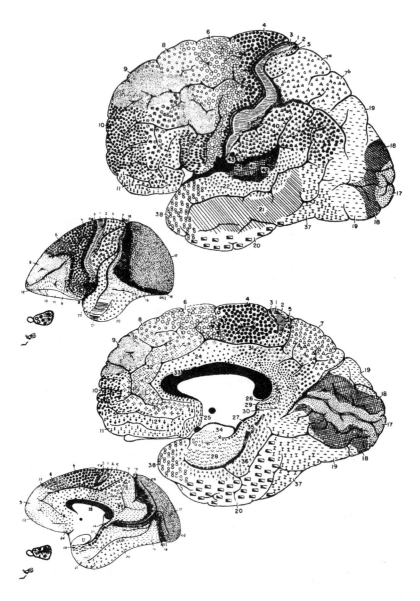

FIGURE 1. Lateral (*upper part*) and medial (*lower part*) views of the cerebral hemispheres in (*from left to right*): mouse, macaque monkey, and human. Individual cytoarchitectonic areas in monkey and human are reproduced on the same approximate scale. Shown in the lower left is the flatworm and the fruit fly, two invertebrate models that have been extraordinarily useful in identifying genes that have been conserved during evolution and whose function therefore can be tested in rodents and primates. Details are described in the text. Adapted from Brodmann (1909).

FIGURE 1 also illustrates how greatly the surface of the cerebral cortex has expanded during evolution. I have selected three mammalian species for this figure: human, because understanding the human cortex is our ultimate goal; mouse, because it is a very versatile genetic and experimental model system; and the macaque monkey, because it represents, so to speak, an evolutionary bridge between the mouse and the human. Cerebral cortical expansion in these three species does not represent a continuum; rather, they represent "snapshots" during an evolutionary process that took millions of years.

Actually, the figure takes evolution back further, all the way to two small invertebrates, the fruit fly and the flatworm (shown, in scale, at the bottom of the figure). I placed them in the same illustration in order to remind us of the new experimental tools that I just alluded to. We can, for example, take a gene first identified in the fly or worm, and knowing from the structure of that gene that it was preserved during millions of years of evolution, delete that same gene from a mouse and thereby determine the function of that particular gene in the rodent nervous system. And by extension, we can validly surmise the function of that particular gene in humans. We can also introduce selected genes into nerve cells of a monkey embryo, label the cells that have been thus altered, and then observe changes in the development and function of that monkey's brain. Alternatively, we can proceed in the opposite direction: take a gene that was identified in the Human Genome Project described by Francis Collins earlier, and then either delete that gene from a mouse embryo, or insert it into a mouse embryo—and thereby, again, define the role of that particular gene in the development of the mouse brain.

Several other important points are illustrated in FIGURE 1: (1) During evolution, cortical areas do not expand uniformly across species; some areas get relatively larger than do others. For example, the primary visual cortex constitutes 15% of the total cerebral cortex in monkeys, but only 3% in humans—making way, so to speak, for expansion of other regions that are important for higher brain functions; an example would be the development of areas that associate the frontal with the parietal lobes. (2) New functional areas are introduced during evolution, the speech area in humans being the most obvious example. (3) And finally, the cerebral cortex expands mainly in surface area rather than in thickness.

The remarkable new techniques that I have mentioned, plus similar advances in neuroanatomic methods, have helped us to understand—at the level of the cell and of the molecule—how the cerebral cortex is created, both during the development of an individual (ontogeny) and during evolution (phylogeny). We now have quite good insight into how genes govern the complex assembly of neurons that results in our cortex with all its functional maps. A concomitant of that insight is the ability, at least the potential ability, not only to meddle with the development of the brain, but also to treat certain neurologic disorders.

The state of technology at the time of Brodmann permitted him to present only a static picture of nerve cells, as shown in FIGURES 2A and 2B. Then the advances in neuroanatomical methods—histochemistry, immunocytochemistry, autoradiography, electron microscopy, combined with various tracer methods—allowed us to determine precisely where in the cerebral cortex each class of neurons projects (Figures 2C–2E). These approaches created the concept of synaptic circuitry: we were able to determine that nerve cells, which project to specific, often distant targets, communicate with each other. Exquisitely small in size and about 10^{15} in total

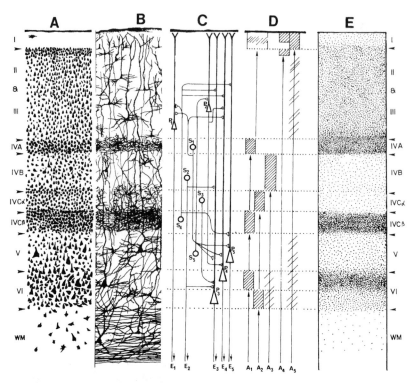

FIGURE 2. Composite diagram of the cellular organization of the visual cortex as obtained with several methods. (**A**) and (**B**) show two methods that were available to scientists at the turn of the century: cellular dyes and silver impregnation, respectively. (**C**) and (**D**) display various outgoing (efferent, E_{1-5}) and incoming (afferent, A_{1-5}) axons of pyramidal cells (P_{1-5}) and stellate cells (S_{1-5}); note that each cell has a different set of connections, depending on its position. (**E**) shows distribution of the alpha$_2$-adrenergic receptor as exposed by ^{3}H-clonidine binding in area 17. Modified from P. Rakic *et al. J. Neurosci.* **8:** 3670–3690 (1988).

number, the synaptic junctions in the human brain are the principal means by which we record our experiences. And even though our experiences differ, the basic pattern of the synaptic connections, no matter how numerous and complex, are remarkably

---

➤

FIGURE 3. (**A**) Three-dimensional illustration of the developmental events and types of cell-cell interactions occurring during the early stages of corticogenesis. Details are described in the text. Abbreviations: MA = monoaminergic input; NB = input from nucleus basalis; TR = thalamic radiation; CC = cortico-cortical connections; VZ = proliferative ventricular zone; IZ = intermediate zone; SP = subplate zone; CP = cortical plate; MZ = marginal zone; MN = migration of neurons; RG = radial glial fibers; E = embryonic (gestational) day. Modified from P. Rakic, *Science* 241:170–176 (1988). (**B**) Fluorescence image of a migrating cortical neuron showing the neuron (MN), an embryonic radial glial cell (RG), and a junctional molecule that attaches the neuron to the glial cell. Reproduced with permission, from Anton *et al. J. Neurosci.* **16:** 2283 (1996).

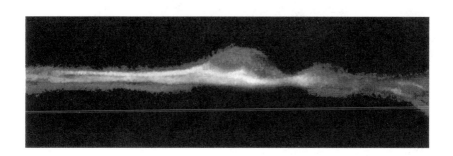

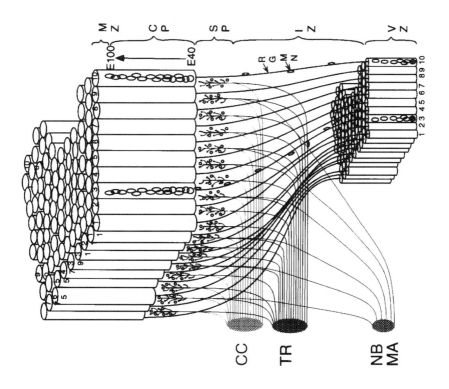

similar in most individuals. That fact prompts us, as developmental biologists, to ask how the shape, location, and synaptic connections of neurons are brought about so reproducibly. As I will show, we have been able to answer these questions, at least partially, through the techniques of molecular biology. These techniques allow us to identify the regulatory and structural genes, and their products, that determine production, migration, and connections of neurons, as well as the signaling apparatus essential for cooperation among neurons, to decipher the biological basis of our mentation.

By using specific molecular probes that either label DNA or control its replication during cell division, one can determine exactly when a given neuronal class is formed. We now know that each population of cortical neurons is formed at a specific time during gestation. For example, by varying the time when probes are given to pregnant monkeys (and hence to the brain of the embryo), we can determine which population of neurons is formed on which day of gestation. Remarkably, we found that the formation of cortical neurons in primates stops at mid-gestation. That fact causes me to digress for a moment, to ask what biological function might be subserved by this unique feature of the brain. Most other organs can regenerate their cell populations even during adulthood. For example, the skin and gut renew their cell populations several times a year. My skin today is not the skin that I had last summer, yet my cerebral cortex today contains the very same neurons that I had as a resident when I posed the question about the Brodmann maps to my professor. It is, in fact, the reason why I can remember an event that occurred many years ago. In the brains of fishes, frogs, and birds—even in the brains of some non-primate mammalian species—there is considerable renewal of nerve cells; but in primates, this capacity is preserved in only a few specific regions of the brain. The evolutionary significance of the drastic reduction in the capacity for neuronal renewal may be that it promotes the survival of our species: We store our acquired knowledge, our experiences, in our neurons and in their circuits. If we were to replace our old cortical neurons with a new set, we would also lose our personality and all that we had learned, and we would have to go to college every year!

Back to development of the cerebral cortex. Our ability to label the progeny of original nerve cells has revealed another remarkable fact: Cortical neurons do not originate in the cortex itself. Rather, they are "born," or generated, at the inner surface of the cerebral ventricle—in the proliferative ventricular zone (VZ in FIGURE 3) —near the center of the embryonic brain; and from there, after the last cell division, they migrate to the appropriate position in the cortex (cortical plate [CP] in FIGURE 3). They migrate along transient scaffolding formed by elongated fibers of non-neuronal cells, called radial glia (RG), which, like a "neuronal highway," enable cells to find their proper addresses in the future map of the cerebral cortex. Early in gestation, the neuronal "journey" is very short and relatively straight; and then, with increasing gestational age, new populations have to negotiate more and more complex pathways.

After arriving in the cortex, neurons become layered on top of one another, thereby forming vertical columns, or parcels (CP in FIGURE 3). Although one of the most prominent features of the cerebral cortex, especially in primates, is the formation of these parcels, we did not know until recently what determines the association of a particular neuron with a particular parcel. Now, however, we have been able to trace the allocation of neurons into specific parcels by inserting marker genes into cells at the ventricular zone (VZ in FIGURE 3) and following the route of their "direct descendant" cells into the cortex. We thus can trace the lineage of a neuronal population ("born" on a certain embryonic day) to specific areas in the cerebral cortex (FIGURE 3B).

FIGURE 3 is a simplified three-dimensional depiction of the process. It shows the proliferative zone (VZ) on the cerebral ventricle, where cells are generated, and the migration of neurons (MN) along the scaffolding of radial glial fibers (RG) to their final position in the cortical plate (CP). The oldest layer of neurons is situated at the bottom of the cortical plate, and then progressively younger generations of neurons are layered on top of one another. Consequently, the cells generated last will always be found at the very periphery of the cortex. The importance of this developmental process is reflected in a certain strain of mice, which has a spontaneous genetic mutation that interferes with the order of "stacking"; these mice manifest defects in cerebral function. It is a fascinating and remarkably dynamic process, which I like to call "biological necessity," for it seems essential and predetermined that each new generation of neurons be layered on top of the preceding generation. Just as we stand on the shoulders of our ancestors, so do our younger cerebral neurons pile on top of their earlier generations.

If the stacking process is to proceed in an orderly fashion, there must be an exchange of information between the newly arrived cells and those that preceded them. We suspected that this exchange might be implemented via surface molecules that mediate recognition of specific cell classes, as well as through an energy-requiring migratory process. But only recently could this hypothesis be tested experimentally. Now, by applying a combination of fluorescence microscopy, confocal laser microscopy, and time-lapse photography to various *in vitro* tissue preparations, we can actually follow cells as they migrate along the glial scaffolding to their specific place in the cortex and test the role of various molecules in the process—and, by implication, in certain neurological disorders. A working model of the process, which involves recognition and adhesion, is shown in FIGURE 4. It is a somewhat complicated process, involving many compounds, and I shall here present only a skeletal description.

Gerald Edelman spoke earlier about adhesion molecules that are homotypic (i.e., mirror images, like our two hands) and are responsible for making cells stick to one another and thereby to move as a group and associate in a common function. It turns out that the brain also contains several pairs of heterotypic molecules (i.e., dissimilar compounds, much like those involved in the association of antigen with antibody), which are responsible for recognition. According to the working model, initial interaction between migrating neurons and heterotypic recognition molecules (RM in FIGURE 4) in the ventricular zone results in the selection of a specific migratory pathway. This step is followed by adhesion to homotypic adhesion molecules (AM in the figure). Then, by a cascade that involves many steps—specific receptors (NMDA) and channels (Ca^{++} Na^{++}) on the cell surface, calcium as an intracellular messenger ($[Ca^{++}]$), microtubules (MT), actin-like contracting elements (actin), and phosphorylation for energy (Tyr-p)—the neuron with its nucleus (N) is transported along the glial fiber (RG) to the cortical plate in the cerebral cortex (for orientation, compare with FIGURE 3).

The mechanisms for movement of neurons in the fetal brain (as depicted in FIGURE 4) currently make up a very active area of investigation. Even at the present state

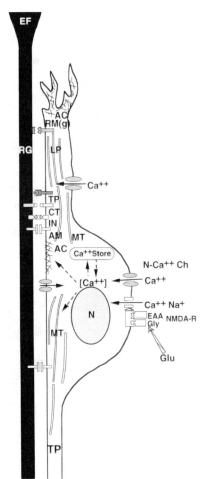

FIGURE 4. Cascade of the numerous cellular and molecular events that take place during the migration of postmitotic cells from the ventricular zone to the cortical plate (VZ and CP, respectively, in FIGURE 3). Details are described in the text. Abbreviations: AM = homotypic adhesion molecule; EAA = excitatory amino acid; Glu = glutamate; Gly = glycine; LP = leading process; MT = microtubule; N = cell nucleus; TP = trailing process; RG = radial glial fiber; RM = gliophilic recognition molecule; Tyr-p = tyrosine phosphorylation; Na^+ = sodium; Ca^{++} = calcium; $[Ca^{++}]$ = intracellular concentration of calcium; N-type = voltage-gated receptors/channels; NMDA = ligand-gated receptor; Actin = actin-like contractile proteins; catenin = cytoplasmic protein engaged in adhesion. Modified from P. Rakic *in* Research Perspectives in Neurosciences, edited by A.M. Galaburda and Y. Christen, Springer, 1997, pp. 81–89.

of our incomplete knowledge, these mechanisms are helping to explain the pathogenesis of certain neurological disorders, such as some forms of childhood epilepsy, certain aspects of mental retardation, schizophrenia, and developmental dyslexia. They also have shed light on the malpositioning of nerve cells that occurs when an embryo is exposed to substances such as cocaine or alcohol, or to harmful agents like viruses or ionizing radiation. Let me give you two examples.

The first example has particular relevance to our drug-oriented society. There is experimental evidence that exposure of monkey embryos to cocaine affects brain development, because neurons that are generated on a specific gestational day do not arrive at the right time and in the right place within the cerebral cortex. Because the neurons become situated in the wrong position, they fail to develop appropriate synaptic connections. Consequently, the brain of the monkey that was exposed to cocaine is not going to be as effective as that of the normal monkey—it will not realize its full functional potential. This fact was discovered in an experiment on an animal model, rather than on the brain of a patient at autopsy, because one cannot utilize radioactive tracers on static, dead tissue. However, the results can be validly extrapolated to humans. A frighteningly large percentage of children in this country are products of pregnancies during which the mother was exposed to cocaine. Some well-intentioned people advocate that we put more resources into specialized education for the victims of such pregnancies—give them more attention and love—in the hope that then everything may be fine. This is currently the topic of a major debate in the allocation of scarce educational resources. But unfortunately, no amount of training will entice misrouted cells to move into the proper position. A brain damaged by cocaine during intrauterine life cannot be fully rehabilitated, and that sad truth needs to be made clear to anyone who thinks that occasional use of cocaine during pregnancy may be acceptable.

Similar examples can be cited for other substances or agents, such as alcohol and viruses. And particularly damaging are toxic substances and ionizing radiation, whose concentrations in our atmosphere are increasing at an unacceptable rate in this industrial world.

My second example concerns ionizing radiation. About 10 years ago, I received a call from Dr. William Schull, an epidemiologist from Houston, Texas, who was phoning on behalf of the International Commission on Radiation Protection, a subcommitteee of the United Nations Scientific Committee on Atomic Radiation. He was inquiring about a cohort of Japanese victims of the Hiroshima and Nagasaki nuclear bombs, specifically, about individuals who were fetuses between weeks 10 and 17 of gestation at the time of the blasts. These victims were in their fifth decade of life at the time of Dr. Schull's phone call to me, and they had major problems with higher brain functions: They were institutionalized and could not keep steady jobs. Other victims who were irradiated at the very same distance from the blasts, but were exposed at earlier or later stages of gestation, had other health problems but not those associated with higher brain fuctions. The subcommitteee was wondering if I, as a neuroembryologist, could explain this apparently very selective effect.

So I went back to my doctoral thesis (which had dealt with the development of the human brain), and I concluded that these Japanese patients had been exposed to radiation during the particular phase of their embryonic development when neurons destined for the superficial layer of the cortex are produced and migrate. These neurons, after arriving in the cortex, normally form connections between different cortical regions as well as between the two cerebral hemispheres. I was therefore able to give Dr. Schull some specific predictions: first, these patients will probably have a thinner than normal cerebral cortex, due to depletion of the superficial layers; second, they will have a smaller volume of white matter and a thinner than normal corpus callosum, due to a decrease in the number of axons originating from the superficial layers; and third, they will have ectopic nerve cells dispersed in the white matter below the cortex, because the migration of these cells was curtailed.

Dr. Schull's initial reaction was to doubt my predictions, because a physicist on his committee had opined that a short blast could not account for the disorders as observed after so many years. A few weeks later, however, Dr. Schull called again to report that a Japanese neuropathologist who had reexamined the autopsy tissues of one of these patients had confirmed all three of my predictions. Subsequently, the findings were confirmed in six additional patients, using magnetic resonance imaging. Naturally, I was pleased, not just because I had been proven correct, but more so because this example illustrated that, if we understand how brains develop, we can make accurate diagnoses. It is, of course, always satisfying to scientists when their basic research has applicability to clinical situations.

There was an ironic ending to this tale. When Dr. Schull had phoned me with the results of the pathological report from Japan, he invited me to become a member of the United Nations Scientific Commission on Atomic Radiation Protection. Since I knew that this UN agency was headquartered in Vienna, Austria, relatively close, that is, to where my mother lives, I gladly accepted. And right after accepting, I learned that the next meeting of the subcommittee would be held in Houston, Texas!

Back to FIGURE 1, which reveals an additional fascinating fact: that although the cerebral cortex in various mammalian species differs considerably in respect to surface area, it does not differ very much in thickness. The number of neurons in the cerebral cortex is approximately 100 times greater in the macaque monkey than in the mouse, and about 1,000 times greater in humans than in mice. But despite this large expansion, cortical thickness remains similar. Understanding how, during phylogenetic and ontogenetic development, the increasing number of neurons was accommodated without a great increase in thickness may yield insights into the evolution of our mental capacity. Let me share with you some ideas based on experiments in embryos.

The *radial unit hypothesis* proposes that the developing cerebral cortex is composed of a large number of radial units, groups of clonally related neurons produced at the same site in the proliferative zone (VZ in FIGURE 1). The hypothesis proposes further that the genes that control the number of founder cells in the VZ may set a limit on the size of the cortical surface. For example, a minor increase in the duration of the embryonic period during which the cells are formed within the proliferative zone could result in a large increase in the number of founder (progenitor) cells that form radial units (FIGS. 5C and 5D). Since proliferation in the ventricular zone initially proceeds exponentially because symmetric cell division predominates (FIG. 5A), an additional round of mitotic cycles during this phase doubles the number of founder cells, and, consequently, the number of radial columns. Accordingly, fewer than four extra rounds of symmetric cell division before the onset of corticogenesis can account for a 10-fold difference in the size of the cortical surface. This can be achieved by postponing the onset of corticogenesis by only a few days. After the onset of corticogenesis, the mode of cell division becomes predominantly asymmetrical (FIG. 5B). Calculations based on the radial unit hypothesis predict that the prolongation of the ventricular proliferative phase by approximately two weeks (in humans, as compared to macaque monkeys; FIG. 5C) should enlarge the cortical thickness by only 10 to 15%. That is actually what is observed. This difference has profound functional consequences.

An additional mechanism that may influence cell production within the ventricular zone, perhaps surprisingly, is the extent of cell death, or apoptosis. Some cells have to die in order to let the brain develop normally; apoptosis is not haphazard, it is programmed by genes. This fact was illustrated in some recent experiments of ours, in which we reduced apoptosis in mice by inactivating certain genes that cause cells to die. In an earlier session of this symposium, David Botstein and Francis Collins emphasized that scientists can often make the biggest strides, even in humans, by working first with relatively simple biological models. The search for genes that

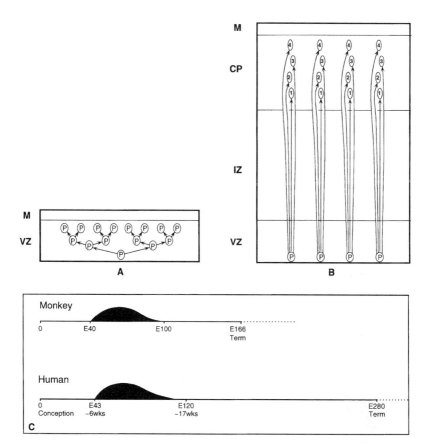

FIGURE 5. (A) Schematic model of symmetric cell division, which predominates before embryonic, or gestational, day 40 (E40). At this early embryonic age, the cerebral wall consists of only the ventricular zone (VZ), where all progenitor cells (P) are proliferating, and the marginal zone (M), into which some cells extend radial processes. As shown, symmetric cell division is exponential; it causes rapid, horizontal, lateral spread. **(B)** Model of asymmetric cell division, which becomes predominant in the monkey after E40. During each asymmetrical division, a progenitor cell (P) produces one postmitotic neuron that migrates rapidly across the intermediate zone (IZ) and becomes arranged vertically in the cortical plate (CP) in reverse order of arrival (1, 2, 3, 4); a second progenitor cell remains within the proliferative zone (VZ) and continues to divide. **(C and D)** Periods of origin of cerebral neurons during gestation in macaque monkey **(C)** and human embryos **(D)**. Reproduced with permission from P. Rakic, *Trends in Neuroscience*, **18:** 383–388.

control cell death is a case in point, for such genes were first identified in yeast, fruit flies, and flatworms. And because biologically useful molecules tend to be preserved during evolution, we could use the same genes that we identified in those simpler organisms, transplant those genes into mice (so-called transgenic mice) or into monkeys, and then examine the function of those genes as we manipulate them during the production and migration of nerve cells—that is, as we delete those genes, over-express or underexpress them, or express them differentially.

In the example shown in FIGURE 6, mice lacking the gene that is essential for cell death showed an increased number of founder (progenitor) cells, which in turn resulted in expansion of the cortical surface area. FIGURES 6A and 6C show the embryonic cerebrum of a normal mouse where the critical gene, called caspase-9, is present, and FIGURES 6B and 6D, the cerebral cortex of a mouse where that gene was absent. The latter shows more proliferating, darkly stained stem cells, and a larger cerebral cortex, which has induced the formation of sulci and gyri by which the much larger surface area is accommodated. Such convolutions are not normally seen in mice, but usually only in species that have larger brains, such as primates. Thus it almost looks as if the cortex of the mouse without caspase-9 is attempting to recapitulate evolution and generate a larger, convoluted cerebrum that is typical of monkeys or humans.

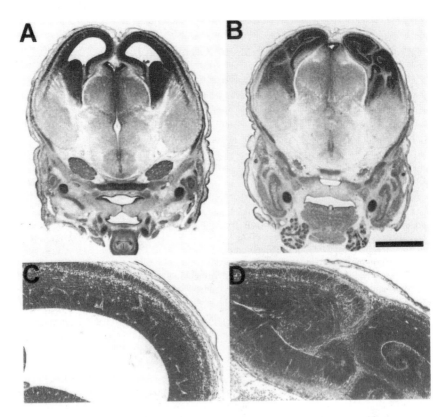

FIGURE 6. Histologic sections across the cerebrum of mouse embryos in which the gene, caspase-9, was present (**A** and **C**) and from which caspase-9 was removed by genetic engineering (**B** and **D**). Details are described in the text. Reproduced, with permission, from Kuida *et al.* *Cell* **94:** 325–333 (1998).

Many people, seeing the experiment shown in FIGURE 6, ask, "Is the mouse on the right smarter? Is modern science now able to create a 'mighty mouse'?" Well, as you know, bigger is not always better, and in this instance, more brain cells were not good for the mice that lacked caspase-9; most of them died before birth. During evolution, mutated cells that last must have functions that aid survival of the species—and the selection process takes millions of years. Thus, to create a "mighty mouse" in the laboratory, I would need grant support for at least a million years. More seriously, I selected this experiment mainly to illustrate the remarkable power of molecular genetics and molecular biology, for here we utilized a gene first identified in a flatworm in order to better understand brain development in mammals such as monkeys and humans.

These are scientific tools that Brodmann probably never even dreamed of having! However, in the near future, not the far future, we may well be capable of constructing larger brains at will, not only by preventing cell death but also by stimulating cell production. I am not at all sure that that will be a desirable capability, but I certainly think that it will be possible. Unraveling the mysteries of the cell cycle and neuronal production is currently a very hot topic in developmental neurobiology. My former graduate student, Richard Novakowski, now a professor at the Robert Wood Johnson Medical School in New Jersey, was involved in designing an experiment about the cell cycle that will be carried out on the shuttle flight into space [April 1998], a flight, by the way, that was dedicated in part to the neurosciences. One of the payload specialists running the Neurolab on that flight will be a faculty member of Dartmouth Medical School, Dr. Jay Buckey.

Determination of cerebral size is not, however, the entire story of brain development. As I mentioned earlier, one of the most prominent features of the cerebral cortex is its parcellation into different cytoarchitectonic areas that subserve motor coordination, specific sensory modalities, and even complex cognitive functions such as language and facial recognition. At present, it is not known how such areas have emerged in evolution. At the core of the matter is a simple question: Is the pattern of cortical parcellation specified by a set of axons coming from initially equipotential cells in the lower brain centers, or does the embryonic cortex contain some cues that attract afferent axons from the lower brain centers to their appropriate positions in the developing cortex? The answer appears to be "both," and it has been formulated in the so-called *protomap hypothesis.*

This hypothesis suggests that specific cortical areas emerge through synergistic interactions between intrinsic, genetically determined developmental programs in cortical neurons, and extrinsic signals supplied by subcortical structures. According to the hypothesis, the neurons of the embryonic cortex, including neurons in the proliferative ventricular zone, set up a primordial, species-specific map of areas that preferentially attract appropriate afferents. Both processes have now been supported by experimental evidence. It has been found, for example, that many genes are expressed in a region-specific manner prior to, or in the absence of, input from the periphery—suggesting that the selective process of evolution may occur in the cerebral cortex itself. In addition, however, it appears that afferent signals arriving from a variety of extracortical sources come into play to determine the size of the various areas, as well as the molecular, cellular, and synaptic characteristics of the adult cerebral cortex. For example, the size of the primary visual cortex is regulated by afferents originating from a single thalamic nucleus. Advanced methods in experimental embryology and molecular biology have revealed several candidate molecules, transcription factors (proteins) that may be involved in the determination of the cytoarchitectonic areas, a process known as "early cortical specification."

Production and allocation of neurons to specific locations (FIG. 3) is only a first step in the development of the brain. The next step is the formation of appropriate connections, called synapses. It is generally agreed that the formation of synaptic connections proceeds in two phases: in the first, connections are formed by a guidance cue; and in the second, the connections are fine-tuned by competititve interactions and selective eliminations of synapses, which depend on activities by the individual.

I will elaborate here on the second phase, in order to link my presentation to Gerald Edelman's concept of neuronal Darwinism. Studies in embryonic monkeys have shown that neurons and their axons are overproduced in the cerebral cortex during early stages of development. Studies of the developing visual system can illustrate this point. In a fashion very analogous to what Richard Axel showed for the olfactory system, cells that serve specific functions in the visual system, such as those that distinguish color, make precise connections to the part of the geniculate that specializes in color, and then transmit the message to the cortex. The pathways and connections for each color are determined very precisely by genes. These studies have also shown that axonal connections are initially less precise in the brain of the fetus than in that of the adult, and that there is some overlap of synaptic connections before segregation of these connections into discrete neuronal territories takes place. The final, precise connections shown in FIGURE 2 are formed partly by rearrangement of axonal terminals at the local level, and partly by selective elimination of nonessential cells and their connections. There are, for example, about 30 to 40% more neurons in the monkey visual cortex during the second half of pregnancy than there are in an adult monkey, and more than 50% of the axons in the optic nerve or callosum are ultimately eliminated. The functional significance of these losses is not fully understood, but the prevailing hypothesis is that activity-dependent functional validation plays a critical role in determining which neurons, axons, and synapses are retained.

After birth, in both macaque monkeys and humans, synaptic density increases rapidly until it reaches a peak in early childhood (FIG. 7). The peak is followed by a rather dramatic decline, which occurs mainly during sexual maturation and ends at puberty. Thereafter, the density of synapses remains at the same, adult level, until senility, when it begins to decline.

Synapses are numbered in trillions, and therefore the magnitude of the losses is stunning when expressed as actual rates: more than 20,000 synapses lost per second in the entire neocortex of the macaque monkey, and approximately 100,000 per second in humans, where the period of sexual maturation is longer and the cortex is 10 times larger. How do these findings relate to Gerald Edelman's postulate of Darwinian selection? There is, indeed, competition among neurons, and it is effected through elimination or retention of synapses. Furthermore, the competition has to be among synapses that have already been formed; those that are functionally validated stay, and those that are not used are lost.

Synaptic loss contributes importantly to human variability. The process and its dependence on activity were beautifully demonstrated by Hubel and Wiesel in a classic experiment on the developing visual system of primates. They closed one eye

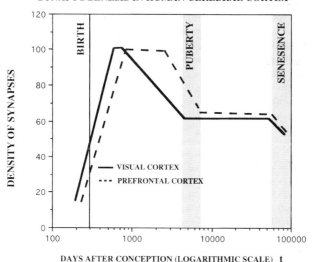

FIGURE 7. Changes in the relative density of synapses in the human cerebral cortex as a function of days after conception. Based on the data of Huttenlocker and Debholkar and reproduced from Bourgeois *et al.* in *Cognitive Neuroscience*, 2nd ed., edited by M.S. Gazzaniga, MIT Press (1999).

of newborn monkeys during the critical period immediately after birth, and found that the connections subserving the remaining, functional eye projected onto the territory that is normally occupied by the closed eye. The pathways for the eye that was closed atrophied, and the synapses within those pathways eventually disappeared, while those that served the functional eye—that is, the pathways that continued to work and therefore were presumably useful for the organism—were strengthened and flourished. Thus, one's experiences (such as loss of an eye) modify our genetic endowment to form different combinations of synaptic connections. However, insofar as changes can be made only within the genetic constraints with which we were endowed, the selective process apparently cannot produce something totally new.

Earlier in this symposium, David Botstein stressed the importance of the basic sciences in biomedical education—the importance of understanding scientific principles rather than just memorizing facts. I hope that my presentation has underscored this importance by illustrating how elucidation of the basic principles of brain development promotes our understanding of the human mind and therefore our ability to deal with hereditary and acquired disorders of the brain that arise from defective production, migration, or maldevelopment of neurons.

Many researchers in this field dwell on the enormous suffering—to individuals, families, and societies—that congenital malformations and mental retardation can cause. I tend to see the optimistic side of things: Having worked on brain development for more than three decades, I marvel at how well our brains develop, especially when one considers how many things could go wrong. And so I say to you, "Be happy with your brain as it is, because this is the only one you have!"

There is an additional reason for optimism: With the completion of the Human Genome Project and the further development of the extraordinary tools of molecular genetics and cellular biology, scientists will be in a position to prevent and cure most congenital malformations. The activity-dependent competitive interactions that occur in childhood may perhaps be used to fine-tune synaptic connections. For example, our educational system, which postpones intensive intellectual exercise until later stages, may not be optimal biologically, since synaptic stabilization occurs during the first 12 years of life. It is well-known that early childhood is often the critical age for the creation of top musicians and athletes, and there is reason to believe that cognitive skills are also set up at this time. One major challenge for the next century will be to unravel the cellular and molecular mechanisms involved in synaptic stabilization.

Let me close on a note of humility. When I entered the field of developmental neurobiology, many of my colleagues, and I myself, were convinced that the basic mechanisms of brain development would be understood within our lifetimes. However, the more I learned about this subject, the more humble I became. To paraphrase Haldane: The universe is not only queerer than we have supposed, it is even queerer than we *can* suppose. Similarly, I now recognize that the development of the nervous system is not only more complicated than we had imagined, but it may be even more complicated than we *can* imagine. What we have yet to learn may ultimately be of enormous significance, as it may equip us to deal with the compelling problems that face humanity in an uncertain universe.

Modern Phrenology: Maps of Human Cortical Function

MARCUS E. RAICHLE

Professor of Radiology, Neurology, and Neurobiology, Washington University School of Medicine, St. Louis, Missouri 63110, USA

I feel a bit like a U2 pilot who flies at high altitude and sees rather gross maps of the world. I'm going to take you, if you will, to a kind of high altitude from where you will get a look at the brain that is very different from the picture that Gerry Edelman and Pasko Rakic have presented. I would like to give you a feel for the kinds of data we obtain, how we interpret those data, and how they shed light on the topic that is the focus of our research, which is the relationship between the brain and behavior.

Neuroscientists have available today a whole array of neurobiological tools (ranging from those of molecular biology to various imaging techniques) with which to examine the function of the brain. These techniques can probe everything from single molecules to the living human brain on time scales ranging from a few milliseconds to an entire lifetime. But if we want to explore what the living human brain is doing, especially the normal living human brain, the number of tools that we can bring to the task becomes substantially less than the entire array available. In fact, we are then really limited to the various imaging techniques, plus the more venerable electrical tools such as the EEG (electroencephalograph) and the ERP (event-related potentials), and their more recent derivative MEG (magnetoencephalography).

There have been three major players in the imaging field. Computerized tomography (CT) is the technique that started the imaging revolution over 25 years ago; it changed not only the way we practice clinical medicine but also the way we now obtain data on organs of the human body. As you know, with this technique one can take virtual anatomical slices of the body and of organs, such as the brain. Invention of the CT was followed in rather short order by the development of positron emission tomography (PET), which is an extension of the technique of autoradiography—that is, a technique in which molecules within the body are radioactively labeled so that they emit radiation that can be recorded and quantified. Depending on what kind of molecule is labeled and where within the body it is located, one can derive all sorts of quantitative inferences about the function, the biochemistry, the metabolism, etc. of the organ being studied. Finally, magnetic resonance imaging (MRI) is an even more recent development, which operates on completely different principles but also yields both anatomical and functional information. With MRI, the behavior of molecules and atoms is discerned from their unique behaviors in high magnetic fields.

In this presentation, I would like to share the kind of functional information that comes from PET and MRI. Although I will show primarily PET data, I would like you to understand that very similar information can be obtained now with MRI.

Let's address first the question of how we make a connection between what we see by an imaging technique and what the brain is doing. The link is a surprisingly simple, yet poorly understood one that was discovered more than a hundred years ago by a very enterprising Italian physiologist named Angelo Mosso. One of the two subjects that he studied was a gentleman who had a neurosurgical defect, which left him essentially like a child, with an open fontanel. Anyone who is a parent knows that an open fontanel is an area on top of an infant's head where the skull has not yet fused, and which pulsates. Likewise, if you have an adult patient, as did Mosso, with a neurosurgical defect where there is no bone beneath the scalp, you can see the pulsations. It was of great interest to Mosso and others to know why the brain pulsated—it was not clear at the time that the pulsations represented heart beats—and so Mosso developed what was at that time an elegant recording device to study the pulsations.

Although one of the suspicions was that blood flow to the brain caused the pulsations, nobody was sure. To test this possibility, Mosso recorded simultaneously over an artery in the wrist and from over the bony defect. On one occasion (related in a marvelous but largely overlooked book written by Mosso, entitled *Ueber den Kreislauf des Blutes im menschlichen Gehirn,* Leipzig, 1881), he was recording near noon when suddenly the clock struck 12:00 and the church bells rang—and the recording over the brain changed very abruptly.

Of course, Mosso realized that it was customary to say a prayer at noon, and here's this poor fellow (his subject) strapped into an experimental setup, which made it a bit awkward for him to pray. So Mosso simply asked the man, "Should you have said a prayer?" And again, up go the pulsations over the brain! And then Mosso did a most ingenious thing: He performed what I would say is the first cognitive activation study recorded in the literature, a task of mental arithmetic: he simply asked the gentleman to multiply 8 by 12. Up went the pulsations over the brain when he asked the question, and up again, slightly, when the subject gave the answer. From this observation, Mosso drew an important and correct conclusion, namely, that the circulation to the brain changes in relationship to its function. Although we have many times replicated these important observations over the past hundred years, we still do not know precisely why a change in brain activity leads so reliably to local changes in its circulation of blood.

What would a modern-day view of this phenomenon look like? To answer that question, let's take a stimulus that is guaranteed to change things in the nervous system very dramatically: stimulation of the visual system with bright flashing lights. During the control situation, we have the subject look at a tiny dot in the middle of a screen, while we record the blood flow in the subject's brain. With PET, the latter can be accomplished simply by injecting some radioactive water, and in less than a minute we have a map of the circulation to the brain. Then we stimulate the subject's visual system by projecting onto the screen a checkerboard that reverses at a precise

→

FIGURE 1. Two positron emission tomography (PET) images of blood flow (top row, first two images) obtained during visual stimulation (labeled "Task") and simply resting quietly with eyes open (labeled "Control"). These images were obtained from a single normal adult human. The brain is oriented such that the nose is at 12 o'clock and the left side is to the reader's left. The difference between these two images, obtained by subtraction, is shown in the top row on the right. Noteworthy is the large increase in the back of the brain in the area of the visual cortex. The second row presents a series of five subtraction images taken from different individuals. Finally, in the third row, the images from all the individuals shown in the second row have been averaged to produce one composite image. This imaging strategy is the basis for the images shown in FIGURES 2 and 3.

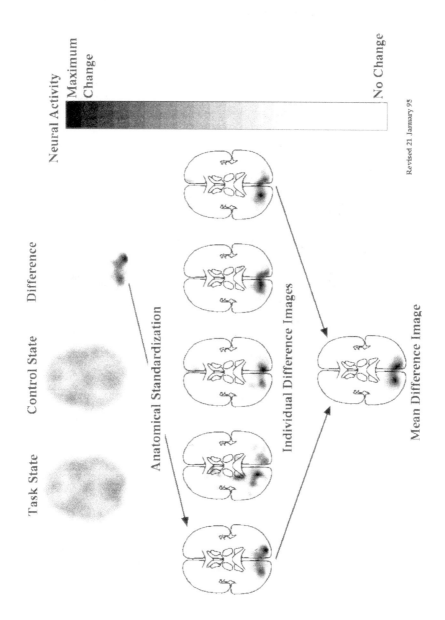

Revised 21 January 95

frequency—a visual stimulus so powerful that it is almost like hitting the brain with a sledgehammer.

FIGURE 1 shows what these results look like on PET. Superimposed on the slices of the brain are shades of gray, which reflect the circulation to various areas of the brain: the darker it is, the higher the circulation. You can spot the areas that are "lit up" during visual stimulation—in the back of the brain, where the visual system resides (image labeled "Task" in FIGURE 1). But the lighting up is not obvious until you subtract the image during the control situation from that during stimulation. And when you do that, the difference between the two states becomes obvious and highly localized. It is this comparison—stimulated state minus control—that is applied in both PET and MRI; the comparisons are usually either average responses for an individual, or averages for a group of individuals. Compared to the elegant techniques of molecular biology that have been presented to you, this kind of information gathering may seem a crude sort of measurement; in fact, however, PET and MRI are remarkably reliable and precise methods that yield very good and useful information on what the brain is doing that can only be appreciated at this level of resolution.

The title of my talk contains the word "phrenology," which, as a concept, has acquired a somewhat bad reputation. The notion of phrenology was that there were areas of the brain that were concerned with observable human functions—that things like mathematical competence, love, and other whole human behaviors were instantiated in certain locales in the human brain. In today's neurobiological world—for example, the kind of work presented by Gerry Edelman and Pasko Rakic and Richard Axel—that notion may seem simplistic, and one would have thought that it had died out. But I'm afraid it hasn't. In fact, the concept was portrayed very recently [1997] in *The New York Times Magazine*, accompanying a story about the kind of work that I do; the map of the brain that appeared on the cover showed areas for cognition, language, smell, taste, and so forth—even for cognitive behavior, such as making the correct change, separating the laundry, and choosing the quickest line at the supermarket!

I would like to disabuse you of this naive notion of phrenology; we no longer think of discrete areas in the brain that instantiate an entire behavior. Rather, we think of these areas as elements underlying the behavior. The analogy that I like is of the brain as a symphony orchestra, in which a finite number of elements (the instruments and their player) can be combined in an almost infinite number of ways to create a very large number of unique products. In a similar way, I see the brain as having—despite its billions of neurons—a finite number of processing elements, each of which contributes in some unique but probably fairly fundamental way to the expression of a behavior; and the great complexity of that behavior arises from the way in which those elements combine. I'm going to say very little about the individual elements and what they do today; instead, I want to give you a sense of what the orchestra that's playing looks like. You might think of the experience like going to a live concert rather than listening to a CD.

Let's consider a very simple example, namely, how single words are processed. I could have chosen any of numerous other examples, but I'm comfortable with this one; it will give you a sense of how we proceed with an experiment, how we interpret the results, and how those results might change our current concepts of the brain.

Paul Broca, a very famous anthropologist/surgeon in Paris, made a fundamental contribution to our understanding of the organization of the human brain when he observed a patient who had difficulty with language. The patient had had a stroke on the left, near the front of the brain, and he became known as "Tan" because the only response he could give to a question, any kind of question, was "Tan." Through his ingenious investigations of this neurological limitation, Paul Broca stimulated a whole series of studies, spanning the ensuing century and more, about how a person might process a single word.

For example, how does a person speak a written word? You see the word "car" and then you say it. What is involved in this seemingly simple task? From what I said earlier in explaining PET imaging, it won't surprise you that the visual system, in the back of the brain, might be a participant. Information is then passed forward to Wernicke's area (named for Carl Wernicke, who first described the consequences of lesions in that part of the brain). In Wernicke's area, the signal is processed into a phonological code—because you learn language by hearing it first—and then the coded message is passed forward into Broca's area, where further processing takes place, and finally up to the motor cortex, and you say what you see; or perhaps more accurately, what you saw.

The elucidation of that cascade—from the visual cortex, to Wernicke's area, to Broca's area, to the motor cortex—was based entirely on damaged brains, usually patients with strokes. That fact raised a question: Does a normal brain work that way as well? We and others doing brain imaging in normal brains with MRI and PET have tried to answer that question. One way to start would seem to be to display a word on a screen and have the subject say it, and then to compare the imaging during that process to the imaging while the subject is doing nothing. But that might miss a lot of steps: the perception of the word; the speaking of the word; possibly thinking about the meaning of the word. What you really want to do is to find out which parts of the brain are concerned with each of those steps.

So we started by imaging the process of reading a single word, and we did that by imaging a series of tasks, and subtracting one from another in a hierarchical fashion. The tasks included lying in the imaging machine with eyes closed; opening the eyes and looking at a blank screen; and looking at a simple noun on the screen, but not verbalizing the noun.

Thus the initial questions were: What happens in the brain when a word appears —a complex stimulus that contains information (the noun)? What does the nervous system do with that stimulus even if the subject is not asked to do anything about it? Once you've answered those questions, you have something to subtract from the imaging during the next task; and the next task; and the next—to peel things out, until you ask the subject to read the word that's on the screen. In this stepwise fashion, you might be able to identify those areas in the nervous system that are concerned with the entire, though still pretty simple, task of speaking a written word. The results of such a "peeling" process are illustrated in FIGURE 2.

For most of us who use our native language, reading words that are common to us, and even speaking those words, is a pretty easy and automatic task. But if we add just one further element to the task, it can become quite complex and far from automatic. For example, if instead of just reading nouns as they are flashed on the screen, we ask the subjects instead to generate a use or a verb for that noun, perhaps one every second or second-and-a-half, it becomes an exceedingly difficult and novel task to perform. The new task involves a lot of interesting and complex and debatable linguistic properties, but the thing that I would like to focus on right now is that it becomes a difficult and, I would like you to believe, non-automatic task. Let me illustrate this point by walking you through the experiment—from just opening the eyes to coming up with a use or a verb for the noun—by showing you what the brain is doing at each step (FIG. 2).

During the experiment, the subjects lie in a scanner, initially with their eyes closed, but then they see either a little white dot on the screen or a very simple, common English noun. So, to begin with, as the subjects open their eyes, there is activity in the back of the brain, in the visual system. And then, as we slice down from top to bottom, so to speak, through the brain, areas in the visual apparatus appear active just from simply opening the eyes and looking at what is essentially a blank screen.

Next, if we project a word on the screen—and even though we do not ask the subjects to do anything with that word—many additional areas become active. (Bear in mind that we have already subtracted the activity reflecting the preceding task of opening the eyes and looking at a blank screen.)

We then ask the subject to read the word, and now areas in the motor system become active, and they include not only the primary motor cortex but also motor areas in the cerebellum.

Up to this point there are no great surprises in this process, with the possible exception that there appears to be no activity in Broca's or Wernicke's areas (see FIGURE 2; activity would have been predicted in the column labeled "$Z = 0$," on the left side in front and back respectively). Thus the standard model, which states that reading a word involves Broca's and Wernicke's areas, is probably wrong; apparently, other operations are required to bring these areas into play.

So let's have a look at another operation, and that is generating verbs for the nouns. Thus, if the subjects see the noun "car," they might say "drive"; or if they see "knife," they might say "cut." With this additional task, areas in the left frontal cortex become active, as does another area along the midline called the anterior cingulate (compare the images for reading words and generating verbs in the column labeled "$Z = 0$"). But what really surprised us is that now the cerebellum was even more active, even in a task that was purely cognitive ("$Z = -20$" in FIGURE 2). (Again, bear in mind that we have subtracted all preceding activity, so we are seeing just those parts of the brain that are concerned with the additional cognitive operation of providing verbs for the nouns.) So the involvement of the cerebellum was, in itself, an interesting new observation. Prior to this, brain scientists and physicians had associated the cerebellum only with the motor aspects of our behavior.

At this point, I hope you get the sense of how one can use imaging techniques to identify the parts of the brain that are concerned with certain operations. But you might say, "Is that all there is to it?" And the answer is "No." What I've shown you thus far is that additional areas of the brain become involved as a task gets more complex—going from simply looking at a noun, to reading it, to generating a logical verb for the noun. In the analogy of the symphony orchestra, it's like adding the second violins, the violas, the flutes—whatever is needed to get the job done. But people of-

FIGURE 2. Four different hierarchically organized conditions are represented in these mean blood flow difference images obtained with PET. All of the changes shown in these images represent increases over the control state for each task. A group of nine normal individuals performed these tasks involving common English nouns (see text for details).

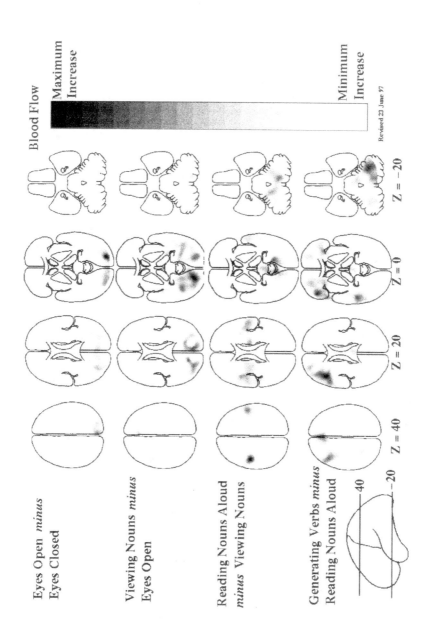

Blood Flow

Maximum Increase

Minimum Increase

Revised 23 June 97

Z = −20

Z = 0

Z = 20

Z = 40

Eyes Open *minus* Eyes Closed

Viewing Nouns *minus* Eyes Open

Reading Nouns Aloud *minus* Viewing Nouns

Generating Verbs *minus* Reading Nouns Aloud

40

−20

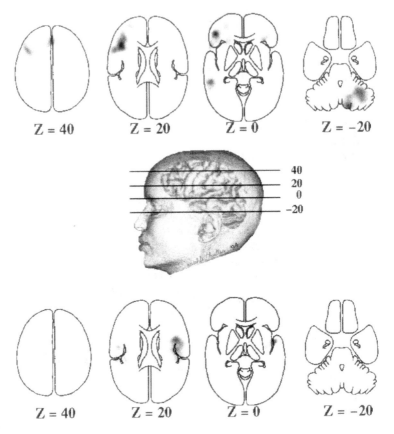

FIGURE 3. Changes in activity resulting from practice on the verb-generation task include decreases (top row) and increases (bottom row) in brain activity.

ten ask, "How do you know that, once a given task has been mastered, the brain still goes through the same progression of steps that led up to that task as it was being learned?" Well, one of the advantages of imaging is that we can answer that question. To do so, we simply had subjects practice generating verbs for a specific list of nouns until they were good at it. This usually took about 10 minutes.

Let me remind you of the experimental paradigm: A subject sees a noun on the screen and says the first word that comes to mind. As I said, that's difficult; it takes a bit of time, and initially the subject is under a lot of stress. But as the task is practiced, the subject becomes increasingly fast—over a matter of just minutes—and at the same time, he or she begins to choose the same verb for a given noun every time that noun appears on the screen. So now the once-difficult task assumes a bit of automaticity, if you will. Soon the subject is very fast, proficient, and unstressed by the whole thing. Once that stage is reached, what is the brain doing? One postulate might be that the same areas continue to be used, but now much more efficiently. That, however, is not what happens.

When the subject first tackles the task, the frontal area, an area in the temporal cortex, and the cerebellum light up (FIG. 3, top row). But 10 minutes later, after the task has been practiced, not a one of those areas is involved. Rather, what has come back on line are bilateral locations in some hidden areas of the cortex known as the insula. These are seen active during word reading ("Z = 20" in FIGURE 2) but are inactive during naive verb generation (not shown). So what you might envision here is that had we practiced verb generation before imaging it the first time, our images would have been indistinguishable from reading the nouns in the first place. I hope that is reasonably clear!

These observations often prompt the reaction "Poor brain, it can only accomplish tasks by stealing blood from one area (remember that blood flow is what our imaging techniques are reflecting) and sending it to the area(s) responsible for the task. It's a plumbing problem, not a neurobiological one." Let me assure you that that is not the case. The imaging techniques can sense and record incredibly small changes of blood flow in the brain, which is capable of doubling its blood flow if need be. Therefore, the imaging techniques are showing us true neurobiological changes not just blood being stolen from one area to supply another. And apparently, those changes (FIG. 3) involve using completely different circuits within the brain as we make a complex task more simple through practice.

Thus, there really were two ways of getting the job done: (1) an automatic system for routine speech output; and (2) a non-automatic processing system that exists in parallel, for more difficult and novel tasks. That fact raises several questions: How can we imagine such a parallel system existing in the brain? Why is it built this way? Why have two systems? One possible explanation could be that we have an "automatic" system for habitual, familiar tasks, as well as for stressful situations, where we are likely to do things in a reflexive way; and we have a more specialized system for processing novel tasks.

If that is correct, we might ask what value the additional (non-automatic) system provides. One way of getting at the answer is to look at a circumstance where the additional system is absent, and that circumstance exists in childhood; infants are born without it. As I showed earlier, the non-automatic system is subserved largely by the frontal cortex, and it takes that area of the brain some time to develop fully after birth. How, then, does a normal young child behave when confronted with the same kind of task?

My favorite paradigm for illustrating the phenomenology was introduced by Piaget many years ago and has been used by many investigators since. In this paradigm, a completely normal, very young child sits in the mother's lap. The mother initially restrains the child's arms while an investigator puts something into one of two wells. The child's vision and attention are riveted on what's going into the well because apparently it is something that interests the child. Once one well has been "baited," both wells are covered by a cloth and the child's hands are released. Normally, the child quickly removes the cloth covering the baited well and retrieves the coveted object.

During most of the trials, the investigator "trains" the child by always putting the object into the same well. And then, suddenly, for the first time, the investigator places the object into the other well, covers each well with a cloth as before, and the mother once again releases the child's hands. The results are dramatic. While keeping his eye fixed on the well where the object was placed most recently, the child's hand "reflexively" reaches for the empty well, to which he had been "trained"!

How can we explain this seemingly paradoxical behavior? After all, this child is perfectly normal, obviously attentive and capable of learning. One way to look at it is that life is complex, and demands that we automate routine tasks rapidly and efficiently as young children obviously do. But life is not entirely predictable, things do change unexpectedly, and therefore we have to have a system that is capable of overriding our habitual and reflexive responses. We have just seen what happens when such a system is absent. In the example used, it had not yet developed. We have also seen just such a system in action in our naive verb generation task in adults (FIG. 2). Other complementary examples exist.

I was struck, for example, by the following marvelous interchange between a linguist father and his daughter; it comes from the famous linguist Martin Brain (quoted in Jackendoff, R.: *Patterns in the Mind,* Basic Books, NY, 1994, p. 104): The daughter says, "Want other one spoon, Daddy." And the father says, "You mean, you want the other spoon?" And the child says, "Yes, I want the other one spoon, please, Daddy." "Can you say, 'the other spoon'?" "Other one spoon." "Say, 'Other; other spoon; spoon; other spoon.'" And then the child says, "Other spoon. Now give me other one spoon!" Of course, one can draw all kinds of conclusions from this interchange, but my take-home message is that we're dealing with an immature nervous system, which is finding difficulty in making an adaptation and changing a habitual response.

Furthermore, this behavior doesn't stop with children. I dare say that every adult in this audience has experienced the consequences of this kind of brain organization. For example, in their book *Absent-Minded* (Prentice-Hall, Inc., Englewood, N.J., 1982—a wonderfully fun read, but a deadly serious work), James Reason and Klara Mycielska cite the following examples: struggling to open a friend's door with your own keys; stepping into the bathtub with your socks on; squeezing shaving cream onto a toothbrush. These reflexive, habitual responses play an immense and mostly useful role in our daily lives. But given the level of unpredictability in our daily lives, we must have a way of overriding the habitual behavior, or we might be in serious trouble!

Sometimes, however, the override we'd hoped for isn't achieved. No matter how much we may wish it, the override doesn't happen, and, in retrospect, we wish we hadn't said or done what we did in the "heat of the moment." It will be important for us to understand how a system that can override habitual responses is itself overridden by our emotional state. A key to that understanding will be to probe the way in which emotions interact with cognition. I do not have time to describe that aspect, except to point out that during the naive verb generation paradigm that I described earlier—the stressful task in which a verb is generated from a noun—among the areas going down in activity is that part of the brain that is concerned with emotion; the area is actually *turned off!* These interactions between cognition and emotion obviously have rather important social implications.

Thus, I hope you can see that modern phrenology is not to find out where certain functions of the brain—say, mathematical competence—are located. Rather, it is to figure out how circuits come together and interact during the performance of human activities—very akin to the analogy of the symphony orchestra that I used earlier.

The brain is going to "look different," physically, during the next several years. Those of you who follow this literature already realize that fact, but most of you do not. The new picture is being driven largely by work coming out of the magnetic resonance world—magnetic resonance imaging, or MRI. Let me end, then, with an example of MRI.

An MRI functional imaging study (usually referred to as *f*MRI for short) looks much like the PET views that I have shown up to now. One of the problems with the human brain is that it is folded, so that if you look at its surface, some 60% to 70% of the brain is not visible. The MRI technique can overcome this shortcoming by "inflating" the brain, just like blowing up a balloon. This eliminates the "wrinkles." And then the balloon is "cut" at strategic points (not actually, but by means of multiple computerized images) to allow the whole surface to be laid flat. Of course, these images will be useful only if you can figure out where in the brain you are, and there are now standardized guidelines for exact localization.

Fortunately, a set of guidelines was developed early in imaging work that enables us to work in standard spaces, so that when we describe responses, we localize them by standard coordinates. That means that all results can be put into databases, stored, and retrieved. In this regard, I hope we can follow the example set by the people working on the genome project; it is admirable that they are willing to share data and file these data in large repositories. As a result enormous amounts of information are available to the entire scientific community. Francis Collins sounded an extremely important clarion call when he warned us against the patenting of much of that information by the private sector.

Over the next decade or so, an enormous amount of information is likely to be generated about the human nervous system. Every experiment yields pictures of the whole brain, even though a given investigator who does the experiment will be interested in only certain specific areas. Thus, we will have lots of maps of the human brain, full of information on how the brain works, that should become available to all.

I submit that if we subscribe to this way of doing things—of sharing new information by placing it in a readily accessible database—we will have an enormous reservoir of information on the human brain that is important not only to neuroscientists and cognitive scientists interested in how the normal brain works, but also to clinicians who have to contend with diseases of the brain.

As yet, none of this kind of imaging includes any information about the electrical circuits that are involved. Gerry Edelman and Pasko Rakic have stressed the importance of timing in understanding how the brain works. Ultimately, will have to include this in the maps produced by imaging, because without timing information, we will not have a complete view of how the brain works. Much work is now being devoted to accomplishing this.

Let me close with a quote from Sidney Brenner, who captured the impact of the unbelievable explosion in techniques for looking at the human nervous system, when he said: "Progress in science depends on new techniques, new discoveries, and new ideas—probably in that order."

SUGGESTED READINGS

1. RAICHLE, M.E. 1998. Neural correlates of consciousness: an analysis of cognitive skill learning. Phil. Trans. Royal Soc. B **353:** 1889–1902.
2. RAICHLE, M.E. 1998. Behind the scenes of functional brain imaging: a historical and physiological perspective. Proc. Natl. Acad. Sci. USA **95:** 765–772.

How the Mind Works

STEVEN PINKER

Director, McDonnell-Pew Center for Cognitive Neuroscience, Massachusetts Institute of Technology, Cambridge, Massachusetts 02139, USA

The human mind is a remarkable organ. It has allowed us to walk on the moon, to discover the physical basis of life and the universe, and to play chess almost as well as a computer. But the brain raises a paradox. On the one hand, many tasks that we take for granted—walking around a room, picking up an object, recognizing a face, remembering information—are feats that scientists and engineers have been unable to duplicate in robots and computers. Nonetheless, these feats can be accomplished by any four-year-old, and we tend to be blasé about them. On the other hand, for all its engineering excellence, the mind has many apparent quirks. For example, why is the thought of eating worms disgusting when worms are perfectly safe and nutritious? Why do men do insane things like challenge each other to duels and murder their ex-wives? Why do fools fall in love? Why do people believe in ghosts and spirits?

Recently, I have been foolhardy enough to try to answer questions like this in a book called *How the Mind Works*. What I will be talking about today comes from that book, which is based on three key ideas: computation, evolution, and specialization.

The first idea is that the function of the brain is *information processing*, or *computation*. Computation involves an age-old problem, one that was raised by Professor Edelman, namely, Descartes's problem of the causation of behavior. If I were to ask you, "Why did Bill just get on the bus?" to answer that question you wouldn't run a neural network simulation and you wouldn't need to put Bill's head in a scanner. You could just ask Bill, and you might discover that the explanation for his behavior is that he wants to visit his grandmother, and he knows that the bus will take him to his grandmother's house. No science of the future is likely to provide an explanation with greater predictive power than that. If Bill hated the sight of his grandmother or if he knew the route had changed, his body would not be on that bus. But this excellent theory raises a puzzle. The beliefs and desires that cause Bill's behavior are colorless, odorless, tasteless, and weightless. Nevertheless, they are as potent a cause of action as any billiard ball clacking into another billiard ball.

How do we explain this seeming paradox? One part of the solution, I believe, is that beliefs and desires are *information*. Information is another commodity that is colorless, odorless, tasteless, and weightless yet can have physical effects without resorting to any occult or mysterious process. Information consists of patterns in matter or energy, namely symbols, that correlate with states of the world. That's what we mean when we say that something carries information. A second part of the solution is that beliefs and desires have their effects in computation—where computation is defined, roughly, as a process that takes place when a device is arranged so that information (namely, patterns in matter or energy inside the device) causes changes in the patterns of other bits of matter or energy, and the process mirrors the laws of logic, probability, or cause and effect in the world. The result is that if the old patterns are accurate or true, or correlate with some aspect of reality, the new arrangements of matter or energy will as well. The cascade gives the device an ability to deduce new truths from old truths, which is not a bad definition of thinking. In fact, the computational theory of mind is the only theory that I know of that can explain how it is that patterns of physical change in a device—be it a computer or a brain, or, for that matter, some extraterrestrial intelligent life—might accomplish something we would dignify with the term "thinking." It's the only explanation we have for how physical changes actually do something we would be willing to call intelligent. It is an explanation of where intelligence comes from.

A few comments must be added to this claim. One is that the computational theory of mind is very different from the computer metaphor that Professor Edelman has alluded to in his presentation. As he pointed out, there are many ways in which commercially available computers are radically different from brains. Computers are serial; brains are parallel. Computers are fast; brains are slow. Computers have deterministic components; brains have noisy components. Computers are assembled by an external agent; brains have to assemble themselves. Computers display screensavers with flying toasters; brains do not. But the claim is not that commercially available computers are a good model for the brain. Rather, the claim is that the answer to the question "What makes brains intelligent?" may overlap with the question "What makes computers intelligent?" The common feature, I suggest, is information-processing, or computation. An analogy is that when we want to understand how birds fly, we invoke principles of aerodynamics that also apply to airplanes. But that doesn't mean that we are committed to an airplane metaphor for birds and should ask whether birds have complimentary beverage service. It's a question of isolating the key component of the best explanation.

Another comment is that the computational theory of mind, explicitly or not, has set the agenda for brain science for decades. An old example from introductory neuroscience classes describes the naive person who asks, "Since the image on the retina is upside-down but we see the world right-side up, is there some part of the brain that turns the image right-side up?" We all realize that this question rests on a fallacy, that there is no such process in the brain, and that there doesn't need to be any such process. Why is it a fallacy? Because the orientation of the image on the retina makes no difference to how the brain processes *information*. Since information-processing is the relevant aspect of what goes on in the brain, the orientation on the retina—and, for that matter, on the visual cortex—is irrelevant; that is why the above is a pseudoquestion. Similarly, the search for the neural basis of psychological functions is guided, from beginning to end, by invoking information-processing. As you know, one of the great frontiers of science is the search for the molecular basis of learning and memory. Well, of the hundreds or thousands of metabolic processes in the brain, how will we know when we've identified the one that corresponds to memory? We will know we have it when the process meets the requirements of the storage and retrieval of information. So again, it is information that sets the interesting questions in neuroscience.

A third comment is that the computational theory of mind is a radical challenge to our everyday way of thinking about the mind, because the theory says that the lifeblood of thought is *information*. That goes against our folk notion that the lifeblood of thought is *energy* or *pressure*. Why did the disgruntled postal worker shoot up the post office? Well, for many years, we say, pressure had been building up until he finally burst; if only he had had an alternative outlet to which to divert all of that energy, he could have released it in more constructive ways. The metaphor is that thought and emotion are animated by some superheated fluid or gas under pressure. Now, there is no doubt that this hydraulic metaphor captures something about our experience. But we know that it is not literally how the brain works: there is no container full of fluid and channels through which the fluid flows. And that raises an important scientific question: Why is the brain going to so much trouble to *simulate* energy and pressure, given that it doesn't literally work that way? I will return to that question later.

Let me continue with the second key idea: *evolution*. How do we understand a complex device? Imagine that you are rummaging through an antique store and you come across a contraption bristling with gears and springs and a handle and hinges and blades. You have no idea how to explain it until someone tells you what it's *for* —say, an olive-pitter. Once you realize what the device is for—what its function is— suddenly all the parts and their arrangements become clear in a satisfying rush of insight. This is an activity called "reverse engineering." In forward engineering, you start off with an idea for what you want a device to do and you go and build the device. In reverse engineering, you stumble across a device and try to figure out what it was designed to do. Reverse engineering is what the technicians at Panasonic do when Sony comes out with a new product. They go to the store, buy one, bring it back to the lab, take a screwdriver to it, and try to figure out what all the little widgets and gizmos are for.

For the last few hundred years, the science of physiology has been a kind of reverse engineering. Living bodies are complex devices and pose questions like "Why, in the eye, do we find the most transparent tissue in the body that just happens to be shaped like a lens, behind the lens an iris that expands and contracts in response to light, and a layer of light-sensitive tissue that happens to be at the focal plane of the lens?" Questions like these can be answered only by the idea that the eye was in some sense "designed" to form an image. We analyze it just as if it were a machine. For centuries, the complexity of the eye and other organs was taken as conclusive proof of the existence of God. If the eye shows signs of design, it must have a designer—namely, God. Darwin's great accomplishment was to explain signs of engineering in the natural world through a purely physical force, namely, the differential replication rates among replicators competing for resources in a finite environment, iterated over hundreds and thousands of generations.

Of course, the eye doesn't just sit by itself, isolated in the skull. Rather, the eye is connected to the brain. In fact, the eye can validly be considered to be an extension of the brain. And that naturally leads us to treat the *mind* as a complex natural device —in this case, a complex computational device—which makes the science of psychology a kind of reverse engineering. Just as in the case of the olive-pitter, we can understand the brain only once we have correctly identified its function. If we thought that the olive-pitter was a wrist-exerciser, we would have a very different explanation for what the parts are for. The crucial place to begin explaining the mind, therefore, is to understand its function. Since the mind is a product of natural selection, not of a conscious engineer, we have an answer to that question: the ultimate function of the mind is survival and reproduction in the environment in which the mind evolved—that is, the environment of hunting and gathering tribes in which we have spent more than 99% of our evolutionary history, before the recent invention of agriculture and civilizations only 10,000 years ago.

The third key idea is *specialization*. The mind is designed to solve many kinds of problems, such as seeing in three dimensions, moving arms and legs, understanding the physical world, finding and keeping mates, securing allies, and many others. These are very different kinds of problems, and the tools for solving them are bound to be different as well. We know that specialization is ubiquitous in biology. The body is not made of Spam, but is divided into systems and organs and tissues, each designed to perform a special function or functions. The heart has a different structure from the kidney because a device that pumps blood has to be different from a device that filters blood. This specialization continues all the way down: to the different tissues that the heart and the kidney are made from, all the way down to differences in the molecules that they are made from. The mind, like the body is organized into mental systems and organs and tissues—a kind of hierarchical differentiation that was beautifully displayed in the functional neuroimaging experiments that Professor Raichle has shown.

I concur fully in a point that has been made several times during this session—namely, that the mind will not be explained in terms of some special essence or wonder tissue or almighty mathematical principle. Rather, the mind is a system of computational organs that allowed our ancestors to understand and outsmart objects, animals, plants, and each other. I will try to give you a glimpse of how three of these organs of computation might be dissected. I will present examples of seeing, thinking, and emotions about people.

Let's begin with seeing. The problem of vision can be made vivid by imagining what the world looks like from the brain's point of view. It is not what we whole, functioning human beings experience, namely, a showcase of three-dimensional objects arrayed in space. Rather, the brain "sees" a million activation levels corresponding to the brightnesses of tiny patches on the retina; the retinal image as a whole is a two-dimensional projection of the three-dimensional world. The task for the visual system of the brain is to recover information about three-dimensional shapes and their arrangements from the pattern of intensities on the retinal image. The brain has evolved a number of tricks for solving this problem, and I am going to talk about one of them—sometimes called "shape-from-shading." Each of these tricks exploits a regularity of optics that is true by virtue of physical law, and the brain can, in a sense, run these laws "backwards" to try to make intelligent guesses about what is out there in the world based on the information that is coming in from the retina.

One important bit of physics is (roughly) that the steeper the angle formed by a surface with respect to a light source, the less light the surface reflects. So as I shine a flashlight perpendicularly to a card, it projects a concentrated, bright spot of light. But when I rotate the card, the beam is smeared across a large area, and any particular part of the area must be dimmer. Now, the shape-from-shading algorithm—a bit of psychology—more or less runs the law backwards and says that the dimmer a patch on the retina, the steeper the angle of the surface in the world. And with that algorithm, the brain can reconstruct the shape of an object by estimating the angles of the thousands of tiny facets or tangent planes that make up the surface.

This process works reasonably well, but it depends on a key assumption. Since it interprets differences in brightness as coming from differences in surface angle, it implicitly assumes a uniformly colored world, or at least a randomly colored world. That means that the process is vulnerable, because surfaces that are colored in clever ways should fool the shape-from-shading module and cause us to see things that aren't there. In fact, it does happen: two striking examples are television and make-up. If alien anthropologists visited this planet, they would be puzzled by the fact that the average American spends four hours a day staring at a piece of glass on the front of a box. Why do we do this? Because the television set has been arranged to violate the assumption of uniform or random coloration. It has been engineered to display a highly *non*random pattern that fools the shape-from-shading module of the brain into hallucinating a three-dimensional world behind the pane of glass.

Another example is makeup. A person who is skilled at applying makeup might put a little blush on the sides of the nose, because the eye of the beholder is attached to a shape-from-shading module that interprets darker surfaces as steeper angles, making the sides of the nose look more parallel and the nose smaller and more attractive. Conversely, if you put light powder on the upper lip, the brain says that lighter equals a flatter angle, which makes the lip look fuller, giving that desirable pouty look that models strive so hard to attain.

More generally, these examples offer an explanation for many of the seemingly inexplicable quirks of modern human thought and behavior. Many illusions, fallacies, and maladaptive behaviors may come not from some inherent defect or design flaw but from a *mismatch:* a mismatch between assumptions about an ancestral world that were built into our mental modules over millions of years and the structure of the current world (which we have turned topsy-turvy by technology in our recent history). It has long been a puzzle for biologists why people do maladaptive things like eat junk food, use contraception (which, when you think of it, is a kind of Darwinian suicide), or gamble. But if you posit that our mental modules assume a world in which sweet foods are nutritious (namely, ripe fruit), in which sex leads to babies (as it tended to do until the invention of reliable contraceptives), and in which statistical patterns have underlying causes, then these activities no longer seem quite so mysterious.

Next, let us turn to the problem of thinking. There is an old puzzle that has worried philosophers and biologists ever since it was pointed out by Alfred Russel Wallace, the co-discoverer, with Darwin, of natural selection. What do illiterate, technologically primitive hunter-gatherers do with their capacity for abstract intelligence? In fact, this question might be more justly asked by hunter-gatherers about modern American couch potatoes. After all, life for hunters and gatherers was like a camping trip that never ended, but without Swiss army knives and tents and freeze-dried pasta. Our ancestors had to live by their wits and eke out a living from an ecosystem in which most of the plants and animals whose bodies we consume as food would just as soon keep their bodies for themselves.

Our species succeeded by entering what a biologist might call the "cognitive niche": the ability to overtake the fixed defenses of other organisms by cause-and-effect reasoning. In all human societies, no matter how supposedly primitive, people use a variety of tools; traps; poisons; various ways of detoxifying plants by cooking, soaking, and leaching; methods of extracting medicines from plants to combat parasites and pathogens; and an ability to act cooperatively to accomplish what a single person acting alone could not achieve. These accomplishments show that the mind must be equipped with ways of grasping the causally significant parts of the world. The world is a heterogeneous place, and it is likely that we have several different intuitive theories or varieties of common sense that are adapted to figure out the causal structure of different aspects of the world. We can think of them as a kind of intuitive physics, intuitive biology, intuitive engineering, and intuitive psychology, each based on a core intuition.

The most basic is intuitive physics, an appreciation of how objects fall, roll, and bounce. The core intuition behind our intuitive physics is the existence of stable objects that obey some kind of physical laws. This is not a banal claim. William James said that the world of the infant is a "blooming, buzzing confusion"—a kaleidoscope of shimmering pixels—and that knowledge of stable objects is an achievement only of late infancy. Yet one of the first things we learn in introductory courses in philosophy is that unless one has an assumption that the multitude of sensory impressions is caused by an underlying stable object, one could experience the blooming and buzzing confusion all of one's life. Indeed, the more we know about the world of the infant, the more we see that William James, at least in this case, didn't have it quite right. The youngest infants that can be tested (about three months old) already are expecting a world that contains stable objects, and they are surprised when an experimenter rigs up a display in which an object vanishes, passes through another object, flies apart, or moves without an external push. As one psychologist summed up the literature: A "blooming, buzzing confusion" is a better description of the world of the *parents* of an infant than of the world of the infant.

But there are many objects that we encounter that seem to violate our intuitive physics. As the biologist Richard Dawkins has pointed out, if you throw a dead bird in the air, it will describe a graceful parabola and come to rest on the ground, just like the physics books say it should. But if you throw a *live* bird in the air, it won't describe a graceful parabola, and it might not touch land this side of the county boundary. In other words, we interpret living things such as birds not through our intuitive physics but through an intuitive biology. We do not assume that birds are some kind of weird, springy object that violates the laws of physics; we assume, rather, that birds follow a different kind of law altogether—the laws of biology. The core intuition of folk biology is that plants and animals have an internal essence that contains a renewable supply of energy or *oomph*, that gives the animal or plant its form, that drives its growth, and that orchestrates its bodily functions. This deep-rooted intuition is found in all peoples and explains why hunter-gatherers are such excellent amateur biologists. Botanists and zoologists who do field work with hunter-gatherers are often astonished to learn that hunter-gatherers have remarkably detailed knowledge about local plants and animals and that their names for these plants and animals usually match the Linnaean genus or species of the professional biologists. These categorizations often involve lumping animals that, from surface appearance, look very different—for example, a caterpillar and a butterfly, or a male and a female bird with different plumage. Hunter-gatherers, using their intuitions about the hidden essences in animals or plants, predict their future behavior. They may, from a set of tracks, deduce the kind of animal and where it is likely to be heading so that they can surprise it at a resting place; or they might notice a flower in the spring and return to it in the fall to dig out a hidden tuber that the flower portends.

They extract juices and powders of living things and try them out as medicines, poisons, and food additives.

The third kind of intuition, different from the first two, is an intuitive engineering. Our species is famous for exploiting and using tools or artifacts, and the core intuition behind tools is their function. If I ask you to define a "chair," you might say it is a stable horizontal surface supported by four legs. But that will not work for beanbags, cubes, severed elephant's feet, and other objects that we can call chairs. The only thing that chairs have in common is that someone intended them to hold up a human behind. The core intuition behind our faculty to appreciate tools involves their *function*, or the intention of a designer. Young children, before they've entered school, sharply distinguish artifacts from living things. For example, in one experiment, children were told that doctors took a raccoon, spray-painted it black with a white stripe down its back, and implanted into it a sack of smelly stuff. The children were then shown a picture of a skunk and asked what it was. Most of them said that it was still a raccoon. But if they were told that doctors took a coffee pot, sawed off its handle, cut a hole through it, and filled it with birdseed, and then are shown a picture of a bird feeder and asked what it is, they say it's a bird feeder. This experiment shows that even young children appreciate that an artifact such as a bird feeder is anything that feeds birds, but a natural object such as a raccoon has an internal constitution that cannot be changed by superficial manipulations.

And finally, people have an intuitive version of psychology. I mentioned earlier that all of us explained Bill's behavior in getting on the bus not by assuming there is some kind of magnetic force that pulls him aboard or that he is a kind of artifact like a windup doll, but that he acts out of beliefs and desires, a kind of entity we cannot help but posit even though it is not directly observable. Again, this ability is displayed early by young children, who can, for example, deduce what an adult knows and wants just from observing what the adult is looking at.

There is evidence, apart from developmental psychology, that our reasoning ability really is divided into these intuitive theories or ways of thinking. For example, the technique of functional neuroimaging, which has been described by Dr. Raichle, has shown that different parts of the brain are active when people think about tools or about living things. Moreover the presumably genetic syndrome of autism can be pretty well characterized by saying that it impairs a person's intuitive psychology: Autistic children really do interpret humans as if they were windup dolls, and have no concept that other people have beliefs and desires.

Misapplications of the four forms of thinking, or a shift from one way of thinking to another, can also explain certain puzzling behaviors and beliefs. One example is slapstick humor. We laugh when someone slips on a banana peel because of the sudden shift from thinking of the person in the usual way (using our intuitive psychology and thinking of him as a locus of beliefs and desires) to thinking of him as an object ignominiously obeying the laws of physics. Belief in souls and ghosts consists of taking our intuitive psychology and divorcing it from our intuitive biology, so that we think of minds that have an existence independent of bodies. And animistic beliefs do the opposite: They marry our intuitive psychology to our intuitive biology, physics, or engineering and allow us to think of trees, mountains, or idols as having minds.

I will now proceed to my final example: emotions about people. The main puzzle about our feelings toward other people is why they are often so passionate and seemingly irrational. Why do people pursue vengeance past the point of any value to themselves? Why do people defend their honor in crazy ways such as challenging each other to duels? Why do people fall head over heels in love? The most common theory, among both scientists and lay people, is the "romantic theory"—the idea that the emotions come from a vestigial force (part of our heritage from nature), and that they are maladaptive and dangerous unless they are channeled into art and creativity. I'm going to explain a very different alternative, the "strategic theory," which proposes that passion is a "paradoxical tactic" wired into us. The basic idea is that a sacrifice of freedom and rationality can actually give one a strategic advantage when one is interacting with others whose interests are partly competing and partly overlapping with one's own. The theory applies particularly well to instances of promises, threats, and bargains. Just to show how unromantic this theory is, I am going to illustrate it by reverse-engineering romantic love.

Cynical social scientists and veterans of the dating scene agree on one thing: that love is a marketplace. There is a certain rationality to love—smart shopping. All of us at some point in our lives have to search for the nicest, smartest, richest, stablest, funniest, best-looking person who will settle for us. But that person is a needle in a haystack, and we might die single if we held out indefinitely for him or her. So we trade off value against time, and after a certain period set up house with the best person we have found up to that point. Good evidence for this sequence of events is the phenomenon called "assortative mating" by mate value: the overall desirabilities of a husband and a wife or a boyfriend and a girlfriend are approximately equally matched, as if each was trying to get the best partner he or she could.

Needless to say, that does not explain all there is to falling in love. There is an irrational part of love, an involuntariness and caprice to it. You cannot will yourself to fall in love. Many people can recall being fixed up with a person who looked perfect on paper, but when they met, they just didn't hit it off. Cupid's arrow didn't strike; the earth didn't move. It isn't a list of desirable traits that steals the heart; it's often something capricious like the way a person walks, talks, or laughs.

Is this any way to design a rational organism? As a matter of fact, it might be. Entering a partnership through totally "rational" shopping poses a problem. If you have set up house with the best person you have found up to a certain point, then by the law of averages, sooner or later someone even better will come along. At that point a rational agent would be tempted to drop a wife or husband like a hot potato. But now think of it from the spouse's point of view. Entering a partnership requires sacrifices—forgone opportunities with other potential partners and the time and energy put into child-rearing, among many other things. Rational spouses could anticipate that their partner would drop them when someone better came along, and they would be foolish to enter the relationship in the first place. Thus we would have the paradoxical situation in which what is in the interest of both parties—that they stick with each other—cannot be effected because neither one can trust the other if the other is acting as a rational, smart shopper.

Here is one solution to the problem. If we are wired so that we don't fall in love for rational reasons, perhaps we are less likely to decide to fall *out* of love for rational reasons. When Cupid strikes, it makes one's promise credible in the eyes of the object of desire. Romantic love is a *guarantor* of the implicit promise one makes in starting a romantic relationship, in the face of the problem that it may be rational to break that promise in the future.

Romantic love is an example of a concept from game theory called "paradoxical tactics," in which a lack of freedom and rationality can be an advantage. An analogy from a nonpsychological domain is the rationale for laws and contracts. When we apply for a mortgage from a bank, the law states that if we default on our payments, the bank has the power to foreclose on the mortgage and seize our house. It is only this law that makes it worth the bank's while to lend us the money, and therefore the law, paradoxically, works to the advantage of the *borrower* as well as the lender. Likewise, leases work to both the tenant's and the landlord's advantage by constraining the freedom of each. In this sense, many passions, such as romantic love, could be viewed as the neural equivalents of laws and contracts. Moreover, by symmetrical logic, if passionate love and loyalty are guarantors that our promises are not double-crosses, so passionate vengeance and honor serve as guarantors that our threats are not bluffs. The problem with issuing a threat, such as "If you steal my goats, I will beat you up," is that carrying out a threat can be dangerous: you could get hurt beating someone up. The only value of the threat is as a deterrent; once it has to be carried out, it serves no one's purposes. Since the target of the threat is aware of that fact, he can threaten the threatener right back by calling his bluff and daring him to go through with the vengeance. How does one prevent one's bluff from being called? By being *forced* to carry out the threat. If we are wired to interpret defiance or trespass as an intolerable insult for which we demand vengeance regardless of the cost to ourselves, that emotion serves as a credible deterrent. One gets the reputation of being someone that people don't want to mess with.

Let me conclude. Earlier I pointed out that the mind seems to be equipped with a certain number of ways of conceptualizing reality, which I called "intuitive theories." How do we go from our everyday "intuitive theories" to the real article in genuine scientific reasoning? I suspect that this unnatural activity called science is another way of misapplying our intuitive theories. In medicine and physiology, we avoid thinking of living things in the usual way—as being driven by a hidden essence or substance, some kind of juice or gel or a quivering mass—and instead think of them as a kind of machinery. That is, we take our faculty of intuitive engineering and apply it to a domain that ordinarily we think of by our intuitive biology. I would like to suggest that a challenge of the next century is going to be doing the same thing for our own minds. As scientists, we will learn to treat our mind not with the faculty of intuitive psychology that we apply every day—as a product of immaterial, inexplicable forces—but, as with the body, as composed of complex machinery that we can reverse-engineer. This prospect is exciting because it will be a realization of the age-old injunction: *Know thyself.*

Commentary on the Neuroscience Session

MICHAEL S. GAZZANIGA

David T. McLaughlin Distinguished Professor and Professor of Psychology, Dartmouth College, and Director, Center for Cognitive Neuroscience, Dartmouth College, Hanover, New Hampshire 03755, USA

JEFFREY J. HUTSLER

Visiting Research Assistant Professor of Psychology, Dartmouth College, Hanover, New Hampshire 03755, USA

> *What is not haphazard, but for the sake of something, is especially characteristic of the works of nature. And whatever has been composed for the sake of something ... has its share of beauty.*
>
> —ARISTOTLE, *Parts of Animals*

Aristotle's words neatly summarize our modern quest to understand the function of the brain and the mechanisms by which those functions are produced. Since this task is remarkably large, the field of neuroscience encompasses many diverse research efforts that each take a unique approach to this difficult reverse-engineering problem. The research focus of four eminent practitioners of modern neuroscience—Gerald Edelman, Pasko Rakic, Marcus Raichle, and Steven Pinker—clearly illustrates this diversity. Although the topics of neural Darwinism, developmental neurobiology, functional imaging, and evolutionary psychology are seemingly unconnected, they do contain many common threads. Surprisingly, these similarities are not restricted to superficial statements about the relationship between brain biology and the complex products of the human mind, but they are founded on fundamental historical debates that reach back through the development of neuroscience as a field and illuminate the paths we will take into the 21st century. These themes include the conflict between localization of function and neuronal holism, and the conflict between biological determinism and biological potentiality. These longstanding issues in neuroscience will continue to shape and push our studies of brain function.

FUNCTIONAL LOCALIZATION

The modern era of neuroscience began in the 1860s, almost a century after Dartmouth Medical School first opened its doors, with the reintroduction of cerebral localization into popular thinking by Pierre Paul Broca (1824–1880). Broca provided limited anatomical evidence that language functions could be disrupted by damage to the inferior lateral frontal lobes. Of interest, he was not the first to suggest that language was associated with the frontal lobes; rather, the true founder of cerebral localization, Franz Joseph Gall (1758–1828), had suggested the concept almost 60 years earlier. Gall's perspective on localization had fallen into disrepute owing to the tenuous nature of the mental faculties for which he proposed specific locations within the cortex. In addition, he believed that individuals with a strong propensity for one of these mental faculties would experience cortical growth that would push out the overlying bone, leaving a personality profile on the surface of the skull that could be read with the fingertips. Phrenology, the name applied to these theories by Gall's favorite student, now seems ridiculous, but at the time it was a major departure from the theories of brain function that had held sway for centuries before. Although Thomas Willis (1621–1675) had implicated the cerebral cortex in such important functions as memory and will in the 17th century, most individuals still held to earlier beliefs that the cortex was either glandular or vascular in its composition. In addition to focusing neuroscience on the cortex as the seat of mental faculties, Gall was a brilliant anatomist and was among the first to propose that the gray matter of the cortex was functioning neural tissue connected to the underlying white matter, and that this tissue is folded in order to conserve space.

History's hero in this drama is not Gall, however, but Pierre Flourens (1794–1867). Through a variety of experimental efforts, Flourens eventually triumphed over Gall by demonstrating that brain functions were distributed throughout the cerebral cortex. Although Flourens devoted significant effort to debunking phrenological claims, in deference to Gall's abilities as a neuroanatomist he once remarked that he had never truly seen the cerebral cortex until he observed Gall separating it from the underlying white matter and unfolding its convolutions. For decades after Flourens's victory, Bouillard, one of Gall's students, maintained that functions could be localized and supported his arguments with numerous clinical cases that demonstrated specific cognitive deficits after localized brain injuries. He was largely ignored, but Broca's announcements in the 1860s were made at the urgings of Bouillard and took their prominent place in the history of neuroscience, not because his declaration of localization was new, but because he was not considered a phrenological sympathizer. More importantly, the scientific community was once again open to considering cortical localization of function as a general principle, a concept that was delayed in history owing to the tremendous backlash following the demise of phrenology some five decades earlier.

The tension between localization of functions within the cortex and mass action has continued to propel the pendulum of this debate back and forth for the last century. Positive evidence about the existence of discrete centers of function came from electrophysiological studies, the neuron doctrine, specific neurological deficits following focal brain injury, and cytoarchitectonics. Evidence against localization of function was also significant and consisted of anecdotal cases that did not fit with localization conceptions, the long-defunct neural reticular theory, and lesion studies in animals, as well as Gestalt theories of biology, psychology, and holistic brain function.

Today, functional localization is again master, but with a wary eye to past mistakes. As Marcus Raichle clearly demonstrates, modern techniques of functional imaging offer an exciting window into the activity of the behaving brain and give us insight into the patterns that may be associated with complex cognitive tasks. But even in the face of this overwhelming technology, we are still confronted with some of the oldest and most fundamental questions surrounding localization of function. What do the areas of activity mean? Do the functional labels we apply to circumscribed regions of the cortex have any utility or validity? Certainly we are closer than Gall when he described more than 30 functional areas, including one for friendship and another for secretiveness, but how close are we? Finally, how localized are functions? In this modern age, few will deny that certain cortical locations are more involved with particular functions than others, but the independence of these cortical locations is still an issue of great controversy. We must guard against the temptation of equating increased activity of certain cortical regions with the task being studied, but we can no longer deny that circumscribed locations become more active depending on the nature of the task. In addition, we are only beginning to gain insight into how blood flow maps relate to the physiology of neuronal activation and how "silent" areas (regions that are equally active in the control and task conditions), and areas that show decreased activity during task performance, contribute to the final behavior.[1]

Raichle clearly underscores this ever-present push and pull between strict localization and functional holism: "We don't view [areas of activation] as instantiating an entire behavior, but rather as elements underlying the behavior itself. There are a finite number of processing elements that exist . . . and each of them contributes in some unique and probably fairly fundamental way to the expression of a behavior. The infinite complexity of that behavior is the way in which those elements combine."

NEURAL DARWINISM AND NEURAL SPECIFICATION

What are the forces that build this marvelously active structure inside of our heads? How are the impossible number of neural interconnections made? Both Edelman and Rakic provide fundamental insights into these questions, but they also reveal another debate in the field between what is genetically specified and what is epigenetic, or a product of activation and environment. This argument over genes is merely a modern-day reformulation of the age-old debate between biological determinism and biological potentiality. Edelman presents us with a view of the brain that is dynamic and not driven by a precise genetic blueprint with prespecified cortical connectivity, while Rakic convincingly demonstrates a highly ordered series of events that serve to construct the complexities of the cerebral cortex during development. These two perspectives are not at odds with one another, but merely underscore two very different aspects of a biological balancing act between what is directly coded in the genes and what arises from nongenetic events that are only loosely constrained by genetic instruction.

The idea that neurons may fight for connectional space is not new. Levi-Montalcini demonstrated in the late 1940s and early 1950s that trophic factors played a significant role in regulating the relationship between target size and the size of the innervating population in the peripheral nervous system.[2] This trophic substance came to be known as nerve growth factor and did not act ubiquitously throughout the central nervous system, but was found only in certain neuronal systems. Other growth factors have since been discovered, but we are still gathering information on chemical substances and their ability to guide and regulate connectivity within the central nervous system. Certainly these chemical substances are coded in the genome, but recent evidence indicates that activity can also play a remarkable role in the specification of neuronal connections. This concept owes much of its beginnings to Donald Hebb, who theorized that during learning, connections that were co-active would become strengthened, while those that were not would become weakened. A wealth of long-term potentiation evidence appears to substantiate this claim, and this same concept has been borrowed to explain the establishment and elimination of connections during development.

Wolf Singer and his colleagues have embarked upon another remarkable series of experiments that elegantly demonstrate that synchronous activation within the nervous system can not only establish connections, but may also be responsible for creating functional coherency out of very noisy cortical background activity. Their studies show that distant cortical neurons that are specialized to respond to particular aspects of a visual scene, such as movement in a particular direction or orientation, will actually synchronize their firing when these properties belong to the same object and will become asynchronous when they belong to different objects. In addition, this cortical synchronization may be directly related to the perceptual saliency of the stimulus, since without the electrophysiological synchronization the ability of a visual stimulus to drive behavior is greatly diminished.[3]

Like trophic interactions, the activity-mediated processes of making connections and regulating their strength are also competitive in nature. Unlike the expression and distribution of trophic substance, these processes are not directly regulated by genetics, except that a very general mechanism that will strengthen connections that are activated together and destroy those that are not may be encoded in the genome.

Darwin's own theory of natural selection almost met with an early demise in the early 1900s owing to important missing pieces: namely, why do species vary and how is this environmentally selected variability passed on to an organism's offspring? Darwinism was saved by the rediscovery of Mendelian genetics (a method of transmission) and the concept of mutation (the engine of genetic variability and change), an event that is now remembered as the "great synthesis." Today we are still struggling with these same issues. Following the synthesis, it was easy to attribute all evolutionary change to random point mutations in the genome; therefore, all change to the nervous system must be encoded within the genes. The DNA was likened to an enormous library filled with volume upon volume of instruction manuals for building a complex organism. Modern studies have shown that the DNA is actually a highly redundant set of instructions, so that our biological libraries are filled with multiple copies of the same book. Despite this repetition, there is still plenty of room for unique instruction, but modern genetics has forced us to come to grips with the fact that the immense complexity of the nervous system cannot possibly be contained within this genetic code. The same genes that hold a seemingly limitless amount of information are still too sparse to contain a precise wiring diagram of the connectional complexity that exists within our brains. Current thinking about what is encoded in the genome and what results from epigenetic factors is diverse. Some theorize that only a limited amount of information specifies the general structure of the brain and that simple instructions about the relative size of regions, coupled with competitive activity and synchronous discharges shape the precision of neural structures from a rudimentary genetic plan.[4] On the other extreme are the numerous specific chemical interactions that continue to be demonstrated for events such as cell migration and axonal guidance. Most modern day neurobiologists echo the sentiment expressed clearly by Pasko Rakic—that connections between brain regions are guided to their final location by molecular clues that are specified by the genetic code, while the final connections that are made both during development and in the mature organism are governed by constant competitive interactions and coincidental firing between neurons. Although extreme views in this debate are perhaps rare, the fight rages on over whether specific genetically encoded changes are at the root of our own unique cognitive abilities, or whether epigenetic factors that are the result of increased cortical proportions are responsible.

EVOLUTIONARY PSYCHOLOGY

Just as evolutionary biologists have argued about what is, and is not, controlled by genes, so evolutionary psychologists must now wrestle with fundamental questions about whether the neural substrates that produce behaviors are adaptive and selected by Darwinian processes. Steve Pinker describes an enticing conception of the mind as an adapted organ whose seemingly maladaptive products, such as romantic love, are actually explainable in the context of evolutionary theory.

Evolutionary psychology has come a long way in constructing explanations for specific behaviors, but controversy still abounds as to whether these behaviors are actually open to selection. The focus on behavior as a target for selection began in the 1970s with E.O. Wilson's publication of *Sociobiology*. In this remarkable volume, Wilson explains the adaptive nature of a number of complex animal behaviors exhibited in such diverse species as bees and primates. Most interesting perhaps is his clear explanation of the work of W.D. Hamilton[5] and J.B.S. Haldane in the realm of the long-standing debate over altruistic behavior. Altruism (an unselfish regard for the welfare of others) appears to be maladaptive on the surface, but in actuality may increase the genetic fitness of an individual by virtue of kin selection or reciprocal altruism. Kin selection postulates that you have a genetic advantage if you help two siblings, since they share approximately 50% of your own genetic makeup, while reciprocal altruism postulates that one may make a sacrifice to an unrelated organism in the hope of gaining help at a later time. Although behaviors such as altruism may be open to natural selection, to be selected they must be passed from generation to generation within the genes of an organism. Since alternative explanations are possible, if these behaviors are not encoded in the genes then natural selection may have no bearing. This does not negate the power of evolutionary explanations, but it forces us to proceed cautiously until evidence of a genetic basis can be obtained.[6] Social Darwinism, the passing on of cultural knowledge that is acquired during the life of an organism, may provide an alternative, nongenetic method of behavioral inheritance, but we are still mired in debate as to whether the fidelity of this process can be maintained over long enough stretches of evolutionary history to exert a lasting effect.[7]

CONCLUSION

Each of these areas of study, as well as the age-old questions they are trying to address, is fundamentally driven by Steve Pinker's closing statement: "Know thyself." This is, of course, not a new injunction but appears in the writings of Plato as *nosce te ipsum* and refers to one of three great maxims inscribed at the temple of Apollo at Delphi (circa 400 B.C.). Our desire to understand our own origins and our own consciousness propels us forward in our quest to answer questions such as "How did I get here?" "What forces made me?" and, most importantly, "How can I possibly be thinking these questions about my own existence?" From this perspective, neuroscience is no different from countless religious and philosophical endeavors that have been with us for centuries. The ability to understand, reason, and solve problems places us in a unique position in the animal kingdom, for only the human species can ever hope to comprehend the tremendous flexibility of its own mind by using the very device it is attempting to understand to solve the problem.

This paradoxical situation may be at the root of the problem's difficulty, but the collective theories of the neuroscientific community and the development of ever-increasingly sophisticated experimental techniques in neurobiology, functional imaging, and computational neuroscience lead us closer and closer to our final goal. It is a primary goal of neuroscience to understand the function of the brain, how the brain is self-constructed during development, and how this complex organ arises out of the seemingly simple processes of Darwinian evolution. Our goals do not, however, stop there. It is not enough to answer these questions, but we must also achieve the insight required to understand the human mind's unique ability to reverse-engineer itself.

REFERENCES

1. RAICHLE, M.E. 1988. Behind the scenes of functional brain imaging: A historical and physiological perspective. Proc. Natl. Acad. Sci. USA. **95:** 765–772.
2. PURVES, D. 1988. Body and Brain: A Trophic Theory of Neural Connections. Harvard University Press. Cambridge, MA.
3. SINGER, W. & C.M. GRAY. 1995. Visual feature integration and the temporal correlation hypothesis. Annu. Rev. Neurosci. **18:** 555–586.
4. HAMILTON, W.D. 1964. The genetical theory of social behavior. J. Theoret. Biol. **7:** 1–52.
5. DEACON, T.W. 1997. The Symbolic Species: The Co-Evolution of Language and the Brain. W.W. Norton. New York.
6. GOULD, S.J. 1977. Ever Since Darwin: Reflections in Natural History. W.W. Norton. New York.
7. SANDERSON, S.K. 1990. Social Evolutionism. Basil Blackwell, Inc. Cambridge.

ADDITIONAL READING

1. DEPEW, D.J. & B.H WEBER. 1995. Darwinism Evolving: System Dynamics and the Genealogy of Natural Selection. MIT Press. Cambridge, MA.
2. EDELMAN, G. 1987. Neural Darwinism: The Theory of Neuronal Group Selection. Basic Books. New York.
3. FINGER, S. 1994. Origins of Neuroscience: A History of Explorations into Brain Function. Oxford University Press. New York.

4. GROSS, C.G. 1998. Brain, Vision, Memory: Tales in the History of Neuroscience. MIT Press. Cambridge, MA.
5. PINKER, S. 1997. How the Mind Works. W.W. Norton. New York.
6. WILSON, E.O. 1975. Sociobiology. Harvard University Press. Cambridge, MA.

Health-Care Session:
The Issue—For Whom and by Whom?

Introduction to the Session

SUSAN DENTZER[a]

Economics Writer and Contributing Editor, U.S. News & World Report,
Washington, D.C., USA

As an alumna and trustee of Dartmouth College, a member of the Board of Overseers of Dartmouth Medical School, and also a journalist who covers health economics and policy issues, I am delighted to be here. Rarely do so many threads of my life come together in such a purposeful way. The title of this session is "Health Care: For Whom and by Whom?" That phrase encapsulates some of the most important economic, social, ethical, and moral questions our society faces.

One of the most special traditions at the Dartmouth Medical School is the annual recitation of the Hippocratic Oath, in its original ancient Greek, by language professor John Rassias. As I've listened to Professor Rassias speak in these mellifluous tones of Greek over the years, I've often thought about something else that has been handed down to us from ancient Greece: the myth of Prometheus.

If you remember your lessons in Greek mythology, the god Prometheus was one of the original "Elder Gods," or Titans, who eventually gave birth to the Olympian gods, including Zeus and his wife, Hera. Moreover, Prometheus was considered the savior of mankind. The name Prometheus means *forethought*; he also had a brother named Epimetheus, which means *afterthought*.

As the god of forethought, Prometheus was very wise, while his brother Epimetheus was scatterbrained. Mythology holds that to these two brothers was delegated the task of making humankind. Epimetheus took the lead. However, because he was so scatterbrained, he set about making the animals first, and to them he gave some of the most stellar skills and characteristics, such as strength to the elephant, swiftness to the cheetah, and courage to the lion. By the time he got around to human beings, nothing good was left over to give.

Epimetheus then turned to his brother to bail him out, presumably appointing him head of a 500-person Human Being Reform Task Force. Prometheus, in turn, set about finding ways of making humanity superior to animals. One of the things he did was go to the sun, where he lit a torch and brought fire back down to earth. Fire, after all, offered humanity the gift of sustaining life, since people could use it for everything from preparing food to defending themselves.

At the same time, though, fire was the classic double-edged sword, if you'll allow me to mix metaphors a bit. It was also the preeminent tool of war and destruction.

[a]Present address: Correspondent, *The News Hour with Jim Lehrer*, 2700 S. Quincy Street, Suite 240, Arlington, Virginia 22206.

Thus it was the essence of humanity's salvation and destruction wrapped up into one single thing.

At this point you are no doubt wondering about the connection between Prometheus and medical school graduation. Well, I'm reminded of Prometheus each June because the world of modern medicine endows these graduates with a power much like Prometheus's fire. Medicine is a tool that we use to make ourselves superior, to live longer than any of our ancestors ever would have dreamed. Yet at the same time, it also gets us into some very perplexing quandaries that may be our undoing.

For example, we have figured out how to spend more on health care than any civilized society might have imagined. We spend so much that we've had to invent a way to manage these expenditures—so we've created managed care, which has had troubling consequences familiar to us all. We've made astounding medical advances, as noted by Joseph Goldstein, from gene therapy to the PET scan, to name just two of medicine's most spectacular recent achievements. But then, recall the stories that Francis Collins trecounted of women faced with overwhelming decisions to make about genetic testing and its aftermath: Whether or not to have such tests in the first place and to potentially become imbued with the knowledge of the particulars of one's impending mortality; whether or not to chop off a breast or excise an ovary or take other extraordinary action in the hope of forestalling illness; whether or not to tell one's own children of their impending fate.

Our medical skills and knowledge are a Promethean tool indeed, and I often wonder whether the graduates have any idea of what they're getting into. Of course, the many stark choices and challenges that modern medicine and health care present to us go well beyond the ones I've mentioned. In this session, we will hear about many other of these choices and challenges in the form of two addresses and a subsequent panel discussion.

The first address is by Dr. C. Everett Koop, who will discuss the top ten issues in health care today. Then we will hear from Professor Philip Kitcher, the Presidential Professor of Philosophy at the University of California at San Diego and author, among other works, of *The Lives to Come: The Genetic Revolution and Human Possibilities.* He will discuss the stark choices that people will have to make owing to advances in genetic research and testing.

The Top Ten Issues in Health Care Today

C. EVERETT KOOP

Former U.S. Surgeon General and Elizabeth DeCamp McInerny Professor of Surgery, Dartmouth Medical School, Hanover, New Hampshire 03755, USA

I am pleased that I have been asked to share with you my thoughts on the top ten issues in health care *today,* rather than—because it's been well over half a century since I earned the right to put that treasured M.D. after my name—to be cast in the role of the old duffer taking a nostalgic look at the good old days of medicine. Although some of you younger folk may think of me as a contemporary of DMS founder Nathan Smith, I still find myself more at home in the immediate future than in the distant past.

And that is good, because the top ten issues in health care today and in our immediate future would have been almost unimaginable in the world of medicine that I first entered so many decades ago. Most of these issues carry compelling ethical questions.

The most vexing issue before the American health-care system at the end of the 20th century is the growth of market-based managed care, and the consequent influence of economic issues on medical issues. It was my privilege to enjoy a 40-year career as a pediatric surgeon at a time when it seemed not only that each day medicine had more to offer the American people, but also that each day more and more Americans gained health insurance, and most health-care providers got paid for whatever they did for their patients.

But then in the 1980s, health-care costs soared, driven up by a variety of factors, including expensive technology, malpractice expenses, physician fees, health-care–worker wages, an aging population, and increased patient demand. And the payer-provider pact came undone when the people who paid for most health care—insurance companies, businesses, and taxpayers—said, "Enough!" Suddenly, economic issues began to play a major role in health care, as more people—insurance clerks, business CEOs, company comptrollers, city treasurers, and a variety of bean-counters—in their combined efforts to hold down costs crowded into the doctor's office to intrude into a relationship that until then had been just between the patient and the physician. These economic issues led to the accelerated growth of market-based managed care at a rate unforeseen by either the supporters or opponents of managed care.

Originally, the impetus for *older* managed-care organizations came from physicians themselves, who wanted the freedom to provide medical care for their patients without the ever-present intrusion of the question of charge and payment for each visit to the doctor, for each test, for each procedure. Some of the first HMOs were truly interested in managing care, in maintaining health, in fostering prevention, in providing only necessary and effective medical intervention. Cost containment was an *unexpected* benefit, not the primary purpose of the health-care organization.

Now, however, too many managed-care companies seem to be interested first in managing costs and only secondarily in maintaining health. The more recently launched managed-care ventures are based upon the expressed rationale that competitive market forces will bring lower costs, higher efficiency, and better quality to health care. And the people behind these ventures tend to come from the world of business rather than from that of medicine.

Now, while I'm a believer in the free-market enterprise American economy, I have some real reservations about the ability of market forces *alone* to do what is best for the health of the American people. Americans, who have spent much of this century fighting the forces of totalitarian states, need to be on guard against the totalitarian forces of the *market*. The most disturbing impact of managed care on the doctor-patient relationship is the way in which managed care can create a financial incentive for the physician to *withhold* necessary medical care from a patient. This creates a very dangerous conflict of interest between the doctor and the patient and threatens to eradicate what little trust remains between patient and physician.

Now I am aware that there are problems in a fee-for-service system, too, with its financial temptation for the physician always to do more to the patient to make more money for the physician. No doubt about it, the abuse of fee-for-service medicine is one of the things fueling the rapid growth of managed care. But at least fee-for-service medicine always allowed the *responsible* physician to act as an advocate for the patient. In some managed-care settings, however, many physicians must choose between their livelihood and their patients.

We must arrest the trend—increasingly common not only in capitated managed care, but also in managed fee-for-service medicine—of taking medical decisions away from doctors and patients, and allowing them to be made by businessmen in insurance companies or in managed-care companies.

Managed care raises real questions: Will managed-care patients of the future find sensitive doctors at long last freed from the financial pressure to order more tests and procedures, freed from the need to practice defensive medicine, freed to do the best as they see it for their patients? Or will managed-care patients find themselves in long lines for short visits, confronting bureaucratic gatekeepers who shunt them to a small number of overworked doctors who see too many patients and who are paid extra to skimp on tests and operations?

Under many managed-care arrangements, the physician's chief obligation is not to her or his patient, but to return a profit to the stockholders in the managed-care company. This amounts to a real, and I hope very temporary, revolution in American health care. Managed care has not yet been sensitive to its obligations to foster clinical research and to offer financial support for the education of the doctors, nurses, and other health-care workers of tomorrow.

The second issue in health care today is the discord in the doctor-patient relationship. What doctors and patients tell me about each other is increasingly disturbing. Patients tell me that they don't trust doctors the way they did in the past, that they find doctors to be impersonal, aloof, difficult to understand, and overly busy. And doctors tell me that their patients are sullen or aggressive, always complaining about the cost of care—even of life-saving care, and that the shadow of litigation darkens every patient-physician encounter, making the doctor even afraid of the person she or he seeks to help. You can see the obvious connections between the issues I raise here, for the growth of managed care hasn't helped the doctor-patient relationship.

Two ways to improve the doctor-patient relationship are the third and fourth items on my list of top issues in health care today: the need to revitalize physician professionalism and then to promote a refined understanding of patients' rights and responsibilities.

As to physician professionalism, society affords certain privileges and compensation to professionals, but it expects something special in return. For example, members of a profession are expected to work not by the hour but until the work is done. But an increasing number of physicians, especially in managed-care organizations, work a shift and then go home. Members of a profession are expected to police themselves, but we must admit that medicine, along with some other professions, has too often coddled the bad apples instead of removing them. And members of a profession are expected to maintain a higher ethic, often confirmed by an oath. I imagine that very few Americans today would say that physicians embody an ethic *higher* than that of the society, as once was the case. The formerly proud and demanding Hippocratic Oath is abandoned or diluted by more and more medical schools each year. Members of a profession are also expected to give something back to society, to donate to those in need. The idea of donating services to society lingers in only a few settings, as most physicians expect to be compensated for every procedure or consultation. Indeed, free care is illegal under Medicare! Finally, and this is the real hallmark of a profession, its members are expected to place the interests of those they serve, be they patients, clients, or students, above their own interests. Managed care will either bury this hallowed hallmark of the medical profession, or this commitment to professionalism will correct many of the problems of managed care.

And along with a refurbished commitment to medical professionalism, a revitalized patient rights movement can force the best from the American health-care system. Patients need to know not only their rights, but also their obligations, especially in this age of shared clinical decision-making. That means the patient must be more informed than ever, informed accurately, and informed sufficiently, but not overwhelmed with information.

This brings me to the fifth issue to be addressed in American health care today, and that is the dramatic explosion in the electronic availability of medical information on the Internet. The Internet will eventually replace journals and conferences in Boca Raton as the place where physicians meet to exchange information, and it will also be the place where patients turn to get most of their health information. But this opens really tough questions about accuracy of information, about privacy, and about confidentiality—questions we are a long way from answering satisfactorily.

Much of the information sought by and available to patients is in the realm of what has usually been called alternative medicine or, as it is also called, complementary medicine. Does the difference between those terms, alternative and complementary, capture both the strengths and the weaknesses, both the appeal and the danger, of this movement? At any rate, this is the sixth issue I shall mention: "Regular" medicine must do a much better job in coming to terms with the appeal of alternative medicine and must come to grips with the reality that one in three Americans involve themselves in at least one form of unconventional therapy. But more than 70% of those people do not inform their physician about their use of alternative or complementary medicine.

Seventh, we need an attitude of both welcome and wariness to greet the increasing number of new biomedical products that reach the market every day. While being leery of the work of quacks and the appeal of fads, we will make great strides as we put to use new vaccines and a host of other products on the horizon such as blood substitutes, called hemoglobin-based oxygen carriers or HBOCs, which will dramatically increase oxygenation rates in tissues and which should significantly improve surgical outcomes, as well as what we are used to experiencing in myocardial infarcts, stroke, and cancer. Similarly, some new drugs may greatly assist Americans in what I hope will be a major campaign to help smokers quit smoking. The final outcome of the tobacco settlement remains in doubt, and while I certainly stand with those who want to keep cigarettes out of the hands—and mouths—of children, I am equally concerned about helping those who *now* smoke in their effort to quit. The effort to encourage kids to say no to cigarettes will keep many from smoking, but I know kids well enough to know that for some just the attempt to discourage them from smoking makes them all the more determined to smoke. However, we know that most smokers—nicotine addicts—truly want to quit, and we have a medical and an ethical duty to do more for these would-be quitters than we have been doing. Quitting smoking prolongs life. We have 50 million nicotine addicts in the U.S. today. At least one-third of them will die prematurely, and poorly, a smoker's death.

Which leads me to the eighth issue, a result of American medicine's dramatic ability to prolong life, and that is the growth in the number of Americans living longer, but with chronic medical conditions. To deal with these folks, American medicine and American society need not only improved skills and therapies, but also an improved attitude to enable this quick-fix culture to deal compassionately and effectively with the long-term problems of the chronically ill and their families.

This topic leads some people to my ninth issue, physician-assisted suicide, which the Supreme Court has now bumped back to the states, where the debate will continue. Although the issues may be heart-wrenching at times, as a physician who took the Hippocratic Oath, I stand against the legalization of physician-assisted suicide. And as an American citizen concerned about the presence of racial prejudice in our society and concerned about new economic incentives for physicians *not* to treat the chronically ill, I fear the impact of physician-assisted suicide on the already-weakened fabric of our society.

To close, I will return to the issue of managed care, which I identified as the chief problem to be addressed in American health care today. I will conclude by saying that in some ways we are on the path to solutions. The growing concern about the problems of managed care are already provoking the historic American pattern of a reemergence of regulation to curb the excesses of the market. The latest genre of pulp fiction, the "HMO horror story," has already produced new laws in a variety of state legislatures, forcing HMOs to increasingly do what patients demand. As we see more and more regulatory restrictions on managed care, HMOs may lose the financial edge that has led to their explosive growth, and we may see a new equilibrium among the health-care players, with patients and doctors regaining what they have lost to business interests. We need a health-care system that delivers to the patient what is medically necessary, not what is profitable—neither the excess of fee-for-service nor the deprivation of managed care. I think we may see a renewed and informed sense of what is medically necessary and appropriate, what is right and fair, and what is in the best interest of the patient, begin to prevail over what is in the best interest of the health-care company's investors. The issues of managed care, of patient rights, of physician professionalism, of health care in America, need their discussion to be lifted from the economic bottom line to the ethical plumb line, to make the best of our economics subject to the best of our ethics. If we do not do this, we may see the worst of health-care economics begin to shape the rest of our society. Indeed, this may already be happening.

I recently heard of a managed-care–company president who was given a ticket for a performance of Schubert's "Unfinished Symphony." Since he was unable to go, he passed along the ticket to one of his managed-care reviewers. The next morning, when the president asked how the symphony had been, the managed-care reviewer, instead of just saying a few words, handed his boss an official utilization review memorandum. It read as follows:

1. For a considerable period, the oboe players had nothing to do. Their numbers should be reduced and their work spread over the entire orchestra, thus avoiding peaks of inactivity.

2. All 12 violins were playing identical notes. This seems unnecessary duplication, and the staff of this section should be drastically cut. If a large volume of sound is really required, an amplifier could be used instead.

3. Much effort was involved in playing 16th notes. This seems excessive refinement, and if all notes were rounded up to the nearest eighth note, it would be possible to employ paraprofessionals instead of more expensive professional musicians.

4. No useful purpose is served by repeating with the horns a passage already played by the strings. If all such redundant passages were eliminated, the concert could be reduced from two hours to 20 minutes.

5. This symphony had two movements. If Schubert hadn't achieved his musical objectives by the end of the first movement, then he should have stopped there. The second movement is unnecessary and should be cut.

In light of the above, it is obvious that if Schubert had given attention to these matters, he probably would have had time to finish the symphony!

Patients in the 21st Century:
The Impact of Predictive Medicine

PHILIP KITCHER[a]

Presidential Professor of Philosophy, University of California at San Diego, LaJolla, California 92093-0302, USA

I want to look a little bit further into the future than Dr. Koop did; I want to speculate a bit more. It is the business of philosophy not so much to deal in fact or factoids, as to think about issues of principle. And, as David Botstein reminded us, that is quite an important thing in medical education today. At any rate, I will try to offer you a way of thinking about the challenges that are likely to arise in the next few decades.

I want to start where many of the presenters in the genetics session left off, with the predicament that we now face because of the explosion of knowledge already happening through the Human Genome Project. In the next few years, lots of gene sequences are going to be known and correlated with various aspects of the human phenotype, which, as Francis Collins noted, is not a trivial matter. Some of these associations will likely not be straightforwardly deterministic and statistical in character, and in some cases, because of a large number of mutable sites in the gene, there will be many ways in which the phenotype varies in response. We will get a lot of information about how human gene sequences correlate with conditions that affect all of us—like diseases, and body build, and even our tendencies toward certain kinds of behavior.

The great hope, of course, is that all this molecular knowledge will translate fairly quickly into ways of treating persons who currently suffer from terrible diseases and disabilities. But the route from gene sequence to treatment is long and uncertain. As David Botstein noted, the genetic code leads you immediately from the gene sequence to the sequence of amino acids in the protein that's coded for by the gene. But that in itself does not tell you much. There is no general way of going from that information even to something as straightforward, or apparently straightforward, as the three-dimensional form of the protein or to ideas about the function of the protein. Nor is there a straightforward road from that knowledge to understanding the causation of a disease condition or what makes the difference between somebody who has a genetic defect and somebody who has the normal genetic condition.

And so this road is fraught with all kinds of uncertainties. It *will* be traveled, in some cases quickly and in other cases much more slowly, with a combination of insight and guesswork—largely aided by comparisons with nonhuman animals. It is important again to stress the role that model organisms will play in the advance of our medical understanding. Meanwhile, much more quickly, within a decade or so, we will have the ability to *test* for a very large number of genetic conditions, even as the interventions, treatments, and cures will arrive more slowly.

[a]Present address: Professor of Philosophy, Columbia University, New York, New York 10027.

I would like to give you a scorecard of where we are, because the recent past may indicate the shape of things to come. Let us look at some diseases whose molecular bases are understood, starting off with one that has been known for about 40 years—sickle cell anemia. When the molecular basis of sickle cell anemia was first discovered, there was much optimism that this would translate very quickly into progress in treating the disease. Well, the truth of the matter is: that hasn't happened. On the other hand, there is a great success story, perhaps as good a success story as comes out of the genetic understanding of disease, in phenylketonuria, or PKU. All children in this country are now routinely tested at birth for PKU, and their lives, if they have the condition, can be salvaged and brought back to relative normalcy through dietary adjustment. These two cases represent the poles of where molecular understanding can take us: not very far in one case and in the other case to a relatively simple way of preventing a dreadful disease.

Now let's look at some more recent cases in which gene sequences have become known through the Human Genome Project. Until very recently, molecular knowledge of Huntington's disease would have translated into very little that could be done. Now, however, there is some hope that there will be therapies capable of dissolving the clumps that form within the cell's nucleus. In the case of cystic fibrosis, molecular understanding has already aided in some progress. But in the case of breast cancer, it was hoped that an understanding of its genetic details might lead to a fairly rapid treatment breakthrough, but it is not obvious, as Francis Collins has noted, that in this case the information is of very much use or that monitoring procedures will be effective. On the other hand, for the various forms of genetically based colon cancer, there is hope that monitoring programs can be introduced that will spare people from acquiring forms of cancer from which they otherwise would have suffered and died.

So the picture is very mixed—and I believe that the future will be mixed as well. To make an analogy I like to use, it's like being offered a lot of free lottery tickets. You'd be very unlucky if some of them didn't turn up winners; in fact, you'd be quite unlucky if none of them won you a jackpot. But you can't predict in advance which of the lottery tickets are going to win. The situation with the genetic understanding of disease seems to me to be rather like that. There will be many more cases of sickle cell anemia in our future, and there will probably be some more cases of PKU in our future, but there will be many mixed cases in which we will make partial progress.

In the meantime, what can we do with our immediate ability to test people for genetic conditions, conditions that predispose them to disease? There are some things that are often overlooked, including, of course, that genetic testing immediately gives us certain kinds of advantages. It refines existing diagnostic tests, enabling us to make faster and more accurate diagnoses; it enables doctors to "disambiguate" symptoms in some cases—to recognize differences between one patient and another patient; and it enables them to see what kinds of medicines would be appropriate for a given patient, tailored to his or her particular condition. But the exciting forms of genetic testing are, of course, the *predictive* ones, and these occur in three contexts: (1) early in life, while people are still asymptomatic; (2) before birth, while the fetus is in the uterus; and (3) even before conception. We can use genetic information to predict, in advance, the qualities of people already born, not yet born, and, in some cases, potential people, who haven't even been conceived yet.

In some of these cases, there are medical benefits—avoidance or lessening of future suffering. We are able to give advice about how to live so as to avoid disease, or at least to reduce risk for disease.

And in all cases, you might think there would be a nonmedical benefit. If you give people information about what they are at high risk for, at least they will have an increased ability to plan their lives. As Nancy Wexler's poignant testimony from patients who know they will get Huntington's disease brings home to us, the knowledge of your fate is not always liberating. For some people such knowledge helps them to put their life in order, while for others the news is crushing. This dilemma is well conveyed in the statistics about Huntington's disease testing: Before the test was available, roughly 70% to 75% of the people who were at risk thought they would want to know. But since the test has become available, only between 17% and 20% of at-risk people actually want to take it.

So if genetic testing is really going to help, it will be very important to insure that those who can get this knowledge are not crushed by it, and that there is adequate counseling and support for them. Francis Collins alluded to the sad truth about the paucity of genetic counselors in this country. Statistics show that if a successful counseling session is one in which doctors think that they have conveyed the information and patients or clients think that they have received it, then 96% of sessions are unsuccessful. One or the other party does not think that he or she has either given or received the appropriate information.

But the biggest difficulties that stem from the explosion of this information were alluded to by Francis Collins. They are issues about what happens to people in a society in which information about their risks and about their conditions flows freely. Here, I would like to talk about three kinds of dilemmas we as a society are going to face in the coming decades. While it would be unconscionably arrogant to give concrete solutions, I would suggest that these dilemmas have to be faced— and faced by thinking about *principles*. These questions are going to require some fairly radical rethinking about features of the medical-social contract.

Here's the first dilemma: As the ability increases for a person to learn about his or her genetic risks—as a woman can now find out, for example, whether she carries one of the mutant breast cancer alleles—other parties in society are interested in that information as well: employers and insurers, for example. As a society our first response to this situation is to declare it none of the employer's or insurer's business. But there is a very simple counter-response: The business of insurance—of medical insurance, as of any other form of insurance—is to correlate the premiums that people pay with their risks. That's what insurance is all about. Underwriters will immediately point out that if you allow people to have information about their risks, information that the underwriters and insurance companies do not have, then the market is in trouble; it will be threatened with collapse because of the phenomenon of adverse selection, of people who are at high risk wanting to buy insurance but seeming indistinguishable from those at low risk.

What to do about this situation? Well, I suggest that we think ourselves back into one of those classic philosophical fictions, the social contract. Often a very good way to be clear about what is fair and just in a society is to think about how you might choose social arrangements if you didn't know what *your* risks were or what the potential threats were to *your* well-being. If you were ignorant of what position you might occupy in a society, how would you choose for the society to be set up? This is a famous device that in recent years has been made extremely clear by the philosopher John Rawls in his conception of the so-called *original position*.

I'm going to offer you a couple of choices in thinking about phenomena associated with medicine. Let's begin with this one. You have to choose a system of medical care that will bind you and your descendants. Your descendants will divide into two groups: (1) the genetically normal (and I'm going to be conservative in saying that 95% of you and your descendants will be genetically normal; other people would put it at only 90%); and (2) the "untouchables" (and I use that loaded term quite deliberately). Five percent of the population, then, will be genetically untouchable: if information about them were given to insurance companies, either they could not buy insurance or they could only buy it at prohibitive cost. This situation already obtains in our society. At present, women who have been diagnosed as carrying the mutant breast cancer allele and parents of children with cystic fibrosis are finding out just how difficult it can be to deal with an insurance company.

Now I will give you two options. Option A is a system very like the one we have: insurance is based on risk, and we can assume that if you are normal, you will have to pay roughly 5% of your net income for your insurance premiums. But if you are untouchable, the figure will be much higher, perhaps even unaffordable, but I will set it at 50%. Option B ups the ante for everybody by spreading out the cost—6% for everyone. Now you don't know—the veil has not yet been lifted—whether you are genetically normal or whether you're untouchable; and you don't know the characteristics of your descendants, who will be bound by this scheme. Which of the schemes do you want to choose? Do you want a system in which you take the risk, and if things turn out all right, you get an economic saving? Or do you want to take the other option and pay somewhat higher premiums to insure coverage for all?

Now, this philosophical device is only a device—it's only intended to bring home to you a certain obvious unfairness that was there before the Genome Project gave us the opportunity to disclose it. We have different propensities, different risks, in our population. It is not our fault if we are at high risk for a genetic disease. So I hope that this exercise in choice may highlight the fundamental moral point that it is unfair to penalize people for genetic conditions and risks that they don't bring upon themselves. And if that is the case, then I invite you, when you think about universal health-care coverage, to consider it not something to be achieved piecemeal, in a patchwork way, which will still bear lingering traces of differentiation according to various kinds of unfairly distributed genetic risks, but rather as an entitlement for all. This is an arena in which conclusions we might have reached by appealing to principles of justice or to compassion can be buttressed by considerations of prudence, drawn from the explosion of knowledge and the birth of predictive medicine.

Let us now consider a second dilemma and a second choice—one that concerns the way in which medical spending is distributed over people's lives. We probably have a vague impression that in the United States quite a lot of money is spent at the end of a person's life, perhaps in the last few months. Now, if the Human Genome Project yields its fruits of great genetic knowledge, then we may have the opportunity to invest funds very early in people's lives and thereby prevent a great deal of suffering.

Let's look at the current situation. It is difficult to obtain statistics on this, but the Harvard medical economist David Cutler has assembled some data about average medical spending by age for the years 1970 and 1987. The principal difference between the two years is that in 1987 there was a much bigger expenditure both early and late in life; and those figures are continuing to increase. What will happen now that we are beginning to be able to intervene more early in life?

Let us reframe some of Cutler's data. A baby born in the late 1980s had roughly a 0.8 chance of surviving to age 65, and health-care spending over the lifetime of that baby would be $281,000, of which $189,000 would be spent after age 65. So, if you do the arithmetic, for a late-1980s or an early-1990s newborn, roughly 67% of the funds would be spent after age 65. Now if we get very lucky with our understanding of genetic diseases and preconditions, we could start investing in programs for diagnosing people for the risks they carry and try to do something about those risks early in their lives. In the future we might get from our pharmacist or doctor that famous CD inscribed with our genotype—and it might be as cheap as the testing itself is likely to become. But the therapies, the interventions, are probably going to be much more expensive.

So this is a second question about the medical–social contract that we have to think about. This time, I will ask you to think about choosing a schedule of medical spending over your lives. What would you want if now you did not know what your risks were in advance but you could choose either to invest in preventive medicine or in reactive medicine? Again, remember that you have to choose a schedule of medical spending that will bind you and your descendants. Now, your descendants will divide into three types: (1) those whose lives can be dramatically improved, like the children with PKU, by early predictive testing; (2) those whose lives can be somewhat improved by early predictive testing, perhaps like those suffering from various genetic forms of colon cancer; and (3) those whose lives will be pretty much unaffected, the lucky ones among us. Let me somewhat arbitrarily—these are squishy figures—divide these types up and say that 5% of the population would have a dramatic improvement, 70% would have a modest improvement, and 25% would be unaffected. Again I am going to offer you two options: One option says the doctor always has a duty to do whatever can be done to rescue the patient; we're going to keep going with reactive medicine. The other option says that these sums of money we're spending late in patients' lives would be better spent by investing early in prediction and prevention. So we will transfer some funds from the late decades to the early decades; instead of allotting $189,000 for people after they reach age 65, we'll only allot $65,000 for that period and we will invest early in prediction and prevention.

When you are thinking about this, you have to ask yourself what you would lose. And the answer is that if this were a rationally pursued policy, the treatments that would be abandoned for the elderly would be those that are the truly heroic ones—the ones that have the least probability of success. So under Option B, if the probability that you will be restored to something like healthy, vigorous, normal functioning fell below a threshold value, probably a very low threshold value, then you would no longer have that treatment available to you. So which of these options do you choose? Once again, the choice is going to be a difficult one, but focusing in this way forces us to think systematically and rationally about what kinds of lives we want to lead, and what kinds of lives we want those around us to lead. Do we want medicine to be available subject to market forces? Or do we want something more rationally designed, something that will allow us to exploit the resources of predictive medicine?

Finally, if you think that the choices I have already offered you are hard and controversial, the last dilemma presents an even harder and even more controversial question. Let us consider the last kind of predictive testing, the kind that takes place before people are born—what I will call extreme prevention. At some point in the foreseeable future of medicine, some conditions will be able to be diagnosed prenatally, but not ameliorated after a child is born by any means that we know. Extreme prevention consists of not bringing into the world infants with those conditions. For those of you who think that terminating pregnancies through abortion is *always* wrong, there will be a very immediate answer to this question. I'm not with you; I think that there are benign current examples that are being practiced in this country and around the world of extreme prevention. There are such diseases as Lesch-Nyhan syndrome, a terrible condition in which boys suffer acute mental retardation and gnaw their lips and finger tips, and Tay-Sachs disease. These are genetic disorders we don't know how to deal with once the child has been born. Our only compassionate way of coping with them is to do what is now being done: prenatal testing and selective termination of pregnancies. The incidence of Tay-Sachs disease worldwide has been reduced by orders of magnitude as a result of this, sparing many people and many families terrible suffering in recent decades. But besides the benign examples, there are also some very disturbing ones: prenatal testing is used in some parts of the world for sex-selection. In northern India and in China, women undergo amniocentesis not to find out whether or not their child has Down's syndrome or some other prenatally detectable disease, but because they want to know the sex. And if it's a girl, they want to terminate the pregnancy.

Lest we think that this couldn't happen here, we have to realize that the tremendous explosion of genetic information that will be available in the next few years will reveal all kinds of conditions and predispositions. And you might say, "Well, let's just let people use whatever tests they want; if they want to find out if their child is a girl, or is brown-haired, or has a 30% chance of being gay, or has a tendency to obesity, or may have attention deficit disorder, or may have some allele that's correlated with low intelligence—let them do it." And there's a rationale for that. It's this: We ought to do the very best we can for our children. And if we can do nothing for them after we bring them into the world, then let's make sure that we bring into the world children who are going to have a decent chance in society. I'm sure the women in northern India aren't moral monsters; I'm sure they say to themselves, "Look, our society is one dominated by prejudice against women. Do I want to see my daughter abused, malnourished, abandoned, with very little chance for a promising future? No! Better to terminate this pregnancy and have a son later." And the same sorts of things can happen anywhere, as a result of an intention to do the best one can for one's kids.

When faced with this argument, there are two responses: One is that this is just a hideous perversion; if this is where the unfolding of genetic knowledge is going to lead, then we ought to want absolutely none of it. If it's going to lead to people trying to design perfect babies, or at least trying to select *against* certain kinds of babies that they *don't* want, that's a terrible thing—it's a rat race that's begun in the womb, and we should have nothing to do with it. The other response is to say this is simply, as the argument suggests, an extension of things we already do. We already try to do the best for our children. Those of us who come from middle-class, professional households already try to give our children all kinds of advantages. What's the difference in taking that one further step back and making sure that we have a child who's got a good chance of a happy and healthy life in our society? I want to suggest there is something right about both these responses. They point to a background condition that is perhaps especially dramatic in the context of Indian society and Chinese society, but that is equally present in our own.

I want to conclude by suggesting that our thinking about these social issues has to be quite systematic and quite radical. If you look into the future, you can imagine a world in which people can be tested for all sorts of things: Tay-Sachs disease, cystic fibrosis, a predisposition for obesity, and perhaps even an allele that affects sexual orientation. (Dean Hamer, by the way, has not, to the best of my knowledge, yet discovered a gene for homosexuality—he's discovered a marker, and of course the concordance rate for homosexual preference in monozygotic twins is only 50%, so genetics is not the whole story by any means. Nonetheless, it's easy to imagine a world in which a test is advertised that "can find out whether your child has a significantly enhanced probability of being gay.") The same obtains for intelligence, though there's surely vastly more to intelligence than some simple genetic determination. Nonetheless, there may well be, in the next decade, correlations between specific places on the genome and children's intelligence. If we live in a society that rewards people very differently—that has very different attitudes towards the bearers of particular phenotypes, which depend on particular underlying genotypes—then there is going to be constant pressure to extend the cases in which we terminate pregnancy, from the very clearly benign and compassionate cases toward the other end of the spectrum. A society that is strongly competitive, strongly individualistic, strongly inegalitarian, and strongly dominated by prejudices is also going to be a society in which parents of the future are constantly facing the pressure to produce only those children who best accord with societal standards.

If, on the other hand, the picture were different, if the expected quality of life for individuals with many different genotypes was approximately equal, if we lived in a world in which children who did not score particularly well on IQ tests could live happy and flourishing lives, if we were prepared to provide serious social services to, say, children with cystic fibrosis, and accommodate their stays in the hospital, then we'd be free from this dilemma.

Finally, let me state the obvious: that the Genome Project did not create these social problems for us. The Human Genome Project is a wonderful explosion of information, full of promise. However, it is being thrust into a society that is marked by profound inequalities and that therefore has the potential to exacerbate those inequalities. The Project is a lightning rod—something that exposes to us background social issues that Americans have wanted to shy away from.

If we are to make the proper use of this medical technology in the coming century, we need to do some serious rethinking about the kinds of opportunities we owe to one another. As James Freedman said at this symposium, in a society that is officially devoted to the ideal of equality of opportunity, we cannot remain content with a situation in which, for example, African-Americans, who have proved that they can succeed in law schools and medical schools (the statistics are there), are in two very populous states of the union no longer attending professional schools in high numbers. There are those who think that we can just muddle on and find pragmatic and political solutions. But I think we also need to stand back and take a more abstract look, a look from a philosophical perspective, and think about the principles that ought to guide our choices. In this somewhat Cassandra-like speech—I apologize for not giving answers—that is what I've tried to do: Not offer you facts, but try to make some of the dilemmas of the future as stark and as sharp as possible and suggest to you some ways of thinking about them.

Questions and Answers

SUSAN DENTZER,[a] *Moderator*
Economics Writer and Contributing Editor, U.S. News & World Report

C. EVERETT KOOP
Former U.S. Surgeon General, and Elizabeth DeCamp McInerny Professor of Surgery, Dartmouth Medical School

PHILIP KITCHER[b]
Presidential Professor of Philosophy, University of California, San Diego

SUSAN DENTZER: Let me turn first to a question for Dr. Koop—a question that goes to the first issue mentioned on his list, that of managed care. The questioner writes: "It is easy, and indeed fashionable, to use managed care as a whipping boy, just as it has been to characterize physicians as motivated primarily by money and the quest for a cushy lifestyle. Shouldn't we be trying to understand the real problems in the health-care system that have promoted the rise of expectations that patients and payers should be getting the right care at the right time at the right price?" And, the questioner goes on to comment, "It is too easy to polarize by using a broad brush to denounce either extreme, and that does little to arrive at meaningful solutions."

C. EVERETT KOOP: The simple answer to the question is *yes*, but it takes a long time to go into all of the intricacies that would lead to a philosophical kind of answer. One of the things that is left out of the vocabulary of those of us who talk about these situations—and I myself left it out of my presentation—is the word "appropriate." The more I look at health-care delivery—the more I look at the plight of human beings—the more I realize that most of our criticism could be directed at the *inappropriate* solutions that seem to be more politically popular, more financially popular, but don't have the perspective of the life of the individual as well as the life of society.

DENTZER: Here's a question for Philip Kitcher. This harkens back to your example of the choices that we might face in an insurance system where genetic "untouchables" would pay 50% of net income as the premium versus a cost of 5% for the rest of society, a cost that would increase to 6% if we moved to a general system where everyone bore the cost. This questioner asks, "What if the increase in insurance that came about by spreading it across the entire group was not just 6%, as in your exam-

---

[a]Present address: Correspondent, *The News Hour with Jim Lehrer*, 2700 S. Quincy Street, Suite 240, Arlington, Virginia 22206.
[b]Present address: Department of Philosophy, Columbia University, New York, New York 10027.

ple, but more like 20% of income? Isn't it impossible to project what the real figures might be, and therefore very difficult to make this kind of calculation?"

KITCHER: I agree that the calculation is difficult to make, but think about it in this way. The increase would be very small if it's assumed that the class of people requiring large sums of money invested in them—the genetic untouchables—is rather small. If you think that the increase is going to be large, it is because you tend to think that the class of such people is going to be large. If the classs were large, the dilemma would be even sharper, because there would be, for each of us, a much more significant chance that either we or our descendants would be the ones deprived of health care. In the end, I'd bite the bullet and say that health is something that is central to the planning and functioning in all our lives—and the fact that we are not responsible for our genetic constitution demands that as a society we have the obligation to spread risks over all. That is the fair and just solution, and the device, the offer of two options, is just a way of getting people to appreciate that.

DENTZER: Dr. Koop, also on your list was the issue of improving professionalism among physicians. What sorts of things, specifically, would you recommend that physicians and other health professionals do to arrest this modern decline in professionalism?

KOOP: I gave five hints to physicians about how they might do that, and I would stand by those. Medicine has lost control of its own profession, which affects the most important part of the physician-patient relationship. I don't know of any other profession where this has happened. I was helpful to the Clintons when they were trying to get the President's health-care reform package through Congress; at one point I was acting as a sort of courier between the White House and Senator Mitchell's caucus, which was trying to hammer out something that could be voted on in Congress. And it struck me one day that I was in a room with 40 people who were deciding the future of a really noble profession, and not a single one of the 40 represented the profession. You couldn't do that to plumbers, you couldn't do it to lawyers, you couldn't do it to paperhangers, but we *have* done it to physicians. So, first, we need to regain control of our profession and the pride that used to go with it, and that entails all those other items that I mentioned.

DENTZER: Professor Kitcher, here's one for you. "Does a person with a self-recognized, treatable, genetically based medical condition, who is covered by a group health insurance plan, have a responsibility to seek treatment for his or her condition in order to reduce the total health cost for the group to which he or she belongs?"

KITCHER: Tricky question. Yes, with rights come responsibilities, and if you're going to develop a situation in which people are given adequate support by society for coping with the problems that come out of their bad luck in the genetic lottery, then one should expect them to try to go along with the program. This, of course, makes for some poignant and difficult cases. I portrayed the PKU case as if it were an unqualified success, but the sad reality is that it hasn't always been an *unqualified* success. First, it is difficult to know how long the PKU diet ought to be administered. Second, there is the economic *cost* of the diet, which in the early days typically had to be borne by the families. Third is the sheer difficulty for teenaged kids to stay on this awful, bland mush at a time when their social life revolves around pizza and Big Macs.

DENTZER: Dr. Koop, you also mentioned the responsibilities of patients—do you want to add something about what you believe the responsibilities of patients to be?

KOOP: I agree that there are responsibilities for patients, which I will illustrate with a personal story. When I was told, many years ago in Philadelphia, before I was Surgeon General, that I would have to have a knee replaced, I also learned that if I lost some weight the symptoms would remit. So I felt I had an obligation to society to lose the weight. I *did* lose the weight, I *did* lose the symptoms, and I postponed my surgery for seven years. I eventually had a very successful knee-replacement, though. I tried to be responsible, but in the long run I spent just as much money and I wish I had spent it earlier.

DENTZER: Professor Kitcher, this questioner relates a sad story about a mother who is 33 years old, who carried her first child to full term and delivered a baby with severe Down's syndrome. Her obstetrician had not thought that at her age she needed amniocentesis, and therefore presumably advised her not to get one. This was the woman's first pregnancy. What are the philosophical and ethical issues raised by an example such as that, particularly since it's quite possible that the woman might have been in a manged-care setting, where amniocentesis would not be encouraged for a woman below the age of 35?

KITCHER: Actually, 35 is simply the point at which the probability curve is steepest. The probability of having a Down's syndrome child goes up in an S-shaped curve, and 35 seems to be the point roughly in the middle. So there's nothing magic about that age. I hope that with the advent of genetic testing, amniocentesis and testing for Down's syndrome will be available to all women who want it, irrespective of their age. But there is an aspect of this case that does present a difficult philosophical dilemma. It relates to something Francis Collins noted earlier. When he was talking about the differences in mutations at various places in the genome, he pointed out how variable the phenotypic effect can be. And with Down's syndrome, we know that's very true. We know that there are very successful persons with Down's syndrome, persons who under greatly improved regimens of support and treatment have managed to do things that used to be thought impossible for those with Down's syndrome: Christopher Nolan wrote a novel, for example, and there have been a number of artists with Down's syndrome. And yet, one doesn't know in advance whether the Down's syndrome will be very severe or whether it will be of the kind that can be supported and translated into really quite a meaningful life. One of the responsibilities of introducing genetic testing generally, and of improving genetic testing for Down's syndrome in particular, will be to give parents a clear view of the range of possibilities and how likely they are to occur.

DENTZER: Dr. Koop, would you briefly address the manner in which traditional and complementary medicine might be integrated.

KOOP: First we have to acquaint allopathic and osteopathic physicians with the broad spectrum of remedies in what we refer to as alternative or complementary medicine. It does not make good sense for regular doctors to be treating patients, if 70% of patients will not share information with them because the doctors are not familiar enough with what they regard as an an alien field to be able to ask questions that will elicit productive answers from their patients. We are not at the beginning of alternative medicine; if you go back to a hundred years ago, we went through the same thing after the Civil War, when alternative medical cults sprang up and for-profit, fly-by-night medical schools offered diplomas, and yet we sorted it out. Today, we are in a much better position to make sense of it because we can subject any alternative or complementary medical treatment to the scientific method and separate the wheat from the chaff—that is the obligation of regular medicine if we feel threatened by alternative medicine. Even in a medical school like this one, there are many well-known therapies that might be called folk remedies, which good physicians use for their patients. The secret of being a healing physician is to use everything available in a particular patient's personality that you can call upon to help in the healing process. Whether it is herbology, prayer, faith, or whatever, good physicians always use it. Until we separate the scientific wheat from the chaff, American medicine should adopt an attitude of kind of practical accommodation toward alternative medicine.

DENTZER: Professor Kitcher, you mentioned that it is immoral to penalize those with genetic defects. But in this age of increased knowledge and access to health information, this questioner writes, "Is it moral *not* to penalize those who appear to choose to increase their health risks (for example, by smoking) and end up costing far beyond their input into the system?" In other words, should we hold those who engage in risky behavior accountable for the financial cost of that behavior?

KITCHER: If you're convinced that the putative destructive behavior is indeed the result of somebody's free decision, and that there is no underlying reason forcing, as it were, the person into the behavior, then accountability is fine. But very often there is serious doubt about this, and I wouldn't want to say that a person should be held accountable unless I were really sure that the decision was a free one.

DENTZER: And in some cases that can be quite confusing, as, for example, when persons with a psychiatric diagnosis abuse alcohol. How do you decide to what extent these illnesses reduce a person's accountablity for the behaviors they may help to provoke?

KITCHER: Exactly.

DENTZER: Dr. Koop, this question speaks to your role in waking us all up to the dangers of tobacco. "There is a new generation of smokers in the People's Republic of China. America's tobacco companies are increasingly seeking foreign markets, and one might predict a major epidemic of lung cancer and smoking-related diseases worldwide as a consequence. How would you advise today's new physicians in the fight against tobacco on the world stage?"

KOOP: It is very difficult, in the arena of the present tobacco settlement, to even talk about the subject. The only reason that a tobacco settlement could be accomplished, behind closed doors in conversations between attorneys general and the tobacco companies, is because the international problem was never mentioned. In case you don't know where I stand on this issue, I will tell you that my last official words as Surgeon General in 1989 were: "I think one of the most reprehensible things that this country does is to export disease, disability, and death to underdeveloped countries in the form of tobacco." There is no question in my mind about that, and it is aided and abetted each time it happens by the United States trade representative, who usually has an office in the White House. The reason the tobacco settlement has gotten as far as it did is that only 8% of global income from tobacco comes from the United States. If you could magically shut off this country's income from global tobacco sales tomorrow, the tobacco world could make it up with just a two-year campaign in China alone. The second day that Dr. David Kessler and I met with our public health group at the request of Congress to form a tobacco policy against which any settlement could be measured, we had 16 e-mail letters, telexes, and FedExes from representatives of foreign countries asking us to please remember that anything we did to curtail sales of cigarettes in the United States would be reflected in more sales and more promotions in their countries, and they asked us to bear this in mind. So all citizens, not just physicians, have to be aware of what we are doing to the rest of the world for the sole purpose of making money. I think it is reprehensible, I think we all should be making a major demand upon Congress to do something about it, and I think physicians should play a great role in this because they are respected on this issue and they can inform their patients to play a role, too.

DENTZER: Dr. Koop, let's take up some questions about financing medical and graduate medical education. "As government support dwindles, and hard-pressed hospitals are unable to provide the support, how should medical education be financed?" And second, "What is your opinion of the proposal to, in effect, reward teaching institutions for reducing the number of residents trained in those institutions?"

KOOP: Let me answer the second part first. What that question refers to, as you know, is that an agency of the government, the Health Care Financing Administration, recognizing that we had too many specialists and perhaps too many doctors in certain parts of the country, asked the hospitals of New York City to reduce the number of residents that they trained. Under the present circumstance, every resident brings to a hospital about $100,000 in income, and for hospitals to give up residents would mean cutting their income considerably. And so the Health Care Financing Administration said, "We will pay you the $100,000 for every resident you *don't* train." It is sort of like price supports for soy beans, tobacco, and so forth. And it seemed to be so appealing to New York hospitals that the rest of the country clamored for it, and now this is to be done over the whole country. I think that is the wrong way to go; I don't think the Health Care Financing Administration has any right in the world to talk to hospitals in New York about how many doctors there will be. We have national boards in this country for every single specialty. Over them we have the American Board of Medical Specialties, and those are the people who should be given the task of saying how many urologists, how many pediatricians, how many endocrinologists we need, and then let the educational system carry out their decision.

The first part of the question I alluded to earlier, when I said that managed care had not become sensitive to its obligation to foster clinical research and to look to the education of the future generations of doctors and nurses. The two outside sources that most medical schools look to for income for education are the so-called profit or non-profit hospitals, and the salaries of clinicians are sometimes taxed by the dean, sometimes by some other method; but a portion of that income properly goes to the medical school, as does a part of the income from the hospitals. But now, because of managed care, fewer beds are occupied, beds are being closed, operating rooms are being closed, and the cushion that provided the largesse from hospital to medical school is disappearing. In a similar fashion, the so-called excessive income of some specialists is also diminishing, for the same reason, and therefore medical schools face a very serious problem in financing. If managed care does not volunteer to do this," the only thing to do is to tax managed care in some way, so that the same amount of money flows to medical education as did before.

DENTZER: Professor Kitcher, are there ethical and moral principles we should keep in mind as we sort out the question of financing medical education, and graduate medical education in particular?

KITCHER: The principal thing that concerns me is that people all around this country—people who come from different backgrounds—should have care provided for them by individuals who are sensitive to their specific needs, who understand their problems, and who are capable of coping with the tremendous alienation that modern medicine can sometimes bring. This problem has shown up in the context of genetic testing, but it is a much more general problem as well. There are different groups in this country who either have very little access to medicine, or who, when they do get access, feel that they are in the presence of authorities who represent a completely different culture. In thinking about the financing of medical education, I would like to see concern given to the distribution of medical resources throughout the country.

Rationing: The Bitter Pill—Panel Discussion

SUSAN G. DENTZER,[a] *Moderator*
Economics Writer and Contributing Editor, U.S. News & World Report

LONNIE R. BRISTOW
Past President, American Medical Association

DANIEL J. CALLAHAN
Director of International Programs, Hastings Center

ROBERT G. EVANS
Professor of Economics, University of British Columbia

RUTH PURTILO
Director, Center for Health Policy and Ethics, Creighton University

WILLIAM L. ROPER
Dean, School of Public Health, University of North Carolina at Chapel Hill

SUSAN DENTZER: Continuing on the theme of Promethean choices, one of the terrifying realities for today's medical students is our ability to do so much for so many people—provided that someone is willing to pay for it. And if someone is not willing, or if we do not have enough of what we want to give out, we ration it. The discrepancy between what we are able to do in medicine and what we are willing or able to pay for is presumably going to intensify the need for rationing in the years ahead.

We all know that health care is already rationed: By denying insurance coverage to certain people, we effectively withhold care from an enormous number of citizens, particularly those at the low end of our income spectrum and those in certain racial groups. At the same time, we spend more than any other nation in the world on health care, and are likely to continue to do so in the future. The recent Congressional Budget Office analysis looked at current health-care spending trends, and attempted to make predictions about those trends. This year [1997] we are facing a federal budget deficit of about one-half of a percentage point of gross domestic product as a consequence of a very successful effort to reduce the rate of growth of federal spending

---

[a]Present address: Correspondent, *The News Hour with Jim Lehrer*, 2700 Quincy Street, Suite 240, Arlington, Virginia 22206.

and a very brisk period of economic expansion over the last few years. However, if we look at the rate of growth of our overall entitlement spending—programs like Social Security, Medicare, and Medicaid—and particularly the fast rate of growth of the health-care component of those programs, Medicare and Medicaid—and we extrapolate that into the future, the Congressional Budget Office predicted a deficit in the year 2050 of somewhere around 24% of gross domestic product. That would be a quarter of the size of our economy in that year, or around $10 trillion annually in current terms, again, largely because of the growth of Medicare and Medicaid.

Herbert Stein, who was chairman of the Council of Economic Advisers under President Nixon, has said that something that cannot go on forever *will* stop, and presumably the growth rate of health-care spending *can't* go on forever and we *will* have to find some way of at least lowering the rate of growth. But how do we do that? This raises many questions. How do we call a halt to the growth of health-care costs when it is producing so much of value? The Harvard economist David Cutler has looked at Medicare outlays, for example, on the treatment of heart attack patients. These outlays are increasing by leaps and bounds; we're spending billions more annually on this form of health care. But these treatments are so efficacious that the unit cost of buying an extra month of life for a Medicare patient who has had a heart attack is actually decreasing. A lot of people are walking around today, spending extra months with their grandchildren, because of the billions of dollars we're spending on heart attack treatment. As a society it is not easy to tell those people that those extra months of life aren't really worth it.

Some years ago, the then-governor of Colorado, Richard Lamm, got into trouble by, in effect, telling senior citizens that they had "a duty to die and get out of the way." Few politicians have made the same mistake since. It is one thing to talk in the abstract about a certain class of patients—the elderly, the severely disabled, the low-income, the uninsured—who are more or less deserving of costly medical care, but it is yet another to look a dying person in the eyes and say "No more care." And regardless of what you think of the contributions of Princess Diana, the global outpouring of grief following her death gives a sense of the enormous value that it is possible to place on one human life.

Do we have to ration health care? Or do we just have to reallocate it, since we spend more than any other country? At Dartmouth we have an excellent testimony to the way we use our medical resources, in the form of the *Dartmouth Atlas of Health Care*, now in its second edition. This is the work of Dartmouth's Jack Wennberg and his crew, and presents some disturbing realities about health spending financed by Medicare. It suggests that we spend so much in such an irrational way that simply distributing the funds more rationally could probably avoid rationing. Instead, coverage could be spread more widely to the people who are now deemed to get less of it. This edition of *The Atlas* concludes that, if the rate of spending in Minneapolis were the standard nationwide—as opposed to the rate of spending in, for example, Miami, where expenditures on Medicare recipients are about $4,000 per patient per year more—we could essentially take the pool of money that we are now spending and cover everybody quite adequately. At the same time, we could also solve the kinds of problems that we face with the Medicare Hospital Insurance Trust Fund. So, do we face rationing decisions? Or do we face reallocation decisions? These are very important questions.

To deal with these and other tough issues, we've brought together a group of experts with a variety of perspectives and with very different roles in health-care delivery and health policy. We will hear from Dr. Lonnie Bristow, who is past president of the American Medical Association and a long-time member of the AMA board of trustees. He has also, incidentally, served as one of the two public representatives in the recent tobacco settlement talks. Next to him is Daniel Callahan, co-founder and former president of the Hastings Center, and the author of many books, including the 1990 *What Kind of Life? The Limits of Medical Progress*. We then have Robert Evans, professor of economics at the University of British Columbia and an astute and regular interpreter, to Americans, of the realities of the Canadian health-care system. Ruth Purtilo is director of the Creighton University Center for Health Policy and Ethics; she also holds an M.T.S. degree from the Harvard Divinity School, was ethicist-in-residence at Massachusetts General Hospital in Boston from 1987 to 1991, and has expertise as a provider of health-care services as well, having in an earlier incarnation been a physical therapist. And finally, Dr. William Roper, a veteran of health-care policy-making in both the public and private sectors. Earlier in his career he served as the administrator of the Health Care Financing Administration and as the director of the Centers for Disease Control and Prevention, and he was most recently in the private sector, with Prudential HealthCare, as the organization's chief medical officer. He has now returned to the sacred groves of academe as the dean of the School of Public Health at the University of North Carolina at Chapel Hill. Welcome to you all!

The panelists will make a few brief remarks to set forth some of their initial perspectives on rationing. Then we hope to engender a very lively debate—like the McLaughlin Group—dissecting these medical rationing issues, though a little bit more politely, I hope.

LONNIE BRISTOW: First, I would like to bring you congratulations from the American Medical Association. We are the young kid on the block, still able to do cartwheels and balance a pencil on the end of his nose as he walks along a picket fence, because we're only 150 years old! When the AMA was formed 150 years ago this year [1997], its major concerns were, first, the ability of physicians to come together and develop a coherent approach, nationally, to the health needs of the American public and, second, to establish a code of medical ethics. Here we are 150 years later, and the subject we are dealing with today touches on both of those concerns—the ability of physicians to come together to develop some national perspective on Americans' health-care needs, and, very importantly, the enhancement and efficacy of our code of medical ethics.

I'd like to illustrate that with a couple of points. First, you may remember a cover of *Time* magazine showing a doctor wearing a surgical mask which, instead of covering his nose, is gagging him; the caption says, "What your doctor can't tell you." This was to illustrate a feature story on what's called the gag rule, which was being applied particularly in managed care in this nation. Specifically, a patient in California, a woman who had breast cancer, was thought to possibly need a bone marrow transplant as a means of treating that cancer. She belonged to an HMO, and the doctor in that HMO properly referred her to the University of California at Los Angeles to get an opinion as to whether or not she was a suitable candidate for that type of procedure. The week that she was supposed to have her consultation, the medical director of her HMO arrived at UCLA and pointed out to the UCLA management that the HMO also had a very large contract with UCLA, and would not look kindly on the sharing of information about services that were not covered by the HMO. Now, that created a momentary dilemma for UCLA. But they, of course, did the right thing and *did* discuss with that patient all of her available options. But it was such a compelling problem that they shared it with the AMA, and the AMA in turn steered *Time* magazine toward exploring this particular issue. Now, as a result, in more than half the states in this nation, legislation has been passed prohibiting the application of gag rules for physicians who are part of managed-care organizations. The underlying basis for those actions is the fact that it is considered by the AMA unethical for a physician to withhold necessary information from a patient who has to make decisions about care.

But do not think that this is a problem localized only to managed care. And by the way, I define managed care as simply being prepaid health care that has contractual arrangements with care-givers outside of a central location. We have had prepaid health care for over 70 years in this country. And before you think this problem pertains only to managed care, let me tell you a more personal story, about a young doctor in gynecologic oncology at UCLA. He was in his sixth year of training after medical school and on call one weekend when a local Veterans Administration hospital beeped him to say that a female veteran had come to the emergency room and was unable to pass her urine, and would he, as the fellow on call, come to see whether he could provide assistance. He responded and found, on examining this patient, that she had a very large tumor, which was the reason for the obstruction. He was able to ease the problem of her passing urine right away, but upon admitting her to the hospital had a conference with the chief of the department of surgery, advising him that the size of the tumor demanded massive surgery that would require a gynecologic oncology specialist to perform. The chief of surgery said that this was not in the budget for this particular hospital and that the operation would be carried out by the surgical department, although they might call in a gynecologist to look over their shoulders and provide advice. This young fellow then went back to the patient, informed her of the difference of opinion that existed about her care, and suggestd that if she was willing, he would discharge her from the hospital, that she could take a taxi over to the county hospital, where he also had affiliations, and that he would arrange to have gynecologic oncology specialists see her and carry out the operation. And that was done; the procedure took six hours—that's how complex it was. A month later, UCLA had grand rounds in that department, and the case under discussion was the one I've just outlined. The case was discussed not because of the complexity of the surgery, nor because of the particular tumor type, but because UCLA wanted to instruct its housestaff that "This is the way we carry out our responsibilities to patients." I point out to you that the VA hospital is not managed care; it's not for-profit. But the constraints of trying to function economically bring us right up against considerations as to how we can avoid making *wrong* decisions about rationing in today's world. And later, I hope that we will be able to explore some mechanisms for making the *right* decisions.

DANIEL CALLAHAN: I have to confess right off that for at least 25 years I have been an enthusiastic supporter of the idea of rationing, and more recently have become fairly enthused about HMOs as well. I have wondered about the genesis for those feelings, and when I recently had a complete medical work-up I learned that the bias toward rationing comes from a break in the number 9 chromosome, and the bias toward HMOs turns out to be an airborne disease. I offer that as a background because I'm only going to say good things about rationing.

I generally believe in rationing because I generally believe that ultimately in this country we need universal health care. And I don't think we will ever get universal health care until we have a medicine that is economically sustainable and affordable. And the only way we will get that, I believe, is by a conscious acceptance of the idea of rationing and, with it, of the setting of priorities.

I am going to give you eight reasons why I think rationing is a good thing. The first is simply that it cannot be avoided. *All* health-care systems ration care. In this country we have done it by ability to pay. It is hard to imagine any system giving everybody everything they want in the name of health care; given the nature of modern scientific medicine, which is inherently expansionary, there is no way that a country can provide everything that is likely to come along. Second, unless controlled in some way, health-care costs will constantly escalate. Some form of rationing is the only way to control costs. That point has been well understood in the managed-care movement, and it is fairly clear that if you do not want to see health-care costs escalate, particularly in double-figure percentage increases, you have to control expenditures. And rationing is the only known way of doing so, whether it is rationing by cost or rationing by regulation. Third, a principal reason for the escalation of costs is the constant introduction and intensive use of new technologies, most of them bringing only marginal benefits at a relatively high cost. Rationing seems the only way to control and manage this kind of obsessive technological imperative. Fourth, Jack Wennberg and his colleagues at Dartmouth have done a great service in demonstrating the enormous and ultimately irrational regional variation and disparity in the provision of health-care services and in the use of technology. An orderly system of technology and outcomes assessment, prodded and driven by the requirement of rationing, is the only way to bring some rational consistency to the use of technology in different parts of the country. Fifth, the most important contribution to population health is a good public-health system and good health habits and behaviors among individuals. The absence of serious rationing in the American health-care system, with an emphasis instead on acute-care medicine, means that it has been difficult to advance the cause of population health and preventive health care. Too much emphasis has been placed on rescue medicine. Only if we consciously accept rationing will we be in a good position to effectively support health promotion and disease prevention. Sixth, and here is a more philosophical kind of point, it is not good to live in a society whose citizens expect to have every need and desire met—it makes people lazy and self-indulgent. Rationing is necessary to remind people of the limits to life and to encourage social solidarity. Seventh, we all need to be reminded of two enduring truths, medical and human: One is that injury, illness, and aging eventually come to us all; we can only forestall them, not avoid them. And the other is that we all die, and no matter what medicine does, it will not save us from that fate. Health-care systems without rationing, dedicated to unlimited individual benefits, seem to tacitly delude us into thinking that, with more research, more progress, more innovation, we can eventually vanquish illness and death. But we can't. Finally, eighth, rationing is a necessary condition for an equitable system of universal health care. It is impossible to have the one without the other. European countries discovered this long ago as they developed their systems of universal health care. Managed care, for all of its faults—and here I would particularly fault the for-profit emphasis—is beginning to show us that rationing can control costs; that is essentially what managed-care organizations are about: they are forms of rationing. Universal health care, if we eventually get it, is going to look like an HMO; that is the only way you can organize systems that provide integrated care in an economically affordable way.

Those are my eight points. A final note: An article in a recent issue of the *New England Journal of Medicine* reported that the Oregon Medicaid plan, which combines rationing and priority-setting, has turned out to be a moderate success. Those of you who followed the debate will recall that there was enormous opposition to the plan; it was thought to be harmful to the poor, thought to be a way of evading the need for universal health care, thought to be a terrible way to deal with health-care problems. But it seems that they have achieved an equitable system of health care for the poor, which does involve the setting of priorities and which does involve rationing but which is working.

ROBERT EVANS: I'd like to begin by recording my agreement, on the fundamentals, with most of what Daniel Callahan has said, because I think we might debate some of the details, and I wouldn't want to sow confusion about more fundamental agreement. The cheery way in which he reminded us that we're all going to croak reminds me of a colleague and former student, Ian Morrison, a Scotsman now working in California, on the cultural relativism of these perceptions. Morrison says that the Scots regard death as something actually quite imminent; Canadians tend to look at it as inevitable; and in California he finds it's simply one of the options.

Cultural background may be quite important in viewing this issue. The notion of rationing has become lost in this country because the word itself has become a missile, a weapon in the struggle over health-care reform: "You *certainly* wouldn't want anything to look like the Canadian system because they *ration* care there" and "They don't ration care in this country, of course, because if you've got the money you can always have it." If the Clintons' proposals were actually Canada-in-drag, as people describe them, then you could expect that folks would be dying in the streets. The idea of rationing simply became part of that political debate, of the effort to reject other ways of organizing the entire system. That debate is now part of the political theater over the appropriate level of overall funding for health care. So it is very difficult to use the word *rationing* because we all have different shades and sometimes different cores of meaning associated with the term. So Daniel Callahan can come out being quite positive about it, while I come out quite negative, and yet we would probably find we agree fundamentally if we could work through the semantics.

"Rationing: The Bitter Pill" is the title of this discussion. The pill is bitter because it's poisonous—watch out, folks! The story told is simple: the advance of technology —led primarily by Americans—is providing ever more benefits for humankind but at ever greater cost, and at some point in the indefinite future, some time in the next century, it will become impossible to bear the costs associated with those vast improvements. And what will we do then? We will call in the ethicists; we will wring our hands; we will try to figure out how to make sure that we get the benefits and somebody else doesn't. This is ethical behavior ... because we're doing it for our children. But in any case, it will be forced on us by the inevitability of technology; technology will dictate this external force—something to do with Prometheus. By the way, Prometheus ended up chained in the Caucasus Mountains while an eagle flew back every night and kept eating at his liver, which probably served him right.

DENTZER: And he wasn't even on the list to get a liver transplant …

EVANS: Right! But, he didn't need it, because a helpful sod had provided him with a liver that kept regrowing. That was the good news; the bad news was that the eagle kept coming back.

Anyway, the logic is simple. But, as H.L. Mencken said many years ago, to every complex question there is a simple answer, and it's neat, it's plausible, and it's wrong. The logic depends on two fundamental assumptions: The first is that the need or capacity to benefit—which technology is presumably continually expanding—is linked systematically and consistently to intervention. In other words, the assumption goes, there is a nice, tight, logical connection between what people out there need and what they're actually going to get. Susan Dentzer has already mentioned the work that has been carried on here at Dartmouth which has culminated in the current *Atlas* and a number of other reports; and if you think there is a tight connection between needs and patterns of care, then you probably have fairies at the bottom of your garden. It is just factually false; there is no basis for that assumption, and in fact there is a basis for thinking that it is *not* true. The second fundamental assumption at work is that whatever the level of interventions that you receive—however loosely, fuzzily, or not at all they may be linked to your needs in some aggregate sense—there is a good connection between the intervention patterns and the costs. Susan has already mentioned that the United States manages to get rid of a trillion dollars a year on its health-care system. And more than $150 billion of that is spent in administrative waste within managed care and insurance companies, on public relations, lawyers, management consultants, even economists. You know these things, and yet you still talk about the inability to afford universal care. Fifteen percent of what you're now doing is complete waste; this would not be tolerated, and is not tolerated, not just in Canada but in any other system in the developed world.

And that is only the beginning. It is also the case, as shown by a number of studies, that you as American physicians are relatively generous to yourselves. Physician incomes, the incomes of more highly skilled personnel, have, in America, been historically much higher relative to the general income level than they are in most of Western Europe or in Canada. In other words, as Uwe Reinhardt at Princeton pointed out a long time ago, you've been very generous in allocating a handsome life-style to providers. The only other countries that come close are places like Turkey and Greece, where the average level of income is so low that it pushes the ratio up. So, Americans are probably spending 30% to 50% more, right now, than other countries would to provide the *same* level of services. And you want to talk about rationing because you can't *afford* it? That is ridiculous.

Now, that's the case at present. In the longer term, would the continuing progress of technology eventually lead you to a situation where you *must* ration even if the present doesn't make sense? The technology does not dictate its own range of application—that's a choice that emerges from your system; it is not forced on you externally. You can choose to go after genetic diseases by intensive research and investigation and genetic engineering, although that probably won't work but would generate a lot of good life-styles for researchers and providers; or you can deal with it the way Tay-Sachs disease was dealt with. But that didn't generate the same level of incomes.

The problem you're dealing with in America is that every dollar of expenditure is a dollar of somebody's income. So the whole income–expenditure loop forces you into finding stories about rationing that will justify continuing expenditure, and forces on you a framework of understanding that sees the country collectively as facing this major problem, this ethical dilemma posed by technology. However, the real issue is that some of you are making out like bandits, while others are being denied care or overcharged for the care they get. Of course, that is not a picture that everybody wants to see portrayed. But that is the picture that is covered over by the inevitability of rationing, and that is why I call it a poison pill.

DENTZER: We may have stumbled on the McLaughlin Group dynamics sooner than we'd hoped!

RUTH PURTILO: If we're going to talk about rationing, we should start by talking about whether we really do want to have a basic level of health care for everyone. And I have heard some consensus on that. I don't agree with Dan Callahan—at least I think it's un-American to believe in rationing. It flies in the face of the American ethos to be faced with that kind of restriction; the idea that we can't do everything for everybody at a cost that we would all like, and thus to believe in rationing, is out of line in terms of the American way.

As a result, the topic of rationing is extremely anxiety-producing. Again, it goes against our grain psychologically as a country to consider placing express limits on what we will do. In situations of great anxiety or stress, one of three things is likely to happen: the first is that you're likely to go back to old solutions, to get the problem out of your consciousness; the second is that you'll deny the problem, or never bring it to consciousness; and the third is that you'll squelch all the disquieting voices that are raising the problem, to shorten the process of dealing with it. And I think we have all three of those responses happening now in our attempt to deal with the necessity of making some hard choices.

My point can be highlighted by focusing on long-term care. I can talk about long-term care out of my own experience—from the aches and stiffness and other nuisances of an aging body and mind, from the axiety of making choices about my own health care, from my experiences as a physical therapist, and, as of 1979, when I completed my doctoral preparation, from the perspective of an ethicist who deals with long-term health-care issues. Long-term health care is an apt test case or challenge to some of the ways we are determining the basis on which we ration. In this emerging era of managed care, there is a growing tendency to look at outcomes and say, "Okay, if we have the positive outcomes, we'll have more evidence-based medicine." At the same time, policies based on outcomes today often do not take into account the complexities—the messiness of long-term care and the more than 85% of us, I am told, who will need long-term care sometime during our lifetimes. Both qualitatively and quantitatively, it challenges our assumptions.

Long-term care has come to our consciousness, in this nation and in all first-world nations, through our sophisticated understanding that increasingly patients present to the medical system with a constellation—a kind of chaotic conglomeration—of signs and symptoms and dysfunctions involving multiple systems that persist over a long duration. Most of these people are not going to die for a long time—months or years. But they're not going to get well, either. Robert Kane at the University of Minnesota, who, with his wife Rosalie, is one of the most persistent and thoughtful commentators and researchers on long-term care, says that he's in favor of using outcomes; he says we're moving in the right direction with the evidence-based emphasis on what works and what doesn't work. But long-term care differs from acute care in that it will have to take as a benchmark of successful outcome not "the person is cured" but instead "the person did as well as he or she could under the circumstances of irreversibly compromised ability." That's not very tidy, he would be the first to concede, as a standard by which to measure success as we usually think of a successful intervention.

As Americans, we have placed value on doing things on our own—on self-determination, autonomy, exercising control over our own lives. Patrick Henry expressed that idea more than 200 years ago when he said, "Give me liberty or give me death." Long-term care truly compromises many versions of what Americans consider their "freedom" or "autonomy," which they equate with their "inalienable right to liberty." And so thinkers like David Hadorn, at the Rand Corporation, and David Orentlicher, a lawyer and a very thoughtful commentator on long-term-care issues, and others are studying the notion of quality of life in health care—as opposed to the notion of mortality, which has defined many of our outcomes-oriented thinking so far. They are showing through their studies that patients who suffer from one of these messy, conglomerate states will be shortchanged every time in our current approaches to defining outcomes. They conclude that we must, instead, bias a successful outcome in the direction of alleviating pain or reducing stiffness or other dysfunction, or decreasing the rate of a downhill slide; otherwise the person in long-term care will always come out lower on the priority list by definition. The move toward emphasizing functional and palliative outcomes is a move in the right direction, but it is still narrowly conceived: Preserving life is still a high priority in outcomes measurement, and most conditions calling for long-term care are not terminal illnesses. They are not life-threatening in a direct sense, but gradually disabling, an ulnar drift and stiffness, for example, or difficulty in taking a deep breath.

So it is important to increase awareness that life-saving interventions tend to be weighted too heavily, the way we're measuring outcomes now, with the effect that persons with no life-threatening symptoms will fall lower in the priority scale. Perhaps we can talk later about what are needed as correctives.

WILLIAM ROPER: In talking about this important topic, I'm reminded of the Southern politician who, when asked his position on an issue, said, "Some of my friends are against it, some of my friends are for it, and I agree with my friends."

We've seen important points being made from a variety of perspectives—ones that I largely agree with. Through the various jobs I've had an opportunity to do, whether in state public health, federal health-care financing, federal public health, managed care, and now academia, I've had a long-standing interest in outcomes research, in evidence-based medicine, in the general topic of quality and effectiveness and value in health care. There's a lot that those words can bring to bear on this issue of rationing, and that is what I want to talk about.

Let me offer just a brief word about managed care. I spent the last four years working for a national health-care management company, and the words "managed care" have been stretched so much to cover such a heterogeneous set of organiza-tional delivery models that they bear little usefulness these days, except to note that managed care, I think, properly means an organized *system* of care. In my view, man-aged care is a *tool,* and like a surgeon's scalpel it can be used to kill or to save a life. The challenge in America today is to figure out how to use this tool, because I don't think we're going to go back to a system of unorganized—unmanaged, if you will—health care.

The first point is that in America rationing is not a future possibility to be debated or avoided, but rather a present reality—indeed, a long-standing reality—to be dealt with. As has been pointed out, eligibility criteria for public programs mean that some people in various age groups get some services and other people in other age groups do not. Lonnie Bristow has just alluded to the rationing in the VA system.

What we are talking about, therefore, and this is my second point, is explicit ver-sus implicit rationing. We have long had implicit rationing, and we are beginning to talk about explicit rationing. In America we will not have all-or-nothing rationing. Rather, the challenge is under what circumstances, for which patients, will certain services be covered, and that is where evidence-based medicine comes to bear. It is carrying coals to Newcastle to come to Dartmouth to talk about a subject that Jack Wennberg and Paul Batalden and Hal Sox and a number of others are world experts on.

Evidence-based medicine has relevance to this discussion because, and here's my third point, that is what Medicare and various health plans are now using as criteria in the decision process of what to pay for. Medicare has long done this using the terms "safe and effective, reasonable, and necessary." I was the administrator of the Health Care Financing Administration when we began covering heart transplants, when they were done in *some* centers; under that theory, we decided they were "safe and effective, reasonable, and necessary" for *some* patients, who had an appropriate chance of survival. And at Prudential, I had responsibility for our technology assess-ment unit, which did this same thing in the private sector: attempting to determine when treatments were no longer experimental and investigational, but ought to be covered on a more widespread basis. However, the whole question of health plans making those kinds of decisions has become very controversial and has been litigat-ed extensively in the courts. The most celebrated cases involve terminally ill pa-tients, most notably women with breast cancer, and the question of whether or not they are eligible for bone marrow transplantation—a potentially life-saving treat-ment for their illness. But, and here's the "but," the only alternative to using evi-dence-based guidelines to decide when and where to do what in medicine is to say that anybody can have anything, or, to put it more bluntly, anybody can have any-thing that they can find a doctor somewhere in America to say that they need. That is the challenge that we face in trying to play this out in the courts.

When I was at Prudential, a group of people reported to me who made decisions about what the company, nationally, would cover and pay for. Usually I would only hear reports about the decisions that this committee made, but occasionally I got per-sonally involved. In one particular case I called long-distance and talked to a woman who was then dying of breast cancer and whose only hope was a bone marrow trans-plant. Over a series of conversations with her, the abstractions went away as I and she, and lots of others, tried to deal with her illness. We do understand that these are not abstract issues for debate, but people's lives that are at stake. I would urge us all, however, not to get caught up in the notion of saying, "This is America and people have a right to care," but rather to say, "Can't we agree that we have a common interest—not just as health professionals but as citizens—in sorting out the best science, bringing to bear that evidence on the practice of medicine, and then helping to make judgments about how we will allocate resources within our health-care system?"

The point I'm trying to make is that rationing is not a *threat* brought to us by managed care; it is a notion as American as apple pie. The challenge that we face is whether we will ration in a way that is thoughtful and scientifically based and yet at the same time is compassionate and deals humanely with people as individuals.

DENTZER: I'm going to take the moderator's prerogative of tossing out some initial questions to get the discussion moving, and I'm going to start with Bob Evans. If I can boil down your prescription for us—the Canadian prescription for how to fix the U.S. system—it sounds like it is two-fold. First of all, get rid of the parasites—the administrators, the scrutinizers, the advertisers, everybody who doesn't particularly add curative value to the health-care system but just makes the business side of it function; get rid of those folks, or at least contain their activities. And second, do a better job of distributing the enormous resources that we already expend. I think that's about it. Not a bad prescription, but who makes those decisions—who does that redistribution? We have already clearly rejected the notion that people from Washington should do it; who do you think ought to do it?

EVANS: You have boiled my points down nicely. I would only offer one or two footnotes: It's not simply the Canadian prescription. Don't get trapped into some kind of bilateral tournament here, between the U.S. and Canada, or the U.S. and Germany, or the U.S. and the U.K. back in the 1950s. The pattern that Canada represents is actually the pattern of the developed world. It's what Joseph White, in a very interesting book he did for the Brookings Institution, called the "international standard."[b] And it is the U.S. that departs from the standard. So it's not simply my prescription. In fact, when Clinton was first elected, *The Economist* magazine—that well-known, pinko, left-wing rag, published somewhere in the mid-Atlantic with an English accent— came out with a piece of advice for Clinton: First, get rid of the private insurance industry. But the private insurance industry also reads *The Economist*, and they thought: First, get rid of Clinton. And the rest is history.

However, yes, you do have a whole lot of people—you called them parasites—who are not adding to the process. That is not to say that you don't need administrators and other people to keep the system running; the $150-billion estimates—and those are American estimates—that I quoted are of the *excess* amount, that is, over and above what it costs to run other systems. In addition, as the other speakers have noted, you are already rationing—you've got money coming out of your ears, and you're *still* rationing. In other words, the two are not connected. It's not a shortage of funds that leads to rationing, it's an organizational set of issues.

Now to the meat of the question: Who does the rationing? Basically, each country has to fight its own way through to this; it's different in each country. In the United

---

[b]Joseph White, *Competing Solutions: American Health Care Proposals and International Experience.* Washington, D.C.: The Brookings Institute, 1995.

Kingdom the national government sets the policy, while in Canada provincial governments run the plans and the federal government supplies additional funds and sets the standards. Each country's political system dictates where the appropriate balance will be. But in America the polity have consistently fought against any concrete scheme for making the system more rational. The American people are consistent in their judgment that the status quo is rotten, as are all the alternatives. And so long as they keep doing that, there isn't any answer to your question. You're not going to get out of this mess until you become so fed up with what you've got that you can emerge from what economists call "the low-level equilibrium trap." In some ways, managed care may be the penalty that the American medical community has to suffer for its own lack of foresight and lack of generosity and statesmanship over an entire generation.

DENTZER: I didn't hear an answer to the question of who does the rationing other than "We have to figure it out."

EVANS: The way your system is set up, rationing will have to be done by the federal government. I know that you are wary of your federal government despite its being crafted by some of the leading minds of the 18th century. But you are still more distrustful of it than any other citizens are of their governments. But I don't see any other place—your states are not strong enough fiscally or in terms of their political credibility to be able to take the role in the way that, say, Saskatchewan did in Canada. I may be wrong about that; I'm not an expert on American politics. But my impression is that you have concentrated so much power in Washington that that's the only place the job can get done.

DENTZER: Lonnie Bristow, one of the aspects of the prescription we've just heard includes the fact that we've allocated some enormously attractive lifestyles to providers in this country, of whom you are one. It sounds like what this Canadian wants to do is to get the federal government to take away your Mercedes-Benz, or at least the ones driven by your colleagues. Are you going to put up with that?

BRISTOW: It does sound like he's saying that. But you've got to realize that Dr. Evans is coming from a nation that has an extraordinary degree of trust in its government, a trust that is not matched in this nation, as he noted. So to back up to your original question, about who should make the choices, I believe, and I think a great number of my colleagues believe, that the best way to make those choices is to put them in the hands of patients. We already have systems in our country that do that. An excellent example is the Federal Employee Health Benefit Program, which gives all federal employees a menu of choices from which they can select what will work best for them and their families. We also have a state, Hawaii, that has had universal health coverage for more than 20 years. That's worked very nicely, thank you. And people there do have choices.

So we do have the capability, within our country, to have universal health care and also to allow individuals to choose the particular insurance approach that will work best for them. Every individual in this audience has a personal set of values, and where you place health care among these values will vary from one individual to another. Some place it higher than education, some place it higher than the home that they live in, or food, or recreation. Having choices allows people to select what which will work best for them and their particular financial situation; it can be done. I expect that the country is moving in this direction. The choices will certainly include HMOs as an option, but as one of several options. There are other approaches that can be used just as well, and as soon as we reach this "menu" approach that the federal employees have already achieved, the rest of us will be as contented as they are. If you'll remember, during the health system reform debates, when the Clinton proposals were put forward, the only group that came to Congress and said, "Whatever you do, don't touch our program," was the federal employees.

DENTZER: So if many of the options that are going to be selected by people are HMOs or managed-care systems, do I hear you saying, "It's okay if managed care takes away my Mercedes indirectly; just don't make it the direct role of the federal government"?

BRISTOW: No, what I'm saying is that the American public deserves a series of choices that would include HMOs, a health IRA approach, and fee-for-service care —all as options so people could select what works best at a given point in their lives. One important change that must be made in our system is that people must be given much more information than they currently have. I believe very strongly that patients ought to know what a service is going to cost before they get the service, so they have the option of deciding whether or not the cost to them is appropriate, in their judgment. That kind of market force would have a healthy effect on our system; fundamental changes of that nature would allow patients to make informed choices, while at the same time preserving for physicians a voice in articulating the important issues that patients should have placed before them in regard to their health-care decision-making. That is why I mentioned the case of the poor woman who had the breast cancer. Patients need to know everything that is relevant and pertinent to their care, and then they, along with their physician, can decide what is going to work best for them.

DENTZER: Daniel Callahan, what about the role of patients? You accorded very little role in your rationing scheme for them to express their preferences, and Lonnie Bristow is in effect saying, "If people want more health care, they should be able to get it."

CALLAHAN: If I were organizing a rationing system, I would do it as a collaborative effort, with patients and physicians together working out the conditions, limits, and guidelines. I would not have it imposed from the top. Instead, the standards should be developed by the people who would be affected by them; I see it as very much a cooperative medical-lay venture. I suppose the question is "Who organizes the overall system?" Here I'm with Bob Evans; ultimately it's the government that's going to lay out the menu and set up the system and put up the money to fill in the cracks. We sort of have what we want now, but a lot of people aren't getting it—the people who are uninsured, the large number who are poorly insured; there's a great deal of insecurity out there. The real question is "What is the relationship between the kind of market approach that Lonnie Bristow has mentioned and government?" And right now the bias is in the direction of the market and there is little talk these days about the role of government; it's as if we forgot all about that possibility. But I hope Bob Evans is right; it's got to come back some day or otherwise a lot of people will fall between the cracks: a lot of people will get all sorts of diagnostic procedures they don't need, and others will continue driving their Mercedeses.

BRISTOW: By the way, I don't have a Mercedes! But I do agree that there's a role for government. I'm not saying that there is *no* role for government. I think government should assure that the public has access to the right kind of information, just as it does with the federal employees. Every year, every federal employee is given a considerable amount of standardized information about the options that are available to them from which they can choose. And then they decide whether or not insurance company A or approach B is most appropriate for them. Our government says to that employee, "Whatever you choose, we're going to provide x number of dollars. If the system you choose costs less than that, you're going to get to keep some of those excess dollars; if it costs more than that, you'll have to put some of your own dollars towards it. But you make your own decision." And what happens is that those various companies and systems have to compete against each other, because broadly comparable information is available to the people so they can make intelligent choices. People buy houses every day, they buy automobiles every day, so they must be intelligent enough and responsible enough to also make good choices about health care. But you have to give them the information in some sort of structured fashion, which is a perfect role for government.

CALLAHAN: I would just add one footnote. we should then introduce into Congress a bill saying that every American citizen will have the right to the same access to health care that federal employees have. Then everybody can make those choices.

BRISTOW: That's an excellent idea.

DENTZER: I want to return to a phrase Dan Callahan used earlier, "marginal benefits." You said that we are in a situation where we have enormous technological advancements that bring only marginal benefits at extravagant cost. Who decides what is a marginal benefit? Is tacking a couple of extra months onto the life of a Medicare patient who's had a heart attack a marginal benefit and therefore one that we shouldn't pay for? Who's going to decide that? We're clearly not comfortable with having people in Congress decide issues like that, notwithstanding your sense that only the federal government can take these things on. Nor do we particularly want Bill Roper's old colleagues back at Prudential, despite his warm and fuzzy feelings about managed care, deciding what's marginal and what's not, do we?

EVANS: That will have to happen, but I would like to see it done on a cooperative basis. The difficulty with the technology assessment movement is that it underestimates the role that values ultimately have to play, because most of the assessments do not turn out to be either absolutely terrific or no good at all. Instead, they're in between; the assessment is, "This will work for some people, some of the time, under some conditions, and it's going to cost x amount of money," and so then you're back into economic and moral questions. You got the data, but the data do not tell you what to do as the next step. I guess Bill Roper has had a lot of experience with that; I'm curious how you did it, in fact.

ROPER: We've clearly said in this country that we're not comfortable with government making these kinds of decisions. And I would argue that we've said we *do* want managed care organizations doing it. That's what the last 15 years have been about. There have been extreme cases that were publicized, and we're seeing the backlash against those situations. But I would argue that not only is that what the American public has said, but that's what rightly ought to happen, policed by appropriate regulation and overseen by the public in the person of the government. But those kinds of decisions are rightly lodged in competing private health plans, so that consumers can make choices. They can choose which plan to enroll in and they can choose to move from one to another if they don't like the care or service or range of options. That is a solution that would work for this country.

DENTZER: But Ruth Purtilo says that her folks, her long-term care recipients, are getting the short end of the stick in any kind of analysis that looks at how much benefit is derived from a given treatment. In fact, if you're talking simply about arresting somebody's decline into decrepitude, if you will, and not necessarily giving them back some function that they've lost, those folks are going to come out very poorly in the calculus. One could presume that a managed-care company might decide not to spend a lot of resources on people whose health status isn't likely to improve a whole lot. Is that what we want? There are 70 million of us baby boomers who presumably are going to need some sort of long-term care in the future; are 70 million people going to stand still until this is sorted out?

ROPER: I hope you are buying your long-term care insurance! The points Ruth Purtilo made are worthy of attention. There's a whole body of work involving quality-adjusted life-years, trying to take other considerations into account beyond just length of life. Now we are being much more explicit about things that formerly we didn't pay attention to. In my new home state of North Carolina, most people think of the Medicaid program as benefiting minority women and their children; however, 79% of North Carolina's Medicaid dollars go to people in nursing homes, and only 21% go to those whom people think of as the typical Medicaid recipient. So we need to be much more explicit when we ask whether people are comfortable about where we are putting our dollars.

DENTZER: Ruth, how would you respond?

PURTILO: I would return to what I said at the beginning—you don't know what a marginal benefit is until you are sure the people who should be defining the benefit are at the table. A lot of good activity in this regard is taking place. For example, many outcomes approaches are now using patient satisfaction scales to help define what a benefit entails. This kind of participatory process is essential as we develop the guidelines for what will happen to a whole group of people. One test would be whether the individuals who are affected are participating directly. Another would be the New England tradition of town hall meetings. For example, the governor of Vermont brings together groups of people for such discussions; there's also the Oregon experiment. It's the American way to try lots of different plans, and in fact the federal government is granting some exemptions from Medicare regulations that will serve as other kinds of experiments. The more broad-based our efforts are, the better. But the key is that they have to be *participatory*.

DENTZER: I'm going to turn now to some of the questions from members of the audience. This one I'll toss to Bill Roper: "There are a fair amount of data now on outcomes analysis of organ transplantation. We can now provide risk assessment for kidney transplants, which have 10 or so important independent variables for graft failure. Included are higher risks for African-American recipients. It is easy to say that outcomes data will permit a basis for rationing, but with actual data we find multiple shades of gray and few discrete cutoffs. Sorting all this out is not simple, especially when we add compassion to that mix." Now, is that something that managed care can handle?

ROPER: Managed care is an institution so heterogeneous that it is hard to talk about. But, yes, I believe that competing health plans are the appropriate locus for those decisions to be made, principally by doctors and their patients, but surely not by government. Applying scientifically sound criteria, like the ones the questioner describes, are the only rational way, I would argue, of allocating scarce resources, whether they be kidneys or livers or whatever else. Admittedly, all sorts of troubling issues are raised. For example, do we give a good liver to an alcoholic? But absent that kind of rational process, we would be saying that "only the famous, or the wealthy, or something else, will be given these organs."

BRISTOW: The questioner has put a finger on a very important point. Rationing has at least two contexts: The first is when you're talking about a scarce resource that is nonmonetary, like organs, available personnel or facilities, and the like; and the second is when you're concerned about the conservation of dollars. In each instance, there are five criteria that need to be applied, albeit with a slightly different twist. These criteria are: first, the degree of benefit that might be obtained; second, the likelihood that benefit might be obtained; third, the duration of any such benefit; fourth, the cost of that benefit; and fifth, the number of people who will benefit. These criteria should be applied regardless of which type of rationing you're talking about, but when it is a question regarding a scarce resource like an organ, then the distribution of it must be extraordinarily fair, and any differences in distribution have to be justifiable by a really substantial difference in one of those five areas—meaning there must be a big difference in degree of benefit, likelihood of benefit, cost, duration, or number of people who benefit.

If you are talking about simply conserving dollars, you would still use the same five criteria, but in this instance it is not a question of fairness in the fashion just mentioned, but rather of making sure there is ample input by the public at the beginning and end of that decision-making process. So this way the public buys into how the criteria are set up and evaluated, and then when the issue or cost comes up in their insurance program, they have already had an opportunity to determine whether that is appropriate for their community.

So those five criteria should be used in either instance; but in the first case, where the resource itself is very scarce, we have to be scrupulously fair about the distribution, even if it comes down to drawing lots, because, as one example, there are fewer organs than persons who need them.

DENTZER: The import of that earlier question seemed to be not only how we distribute kidneys, but also how we make decisions, since the outcomes are cast in so many shades of gray. Bob Evans, do you think that managed care—which is the way we have organized ourselves to make these decisions—is up to that task?

EVANS: In shifting from the Afro-American to the alcoholic, Bill Roper was shifting the ground in a way I would question. First, the alcoholic is presumably somebody who can conceivably change his or her behavior; therefore, it is not an automatic given that the liver will be destroyed. Second, if we believe that the liver *will* be destroyed, a kind of a moral negative attaches to the process of destruction. We think of alcoholics then as having somewhat lesser moral eligibility because we anticipate destruction of the new liver in a way we think is irresponsible. If you substitute "Afro-American" for "alcoholic," neither of these points holds.

Now, can a competitive market handle these questions? Yes, but you might not like the answer it gives. Say I discover that I can sign up with one competitive program that uses in its algorithm for deciding who shall have access to livers, for determining relative expected benefit, some data that are a detriment to Afro-Americans. I'm not an Afro-American; therefore, I'll sign up with that plan; Afro-

Americans won't. The market will segregate us. The marketplace, if it provides complete information, will lead to a fairly obvious sort of selection bias. But selection bias is the Achilles heel of market-based insurance, as was shown earlier by Professor Kitcher. It will kill competitive plans, which is why no other country has used that approach. Perhaps Americans can find some unique combination that will work. My argument was not simply the superiority of Canada's approach, but rather that no other country has gone your route. So as a country you're in an impossible situation if you insist on using the managed-care tool inappropriately.

DENTZER: Bob, we've all read the statistics about how, for example, there are more MRI machines in Seattle than in the entire country of Canada. It is very clear that one of the ways you control the use of health-care resources is by controlling supply of these underlying inputs.

EVANS: Yes.

DENTZER: The point is also made that many Canadians, when told that they have a long wait for a procedure, especially an elective one, hop across the border to the United States. Could the Canadian system exist without the safety valve of America?

EVANS: Indeed it could. The interesting thing about all those people who swarm across the border is that they go so fast you can't see them. It turns out that those claims refer to the "snowbirds," who go to Florida, Arizona, and New Mexico for the winter since they tend to be elderly and retired. If they get ill in winter, they get care down there, which is not the same as going across the border *for* care. There are about seven different reasons why Canadians get care in the U.S.; we have a project to determine the categories and numbers of persons supposedly pouring south to get care that they're being denied in Canada.

It is absolutely true that we provide fewer of the high-tech facilities such as MRI machines than you find in America. But we run the ones we've got a lot harder—and that is in your own literature; Victor Fuchs at Stanford has done a lot of work on that. We just use the machines more efficiently. Of course that's not the whole story—we do fewer procedures overall. However, there is no evidence that this leads to poorer outcomes—and it all comes back to outcomes in the end.

So, yes, we *do* control these procedures. On the other hand, when the difference in overall costs between our two systems is calculated, allocating out the proportion that represents prices, we get as many services as you do. You just pay more. We do get a different mix of services; the critics of our system are quick to jump on that. There are some services where Americans get more per capita than Canadians do; MRI is definitely one of them—it tends to be the high-tech, high-end services where that is the case. On the other hand, Canadians get more primary-care services than Americans do—not surprisingly, because we have 50% general practitioners, where you have gone heavily into specialty-centered practice. This was a deliberate decision taken by the physicians' associations themselves. When you change the mix of personnel, you get a different pattern of care—and again, the research supporting this is being done by Americans, Pete Welch at the Urban Institute and Steve Katz at Michigan. A growing body of research shows that we get as many services as Americans do—it's just a question of the mix. Then the question regarding the mix becomes "Given what we know about outcomes, are we losing ground because of that?" And the answer is no.

The real threat to Canada's system would not be the absence of the American system—it is the *presence*. So much disinformation is generated in the U.S. about Canada, and it drifts across the border like a form of intellectual acid rain. That poses a serious threat.

BRISTOW: I appreciate Dr. Evans's basic point that it is not that Canadians are getting too little care, but that Americans are getting too *much*. But I beg to differ with him on the issue of patients crossing the border for care; 25% of the patients at the cardiac surgery unit of Buffalo General Hospital in upstate New York are Canadians, So there is a steady stream of Canadians coming across the border to get care here.

EVANS: Not *steady*. There *have* been particular crisis times, and you've got to remember that an enormous amount of theater goes on in a politically funded system. So when the cardiac surgeons in Canada decide—and they do decide collectively; it happens provincially—that they're going to put pressure on the provincial government, you will suddenly find referrals to the United States and news stories put into the press. All this drama is necessary because you have to boot fairly hard in a political system to get it to respond. But then, the system eventually responds and a more rational priority system is put in place. That was done several years ago in Toronto, and it has been written up in the literature. And it was done in Vancouver, and again some of the results were published in the *Journal of the American Medical Association*.

So you don't want to get trapped into imagining that a piece of political theater represents the total picture. On the other hand, it is also true that there is a stream—though not a very large one, as far we can tell—of Canadian patients who come down to places like the Mayo Clinic and other centers of excellence in the U.S., as they do from other parts of the world. A lot of that has to do with the fact that we're a small country and a very spread-out country. And when that happens, our governments pay for it.

DENTZER: This question is for Dan Callahan: "Please respond to Dr. Purtilo and her sensitive comments on the need for quality of life for people who are suffering, either because of chronic illness that may take a great deal of time and effort to deal with, or illness that is difficult to diagnose, perhaps due to the rarity of the illness. Would you be willing to just ignore these people?"

CALLAHAN: We ought to put at the very top of our priority lists those services that we ourselves are most likely to need. And since we're all most likely to need long-term home care at some point in our life when we cannot be cured, I would put taking care of those needs at the top of my priority list, and I'd put organ transplantation at the very bottom. I'd flip the current priorities right over. Currently we are heavily oriented toward the *saving* of life; I would reorient priorities toward the *quality* of life. And for the saving of life, I would put the emphasis on population health and prevention programs, and put the individual spending into long-term and home care and the care of the chronically ill who can't be cured. This bias toward a cure, toward the saving of life, is now reflected in our NIH budgets and in the varying levels of prestige we accord certain goals. None of us is going to get a Nobel prize for designing a better long-term health-care system, you can bet on that.

DENTZER: Ruth, do you want to respond.

PURTILO: One of the things that Dan's comments point to is that a good rationing plan needs to include both the sites of care and the people who should be giving the care. Another shortcoming at the moment is that we have not looked as carefully as we can at who else besides physicians could deliver care—could do what physicians are doing, just as well and for a lower unit cost. And again, remember that anxiety and stress play a role here. It's anxiety-producing for me as a physical therapist, for example, because we're learning that some of the things we thought therapists should do can be accomplished pretty well—usually better—by mom at home. If we would reimburse her and give her some respite care, she could provide the care with an extra, important humane dimension; but without support, she will quickly burn out. So I'm agreeing with Dan in suggesting that another yet-to-be-determined variable here is where and who should be providing long-term care, and who should be eligible to receive it.

DENTZER: Let's wade into the question of the role of the for-profit health-care system. This questioner writes: "We speak of rationing, of cost expenditure loops, of limited resources, and HMOs. I'd like to know how the panelists feel about for-profit health care since it reallocates many people completely out of the health-care system. What role will for-profit health care play in the future of health care and in rationing in the U.S.? Is this good health care, rationing, or robbery?" Bill Roper, would you like to try that one?

ROPER: The company I used to work for was, on a good day, a for-profit health-care company. I believe it is perfectly appropriate to operate in that fashion, provided it is done in a way that meets the test of ethics and good business practices. Extraordinarily highly paid executives, people who don't practice business ethically, are not to be tolerated in health care any more than they are to be tolerated in any other part of our economy. But I would argue that the issue of for-profit and not-for-profit is largely an artifact of our internal revenue code: that there are non-profit organizations that have marble hallways and highly paid executives and all the other attributes of for-profit institutions. And lots of my physician colleagues who drive a Mercedes work for not-for-profit institutions. We need to look within ourselves and ask whether we are satisfied with the way the dollars are flowing and how beneficial this is in the long run for society. And finally, for the record, I drive an 11-year-old pickup truck.

DENTZER: But you're now in academia.

ROPER: I've *had* it for 11 years.

DENTZER: Stories have been in the news about Columbia/HCA and the pressure to deliver enormous returns to shareholders—a 20% annual return on investment—that led some people within that organization to probably overbill Medicare. Would this kind of thing be tolerated in Canada?

EVANS: The easy answer is no. But I think that Bill Roper's point is important; unethical behavior or robbery can arise in any institution—it's not strictly a question of whether it's for-profit or not-for-profit.

The main thing I would flag for your attention in the Columbia/HCA case is the *annual* requirement of 20% return on equity; with the magic of compound interest, next year you've got to get a 20% return on an equity that is now 20% larger—or 1.44 times the original equity. And that requirement recurs year after year: That's the magic of compound interest; it is why capitalism is such a dynamic system and such a powerful instrument of change. But it also creates the tremendous pressures that you're now seeing in Columbia/HCA. The real question is a more complex one—how do your capital markets function? Do they permit the survival of organizations that try to balance the interest of shareholders against other ethical considerations? Or do they say that for-profit organizations are solely responsible to the shareholders?

BRISTOW: In response to that question, there are two things to remember: First, the four largest insurance companies in this country have an admitted worth of over a half-trillion dollars. This is an enormous amount of capital, and along with it goes an enormous amount of leverage. Second, the approach that needs to be applied to for-profit managed care is the same one we should apply to not-for-profit managed care: It is essential that the public have full disclosure of certain key items: first, exactly what is covered; second, what is *not* covered; third, the percentage of the premium dollar that's actually expended on providing patient services as opposed to anything else; fourth, the results of satisfaction surveys; and fifth, the scientific basis for what is being used for making coverage decisions. With that kind of information, the average consumer can make an intelligent choice. The public has to have that information, and ensuring that they do is an appropriate role for government. Consumers will know how to choose what's in their best interest once they know the profit margin and the criteria being used for coverage decisions. Are there, for example, any incentives from that managed care organization for doctors to withhold services? That information should be easily available to the public. And with that proviso, the free-market system can work for people instead of against them.

CALLAHAN: I got interested in health-care rationing in this country long ago and was buffeted for years by those who claimed that if we just got rid of the waste and assessed technology better, we would not have to talk about rationing at all. But beginning in the late 1980s, I spent a lot of time in Europe and found that they didn't have the overhead or the Mercedes, and they were trying to figure out how to better manage their health-care systems, and they were still explicitly talking about rationing. Finally, by the '90s, it was pretty clear that there was a major movement throughout the world to turn to the market in order to relieve pressure on government. I understand that a lively debate has broken out in Canada about perhaps letting this deadly snake into the Canadian health-care system, which has had some troubles in recent years. So I'm curious about Bob Evans's feelings about the potential role of the market and for-profit organizations—both in Canada and, more generally, as a worldwide phenomenon.

EVANS: I can answer that pretty quickly. To a large extent, the tide has rolled back in Canada and is beginning to roll back in Europe as well. In both places the enthusiasm for the market turns out to have been based on the market's being a good way of redistributing the burden of paying for health care. No matter what kind of system you have, there are big costs—whether it's 15% of gross domestic product, as in America, or 9.5%, as in Canada. So who pays those costs? Do they get distributed across the population more or less in proportion to income? That is what tax-based financing does. Do they get distributed in proportion to risk of illness? That is what private insurance does. Do they get distributed according to experience of illness? That is what user charges do. What mix of those methods do you use? And the mix that you choose determines how the overall burden will be distributed through the society. So the recurring enthusiasm for market mechanisms in Canada and elsewhere has very little to do with efficiency. That is why some of those private market initiatives are starting to get rolled back now.

BRISTOW: The reason why you can go into any store today and buy a toaster for $22 is because they are not regulated; it is the market that makes toaster-manufacturing efficient. The same is true for television sets, which can now be purchased for

$200 instead of $500. The market works when people have an opportunity to know what it is that they are purchasing and can make their own decisions.

EVANS: And the reason it's a Japanese TV set is because they regulated their market!

ROPER: I will add a point to this discussion of market forces. The remark was made earlier that if we have become a managed-care system, the HMOs need to take responsibility for solving the problems of the uninsured, of funding for research, and of funding for medical education. It is quite appropriate for us as a society to say we'll pool our dollars to solve these problems. And it is quite appropriate to say we will tax all health plans in order to raise the funds to do these things. There are some important technical challenges that Washington health-policy nuts understand about how to apply such a tax fairly across all plans, but managed-care firms are in agreement with this idea as far as health care for the indigent and covering the costs of research are concerned.

But on the issue of funding for education—if I can lob one more grenade—it's beyond me, what the public-policy argument is for taking tax dollars, trust fund dollars, to fund young doctors going into specialties that are already greatly oversupplied. I can understand the public-policy argument for taking tax dollars to train lawyers who are going to spend their careers working for, say, a legal services corporation or a public health agency. But how can we justify taking tax dollars to support somebody who's shortly going to have a pay level of $700,000 a year? The answer to that question escapes me, but we need to seriously address it.

DENTZER: As a closing thought, I'll just note that we may not have made a lot of headway in coming up with definitive answers to these questions, but we have certainly shed light on what questions we should be asking as we grope our way through these issues in the years ahead.

Commentary on the Health-Care Session

HAROLD C. SOX

Joseph M. Huber Professor and Chair of Medicine, Dartmouth Medical School, Hanover, New Hampshire 03755, USA

The topics for the health-care session of this Bicentennial Symposium were well chosen to provoke a rethinking of this complex issue. Many of the ideas discussed either were new to me or were expressed in a more persuasive form than I had heard them posed previously. In this commentary, I will enlarge on several ideas drawn from the two presentations and from the panel discussion; each idea appears in bold-face italic type below, followed by my discussion of that particular point. I will then finish with some ideas about screening the genome, a topic that links the health-care session to the Symposium's sessions on genetics and neuroscience.

A clash of ethical systems is causing much of the pain in today's managed-care–dominated health systems.

This implication of Dr. Koop's presentation is most intriguing. He traced the development of market-driven health-care systems, known as managed care. He registered his concern about health plan rules that tie physicians' compensation to a restraint of health-care expenditures—to guidelines that in effect say "the less you do, the better your pay." This situation puts a physician in an ethical bind similar to that of fee-for-service medicine, in which doing *more* for the patient increases the physician's pay. Which of these two incentives is the more harmful? Some say that withholding care causes more harm than giving care that exceeds the necessary minimum. Others would argue that an elegant, flexibly minimalist approach to health care is medical care at its best. A considered application of "watchful waiting," with careful follow-up, is usually a very sound principle of patient care, as long as it is coupled with a sound grasp of the right time to intervene aggressively.

The lack of consistency between two systems of ethics—the ethics of health care and the ethics of business—is the root cause of much of the pain produced by market-based health-care systems. The ethical principle that is most pertinent to this discussion requires that the physician always give primacy to the interests of the patient. The content of the interaction between the patient and the physician determines whether the encounter was ethical. In business ethics, however, the focus is on understandings related to the transaction itself, rather than on the content of what passed between seller and buyer. If the seller provided accurate information to the buyer about the service or product, the seller acted ethically. A health plan that enforces a maximum of 24 hours in the hospital following childbirth or a breast lumpectomy would say to a disgruntled patient, "Read the fine print. It's all there."

Donald Berwick has called for a new ethics of health care, in which physicians and businesspeople reach accord on ethical principles that apply to health-care organizations.[1] If the three salient parties in market-based health care—physicians, businesspeople, and patients—can agree on the appropriate ethical principles, then some of the present conflict should subside.

Universal, complete knowledge of one's health risks may beget access to health care for all Americans.

The presentation by Philip Kitcher suggested that a solution to this country's universal coverage dilemma could come from an unlikely source. He discussed how increasingly perfect knowledge of one's own genes can affect planning for one's lifetime health expenditures, one's children, and society's preferences for structuring a health-insurance plan. He surmised that the Human Genome Project will eventually lead to a radical rethinking of the medical-social contract. For me, the most provocative part of his talk was its implications for the health-insurance industry.

Health insurance has a social role because people's future medical needs depend on luck. Among those with an equal risk of incurring health-care costs, some will incur costs and some will not, depending on events that occur according to the play of chance. The business of insurance is to relate a person's health-plan premiums to the person's risk of incurring costs, as Professor Kitcher said in his lecture. One-sided knowledge of a health-plan applicant's risk status, if known only to the applicant, destroys the concept of insurance. If people know their risks, but the insurance company does not, people will flock to a plan that offers good coverage for the diseases that they have or will probably get. At present, insurance companies protect themselves from that sort of action by using the pre-insurance examination to predict risk and thus expenditures. The company will raise an applicant's premium to cover the expected cost of the diseases that the person has or is likely to get. Risk-adjusted premiums allow the insurance company to stay in the business of protecting people against the consequences of bad luck.

Much-improved knowledge of a person's risk of developing disease, such as that provided by knowing one's genomic content, will make actuarial predictions of a person's lifetime health-care costs far more accurate than heretofore. A pre-insurance examination will then be a much less accurate way to assess risk than will knowing the applicant's genomic content. So, as long as the right to privacy includes a person's genomic content, the Human Genome Project will create asymmetry in the knowledge that an insurance applicant and the insurance company bring to their transaction. To protect themselves against people who know their genomic content, insurance companies will either raise their rates to levels that average-risk people cannot afford, or they will offer minimal coverage that will have little value. Either response will diminish the social value of health insurance.

This analysis suggests that perfect knowledge of everyone's genes will lead to the end of private health insurance and to a search for other solutions to assure adequate health care for everyone when he or she needs it. Will the American people choose a solution that looks like British- or Canadian-style plans in order to assure universal access to health care? Their response will depend on whether they agree with Professor Kitcher that it is morally wrong to penalize people for genetic conditions and attendant risks that they don't bring upon themselves. However, a person's sense of individual vulnerability may be more influential than moral imperatives. The polls taken at the time the Clinton Administration proposed its health plan showed that the American people placed a very high priority on health-care reform, but wanted to apply any savings to reducing insurance premiums or to expanding benefits, not to extending coverage to the uninsured. Perhaps the Human Genome Project, by reminding more Americans of their own vulnerability to high health-care costs, will drive a political solution to the vacuum created by the decline of traditional health insurance. Will universal access to health care be an unintended legacy of the Human Genome Project? The possibility is worthy of careful thought.

Much of the fireworks in the health-care session occurred during the panel discussion on rationing. Economists define rationing as a process for allocating goods in the face of scarcity. Congress has decided that medical expenditures are too large a share of the federal budget. Other large-scale purchasers of health care have decided that the cost of providing employees with health insurance is adding too much to the cost of producing goods and services. Much of the current angst in health care is occurring because these payers of insurance premiums will not cover ever-increasing premium fees. Rationing occurs when a health insurance plan, faced with limited income from premiums, must decide what services the premium will and will not cover. Rationing also occurs during individual visits with physicians, as described by Asch and Ubel.[2]

We don't need to ration right now, we just need to spend at the level of Minnesota.

The panel was very enthusiastic about one of Dartmouth's own—Dr. John Wennberg's benchmarking studies of per-capita Medicare spending. As a benchmark, Dr. Wennberg chose Minnesota, which is a mature managed-care market that has had time to adjust its physician workforce to the needs of caring for a defined population. The number of primary-care physicians in Minnesota is 93% of the national per-capita number. Per-capita spending in the Minnesota Medicare program is also lower—in fact, the national average is 40% greater than the rate in Minnesota. The 1993 total national Medicare reimbursement for enrollees aged 65 years and older was $115 billion. If the national rate of Medicare spending was equal to the Minnesota rate, the total Medicare outlay would have been only $83 billion, or a savings of $32 billion.[3] Dr. Wennberg has commented on the implications of this finding for access to health care: "Within the savings generated by the judicious use of resources and spending to the level of such benchmarks [e.g., Minnesota], the nation can find the resources to provide access to health care for all Americans."[3]

How does Minnesota do it? No doubt there is rationing in Minnesota, but the public seems to be satisfied with its health care. Perhaps rationing occurs in a myriad of day-to-day patient-care decisions by physicians who accept their role in containing costs and are effective in engaging their patients in this quest. Perhaps it occurs at the level of erecting barriers, such as waiting lists, which slow access to some health services. Evidently, rationing does not take the form of drastic rules that lead to heart-rending denials of service and subsequent public outcry.

Dr. Wennberg's findings suggest that U.S. physicians could provide good-quality health care to far more Americans if they spent at the presumably achievable levels of Minnesota. We need to understand what features of the Minnesota health system make its achievement possible. Even with this knowledge, the potential savings may be out of reach if Minnesotans turn out to be more healthy, to be more economically well-off, to have better genes, or to have different indigenous values—or if the success in Minnesota has depended on unique regional features of the politics of health care and health plans there.

Does demand for excessive health care contribute to health-care costs (the "I want what I want when I want it" syndrome)?

No one took Professor Evans to task for his claim, repeated several times, that America's health-care system is an outlier among developed nations: Everyone else pays their doctors less. Everyone else has universal access to adequate health care. Everyone else spends less on health care. More people in other countries seem to believe that long life is a lucky accident, a blessing, or, perhaps, the result of self-discipline. Professor Evans claimed that Americans act as if a long and healthy life is a basic entitlement. An expectation of unlimited medical care is a concomitant of this belief.

The view that any risk, no matter how slight, is worth reducing at any cost may be a consequence of the economic "good times" many Americans have enjoyed during the past 50 years. In times of plenty, people think of their needs in isolation from the needs of the populace at large. Trouble, in the form of war, a drought, or a disaster, brings out the best in the American people. Those who are pressing to reduce health-care costs haven't convinced the American people that the situation warrants individual sacrifice for the benefit of the common good.

Health insurance has insulated its beneficiaries from the consequences of health-care spending—except, perhaps, for a sense of disbelief and anger upon reading their paycheck stub and realizing the amount withdrawn for health care. But having paid plenty for health insurance, few sick people feel any obligation to make choices that might save money for the health plan. They want everything that might reduce their risk of an adverse outcome, even if the risk is small and the evidence of benefit is tenuous. Physicians have been accustomed to their role as patient advocate, even to the point of acceding to requests to do something that they know to have little chance of benefit. Now, with the pressure to reduce health-care costs, the physician has to assume the unaccustomed role of naysayer.

Instead of providing whatever a patient asks for, the physician must act as if there is a limited pool of money to pay for the care of a whole panel of patients—so that providing one patient with costly, low-yield services hurts another patient. This role, in which the physician becomes an agent of social policy, can undermine the individual doctor-patient relationship. However, if physicians don't accept a central role in reducing unnecessary health care, the health plan will step into the breach. The physician must exercise clinical insight, tailoring recommendations to the requirements of the patient's individual circumstances. Otherwise, the health plan will create rigid rules that further limit the physician's flexibility.

Responding to individual needs is one of the joys of medical practice, making it a constant challenge instead of simply a job. Explaining why antibiotics aren't needed for a runny nose and why a chest X-ray isn't needed for the accompanying dry cough is part of that challenge. Sadly, the explanation often falls on deaf ears, and a partnership turns into a confrontation. The patient is the physician's natural ally. Both are being hurt in the collision between inexorable advances in expensive health technology and payers' determination to contain costs. Each have their role to play in rationalizing health care.

Patients should share responsibility for decision-making at the population level.

The panel seemed to agree that patients should play a far more active role in deciding what health care they should receive for their money. Americans used to make these decisions. Fifty years ago, most patients paid their health-care costs from ready cash, on a pay-as-you-go basis. They had first-hand experience in working with their physician to find an acceptable balance between an increased risk of adverse health outcomes and the increased out-of-pocket expenses that could mean a lean month at the dinner table.

Now, most patients have health insurance. Insured patients have little idea what it means to participate in making trade-offs between added personal cost and added risk. The health plan simply dictates the coverage rules. One way to involve patients in this problem would be to engage them in formulating the benefits offered by their health plan—in effect, to have them design the plan.

What would this role mean? An example might be helpful. Suppose a health plan asks a consumer advisory board for help in shaping the plan's benefit package. (I base this example loosely on David Eddy's Eisle Lecture at the 1998 Annual Session of the American College of Physicians; I intend the numbers to be illustrative rather than accurate.) At one of its meetings, the health plan asks the advisory board to help decide which of three policies to adopt on the use of alendronate for osteoporosis prevention. According to the first policy, the plan would pay for alendronate for any postmenopausal woman, even though most women have a lifetime fracture risk of only 5%; this would add $500 per year to the cost of the plan. The second policy would require the health plan to pay for alendronate for only the small fraction, say 5%, of women who had the clinical characteristics that indicated a 75% lifetime risk of fracture; this would add only $25 per year to the cost of the plan, and women at low risk for osteoporosis who wanted alendronate would have to pay for it out of their own pockets. The third policy would exclude alendronate from coverage; this would mean no additional cost at all, and anyone who wanted alendronate would have to pay for it herself.

The third policy appears attractive on the surface. In effect, it says "Why have everyone in the plan pay for a medication needed by only a few high-risk people? Let people buy alendronate if they want it." This approach is reminiscent of the 1950s, when people often met their health-care costs out of ready cash. But there are two reasons for sharing the cost. First, potential enrollees, especially those who thought they were at increased risk, might prefer a plan that spread drug costs over all plan members. Second, preventing hip fractures could lower the cost of health care for plan members, since the plan would have to raise the cost of the insurance premium for all members if many of them had hip fractures.

To make an informed recommendation, the advisory board would need information. Knowing the costs of the drug and of treatment for a hip fracture; the frequency of hip fractures with and without the drug; the proportion of high-risk patients; and the accuracy of methods to identify them would probably lead to a very sensible decision. The board might also do a survey to find out how potential enrollees felt about the tradeoff between increased costs and reduced hip fractures.

The advisory board is one way to involve patients in decisions that involve a trade-off of cost and risk. There are doubtless others. By one means or another, we must recapture the days when the patient and the physician were in partnership to keep costs down.

The complexity posed by the possibility of screening the genome requires some rules of evidence.

The decision to characterize one's entire genome early in life would be a very complex, individual matter. Many people would seek guidance from broad recommendations that take into account, on a population level, the balance of harms and benefits from screening, diagnosis, and treatment. The framework used to evaluate screening tests by expert groups, such as the United States Preventive Services Task Force, may apply even to as complex a test as a search for mutations in one's entire genome.

Here is how that framework could apply to the case of genomic screening:

The screening test: The test must detect disease in a presymptomatic phase, something that characterization of the allelic constitution of each gene would do uniquely well. The test must not be excessively costly, which is certainly possible given the rapid rate of evolution of biotechnology. A screening test should also have a low frequency of false-positive results. A search for mutations across a large number of genes could lead to many false-positive results. What would be a false-positive result of genomic screening? I define a false-positive result as one that shows an abnormal allele in someone who does not develop a disease that can be a consequence of malfunction of the gene. To measure the false-positive rate of an abnormal allele, one would have to measure the frequency of disease in persons with the allele, a process that would require monitoring over each such person's lifetime. Multiply this requirement over all alleles of all genes, and it is apparent that the task of measuring the false-positive rate of screening of the human genome would be daunting but certainly not impossible.

Diagnosis: In the context of screening for genetic disease, diagnosis is the process of evaluating a patient with an abnormal allele to detect whether disease is already present. For example, someone with a mutation in an oncogene associated with colon cancer might require an immediate colonoscopy to detect cancer and to remove any benign polyps before they became malignant. This person would then require periodic screening colonoscopy. This sequence of screening test leading to diagnostic test leading to intervention would be very tidy for a gene that always leads to disease. But after determining the natural history of many mutations, we may find that many mutations do not lead to disease in most patients. A person who had the allele but wasn't destined to get the disease might undergo periodic screening without any potential for benefit. Measuring the risk of disease associated with various mutations in a gene and the cost and risk of periodic diagnostic evaluation would inform the decision about diagnostic evaluation and monitoring of patients with an abnormal gene. This information should also inform the decision to screen in the first place.

Treatment and health outcomes: Does early detection of a mutant gene alter health outcomes? In other words, if genetic screening makes it possible to detect disease earlier than would be possible by waiting for symptoms to appear, is the earlier application of treatment more effective? The ideal way to answer this question is to perform a clinical trial in which the investigators randomly assign people to receive genetic testing or not receive testing and then measure the death rate from the disease. This approach has given very valuable information when applied to such conditions as breast-cancer screening or colon-cancer screening. It avoids the problem of "lead-time bias," in which early detection of a disease without effective early treatment can lead to a misleading lengthening of time from diagnosis to death without any lengthening of life. A randomized clinical trial is the best approach, but another strategy would be needed for diseases that are so rare that it would be very difficult to identify a sufficiently large pool of trial participants.

Dissecting the decision to screen for genetic diseases emphasizes the complexity of the task of developing a clinical policy about screening for one gene mutation, let alone for characterizing a person's entire genome. It would not be appropriate to screen for a mutation that seldom expressed itself clinically, since carriers of the mutation might undergo monitoring tests that would be costly but could yield no benefit. The task of characterizing the rate at which mutations express themselves clinically over a person's lifetime is formidable, but it is one of the ways that we can realize the benefits of the Human Genome Project while minimizing the potential harvest of added grief and expense.

REFERENCES

1. BERWICK, D., H. HIATT, P. JANEWAY & R. SMITH. 1997. An ethical code for everybody in health care. Br. Med. J. **315(7123):**1633–1634.
2. ASCH, D.A. & P.A. UBEL. 1997. Rationing by any other name. N. Engl. J. Med. **336(23):**1668–1671.
3. THE CENTER FOR THE EVALUATIVE CLINICAL SCIENCES, DARTMOUTH MEDICAL SCHOOL. 1996. The Dartmouth Atlas of Health Care. American Hospital Publishing, Inc. Chicago, IL.

Special Address

Population Growth and Environmental Impact

AL GORE
Vice President of the United States

It is a pleasure to be back on this campus, especially on such a warm evening. The last time I was at Dartmouth, it was so cold, people thought I was frozen stiff. But I have to say, even as a loyal Harvard graduate, that President Eisenhower was right when he said that this is what a college should look like.

For a few centuries now, there has been a rivalry between Dartmouth and Harvard. I recently heard a story about the president of Dartmouth, James Freedman, and the president of Harvard, Neil Rudenstine, that proves that the rivalry is still going strong. It seems that the last time Jim Freedman was visiting his counterpart at Harvard, he noticed a large crimson phone on Neil's desk, and he asked why it was there. Neil grinned and said, "Well, Jim, in case you have forgotten, I am the president of Harvard, and that phone is my direct line to God."

Jim said, "Well, I have to admit that's pretty impressive. Would you mind if I gave him a call?"

Neil said, "Sure, go ahead, but don't stay on the phone too long, because it's long distance."

A few months after that, Neil drove north to visit Jim Freedman here at Dartmouth, and, as he sat down in his office in Parkhurst Hall, he noticed there was a large green phone on President Freedman's desk.

Neil asked Jim, "What is that?"

Jim replied, "Well, Neil, I was so impressed with your phone that I decided to get one, too. I just had it installed, and God and I talk every day now."

Neil was naturally surprised, but he figured he might as well take advantage of it. So he asked, "Since I was kind enough to let you use my direct line, would you mind if I used your phone while I am here?"

Jim handed him the receiver and said, "Certainly, Neil. By the way, stay on as long as you like. Heaven's a local call from here."

Happy bicentennial to all of you!

It has been two centuries since Nathan Smith's dream of a medical school, nestled in this beautiful land, began to come true. Dartmouth Medical School is here—and I quote Dr. Smith's own words—"to promote useful science." He knew then what we all know now: For science to be truly useful, it must go hand-in-hand with our values, the ethical and moral framework that is the foundation of our society. That is why it is so appropriate to mark this milestone by probing some of the toughest ethical and moral questions that will be faced by modern medicine in the first quarter of the coming century.

You've chosen to do so by focusing on an impressive range of issues—genetics, neuroscience, health care, and population growth and the global environment. All of the subjects explored here are destined to change our society in ways that we are just beginning to comprehend. The fact that this celebration looks forward, not backward, says a lot about the strength and vision of Dartmouth Medical School.

I am impressed by the list of speakers at this symposium. It is deeply humbling to be included in such a distinguished group. I use the word "humble" advisedly because I remember Winston Churchill's description of one of his opponents: "he has a lot to be humble about." Not only am I not a doctor, I don't even play one on TV!

But as an elected representative of the people of the United States, I can tell you that there is great public concern surrounding the issues that you have chosen to discuss here. That public concern, in addition to my own personal interest in science, has led me to spend a good deal of time examining some of these same topics—having hearings in Congress and trying to learn from the very able scientists who are part of the federal government.

I want to talk about the environment and the role played by rapid population growth. I would like to begin by trying to put those two issues in a larger context—one that might also pertain to some of the other topics addressed here.

One thing is certain: We live in a unique time, an age of possibility. It is a time when our society is making such rapid advancements that we can barely keep up. We sometimes trip up on the clichés describing the impact of the information age. And our minds are boggled by statistics on the accumulation of new discoveries in many fields—to the point where knowledge is doubling every six to eight months in some specialties. We are on the verge, it seems, of finding the causes and cures for some of our worst plagues and most serious problems. We are making enormous progress in the fight against AIDS, for example, and hope is beginning to emerge from our war on cancer. We are more optimistic than ever before about reducing the burdens that come from afflictions like diabetes, cystic fibrosis, and spinal cord injuries, among others. We are living longer, and, because of the new technologies and creature comforts, our standard of living is higher than we ever dreamed. Some would say we are truly mastering this moment, and in some ways they're right.

But of course it is also a time of great peril, with more people suffering from hunger and diseases and warfare than at any other time in history. And it is a time when we are becoming increasingly aware that the new powers conferred upon us by science and technology carry profound obligations as well. Because we have a much greater ability to affect the world in which we live—the physical Earth itself—we need to transcend some of the ancient habits and behaviors that we've grown up with. We need to become better stewards not only of our environment, but also of science and technology and ourselves.

This raises questions with deep ethical and moral ramifications. How do we ensure that we conduct the best possible science and use it for the best possible end? How do we support the scientific community's ceaseless quest for knowledge while working to ensure that we confront the moral and ethical issues often raised by new discoveries? How do we keep raising our standard of living without damaging our prospects for the future? How do we use the growing powers now conferred on humankind for good and not for ill?

The place to start is with the fundamental recognition that there is something profoundly new in our lifetimes about the relationship between humankind and the Earth itself. That's a sticking point for some people—they ask "How can we have the ability to affect the Earth itself, when the Earth is so vast and we are so small?" But some things have changed to make it so.

A combination of three factors has dramatically transformed the relationship between human civilization and the Earth itself. The first is the rapid growth of the population; the second is the still-accelerating scientific and technological revolution; and the third is a set of philosophical assumptions associated with the modern hero, which have caused many to discount obligations to the future that were once taken for granted.

That assumption, on the part of some, that we can't really be powerful enough to affect the Earth reminds me of a true story from my own education. When I was in the sixth grade, we had a map of the world at the front of the classroom, and it was rolled up on top of the blackboard. When it was time to study geography, the teacher reached behind his desk and pulled down that map. One day a classmate of mine, who had been staring at that map, asked a question. He pointed to the outline of South America, to where it sticks out into the South Atlantic. Then he pointed to Africa and the indentation in its coast on the other side of the South Atlantic, and he raised his hand and asked, "Did they ever fit together?"

And the teacher said, "That's the most ridiculous thing I have ever heard."

That child's creativity was stifled. Of course, we know now that continental drift is a fact. But the teacher was expressing the accepted science at the time, based on an assumption that continents are so big that they obviously can't move.

Yogi Berra once said that what gets us into trouble is not what we *don't* know; it's what we know for sure but just ain't so. One of the things we know for sure, but that just ain't so any longer, is that we cannot have an effect on the entire Earth.

Let me take one by one those factors that, when combined, transform our relationship with the Earth. The first is rapid population growth. To put this in context, you almost have to go back to the beginning of the human race. I don't want to get into a religious argument about when the human race began, because we had a trial in my home state about that, and I am a little sensitive on the matter. But just for the sake of argument, let's assume that the scientific community is correct and that *Homo sapiens* emerged sometime between 150,000 and 200,000 years ago. If you drew a line depicting the population of the Earth beginning with the first two people, that line would be flat for almost all of human history, until the agricultural era began and the line started to go up slightly. By the time of the Roman Empire, there were about 250 million people on the surface of the Earth. By the time Christopher Columbus sailed, there were 500 million people. By the time of the American Revolution, there were one billion people. And by World War II, there were roughly two billion people. In other words, it took 10,000 human lifetimes before we reached two billion people. Yet in my 49 years, we have gone from two billion to more than five and a half billion, and in the next 50 years, they tell us, we will go to eight or nine billion. So it took 10,000 lifetimes for the world population to reach two billion, and a little more than one lifetime to go from two to almost nine billion. That's a profound transformation occurring right now.

There are reasons for optimism about the stabilization of this rapid population growth. In September 1994, representing President Clinton, I led the U.S. delegation to the Cairo Conference on Population and Development, where the world abandoned the old Mexico City policy and crafted a new program of action to improve survival rates for children worldwide. The new program is based on the wisdom that the most powerful contraceptive is the confidence that one's children will survive—especially in developing countries, where large families have traditionally been insurance for old age against the high mortality rate among children. The new consensus also called for the widespread availability of culturally acceptable contraception methods. And it called for the empowerment of women and the participation of women in choices concerning family welfare and childbearing. We know from experience that when those conditions are present for a period of time, there is a shift from high birth rates and high death rates to low birth rates and low death rates. This demographic transition, which has occurred in virtually all developed nations, is occurring right now in many developing nations, so there is cause for optimism. But the continuing momentum in population numbers still presents a challenge.

The second cause of the transformation is the scientific and technological revolution. Let me give you an example. Warfare has been a part of human society since the beginning, but with the emergence of nuclear weapons, the consequences of that old habit were transformed. We had to find a way to change our thinking about warfare. A new pattern—the "cold war"—emerged.

The same phenomenon is evident with chlorofluorocarbons, the chemicals that cause the hole in the ozone layer. These chemicals were not invented until this century, but because they were used in large quantities after World War II, the air we are breathing in this room has six times more chlorine atoms than were present when this room was built. That doesn't have any direct effect on human health, I am told, because the concentrations are still low, but it's a dramatic example of our new ability, because of technology, to have an impact on the atmosphere of the entire Earth.

Now, of course, the reason for concern about global warming is that new technologies—technologies that involve the burning of fossil fuels, hemp, and other materials—have led to a dramatic increase in the concentration of carbon dioxide in the atmosphere. As you know, that thicker blanket of "greenhouse gases" traps a higher fraction of infrared radiation from the sun, and this is gradually heating up the Earth's atmosphere. But although this process may seem gradual to us, in terms of historical trends it's happening very rapidly.

I believe this is an ethical issue. When I began studying it, I looked closely at the evidence that was available, and one of the most compelling studies I found was from Antarctica, where the ice is more than two miles thick. It's been laid down over hundreds of thousands of years in annual snowfalls that are very, very light; there is so little precipitation there that it is technically a desert. Scientists are able to drill cores down through these layers of ice, and when they pull these cores out they can tell a great deal about the atmosphere many years ago. By studying the gases contained in bubbles of air trapped in the layers, they can determine, in particular, changes in the concentration of carbon dioxide and in the temperature. The way they get that information, I am told, is by studying the chemical composition of the different forms of oxygen, a technique that turns out to be quite an accurate thermometer. Just as foresters can read tree rings, these scientists can read ice cores.

You could then take that data and plot the earth's temperature and the concentration of carbon dioxide in our atmosphere against time measured in tens of thousands of years—back to 160,000 years ago. The line representing temperature would show a significant drop during the two ice ages, as well as a significant increase during the period of great warming in between them. Such a graph would also show the fluctuations in the concentration of carbon dioxide, from 190 parts per million during the ice ages to almost 300 parts per million during the warming interval. And you'd see that in the modern era, both lines would start climbing, inexorably and at an ever-increasing rate.

I would like to make two points about this graph, if you can picture it. First, if you looked closely at those two lines—temperature and carbon dioxide levels—you'd see that the two lines seem to rise and fall together. If that classmate of mine in the sixth grade who noticed the complementary shapes of Africa and South America could see these lines, he'd say they "fit together." The precise way they fit together is complex, but the most salient fact is that higher levels of carbon dioxide have led to higher temperatures.

The second important point that could be made by such a graph is that because of the new powers that we human beings gained during the science and technology revolution, we're dramatically increasing the levels of carbon dioxide and other greenhouse gases in our atmosphere. In the graph I've described, the two lines would be rising at a nearly vertical pitch on the far right. It's going to be very hard to keep those increases from continuing; some people are saying they will go much higher still.

Here is the ethical question that I alluded to earlier: If the world's scientific community tells us we are now having a discernible impact on the Earth's climate, and if there is no disagreement whatsoever that continued accumulations of greenhouse gases will drive temperatures upward, is it ethical to assume that this isn't going to cause any serious problems?

I think it is reckless. In medicine, there is an ethical prohibition against reckless human experimentation. I believe this is a reckless experiment with the climatological balance that has existed for the entirety of human civilization. This isn't right, and we need to confront it.

This is also a medical question. Physicians for Social Responsibility, a group that was formed to awaken doctors and the public to the health consequences of the nuclear arms race, is now responding to the issue of global warming. They are working to educate physicians about the health effects of global climate change, and they have launched a series of televised public service announcements about climate change that has already aired in 28 states. They are now circulating a letter that has been signed by more than 1,000 physicians, including four Nobel laureates. The letter is on the importance of global climate change to our environmental health.

Studies show that the impact of global warming on public health can be quite severe. Changing temperatures can have a direct impact on the spread of infectious diseases. Insects that carry disease organisms may now move into areas that were once too cold for them to survive in. Diseases like malaria and dengue fever, to mention just two, are historically associated with the tropics but are now making their way north.

To take one example: In August 1995, a 31-year-old Michigan resident contracted malaria in suburban Detroit. Nobody can say whether it was caused by the warming of the climate, but during the month when he contracted malaria, the average evening temperature exceeded the 30-year average by nearly six full degrees. It might not be coincidental that 1995 has now been officially declared the warmest year since modern records have been kept.

Global warming is also making an impact on our national heritage. Let me use two examples here. Recent reports show that global warming is having an adverse effect on New England's White Mountains by disrupting the fall foliage season. The reasons for this are complicated and have to do with warmer nighttime temperatures and the way they affect the emergence of color and the persistence of bright color in the leaves. This warming is also causing a decline in maple syrup production, a shortened ski season, a dramatic decrease in trout habitats, and severe changes in the productivity of the timber industry. These effects should command our attention, and we all should respond.

Again, to put this in the context of the larger changes taking place, think of the same challenge in connection with another topic at this symposium—recent developments in genetics. The emergence of our new power to change genes offers exciting new prospects, but, as with the other issues, simultaneously creates new ethical dilemmas.

I've always been fond of Thomas Jefferson's statement that our laws and institutions must go hand in hand with the progress of the human mind. President Clinton signed legislation in 1996 to prevent insurers from using genetic information as a preexisting condition to deny or limit health insurance for our citizens. We are supporting legislation to guarantee that those who are self-employed, or who otherwise buy insurance for themselves, will not lose or be denied health insurance because they have certain mutated genes. New legislation we're trying to pass through Congress right now will prevent health insurance plans from using genetic information in any way when determining premiums. We are going to issue a report this fall [1997] detailing our recommendations for preventing genetic discrimination in the workplace—such as using genetic information in hiring or setting salaries or disclosing it without the permission of the individual.

Resolving moral and ethical questions like the ones raised by genetics and global warming will be a major challenge for all of us in the years directly ahead. And that leads me to the final of the three factors that have combined to transform our relationship to the Earth. This last factor, which is the most subtle, but in many ways more significant, is a philosophical shift in the way some view our responsibility to the future. I believe that we need a willingness to work together to insist that when new discoveries emerge, we take the time to carefully analyze the ethical and moral implications of those discoveries and to demand that those implications be taken into account.

Where climate change is concerned, President Clinton and I advocate that the United States go to the international meeting in Kyoto in December [1997] and work for realistic, binding limits on the emissions of greenhouse gases. We will emphasize approaches that are flexible and market-based to create and maintain opportunities to develop the most cost-effective solutions. We are working to develop new energy technologies, and we've asked the leading experts from academia and industry to conduct an intensive review of all of our energy research and development programs, to be completed by October 1 [1997], with recommendations to help us shape a new national energy strategy.

We cannot ever forget what all of the new abilities in human civilization are really for in the first place: to improve our lives and our livelihoods; to improve our health and our well-being; to unlock more of the secrets to longer, fuller, and happier lives on this Earth.

I suspect that it is that prospect—as much as the search for knowledge itself—that drives most of the discoveries that have been made here at Dartmouth and at other, similar institutions. I am pleased that Dartmouth is holding this symposium and, in keeping with its long-standing commitment to bioethics, is taking the time to reflect deeply on the challenges that lie ahead. If science is to achieve its full potential, it must always be fused with ethics and morals and a broader sense of society.

Today's challenges would have been totally unimaginable to Nathan Smith and the faculty of your Medical School two centuries ago: the growth of our population; global warming and climate disruption; the threat of discrimination based on the new discoveries about an individual's fundamental genetic makeup.

These and other challenges are brand new and very difficult. If we are to meet them—as we have met other challenges throughout the course of this nation's history —we have to look at medicine and medical ethics in new and different ways.

This symposium is an important and honorable mark of that process.

World Population Session: The Crisis of Human Crowding

Introduction to the Session

MICHAEL S. TEITELBAUM

Program Officer, Alfred P. Sloan Foundation, New York, New York 10111-0242, USA

I've been asked to moderate this session, which deals with long-term trends in health and population, environment, and migration. I want to kick it off by noting very briefly two striking points: The first is that an American medical school would have the breadth of perspective to include these topics in its bicentennial symposium. These are not topics normally found in the medical curriculum, but they do have powerful connections to trends in mortality and in fertility, and in both directions of causation. This fact alone should reinforce the picture of exceptionalism that I believe correctly has been applied to the Dartmouth Medical School and to the organizers of this symposium.

Second, I want to note the remarkable fact that at least one leading American politician, Vice President Al Gore, who spoke here on these matters, has developed deep personal understanding of these issues. These are matters, as you will see in all of the presentations during this session, that operate not over the next election cycle, but over many decades, indeed perhaps over centuries. And American politics functions on a time horizon of at most a few years—some would say next Monday morning. So it is quite fitting that this particular vice president should have been invited to speak here.

Let me now ask you to consider the world at the time that Nathan Smith was founding this medical school in 1797. At that time, the world's population numbered less than one billion humans. Now [1997] it is nearly 5.9 billion. The main driving force of this six-fold increase over that 200-year period has been a remarkable decline in mortality. It has been caused by a complex of factors: mainly by sanitation and public health initially; by improved nutrition and prosperity; by political stability, whatever you think of the 20th century; and by preventive medicine and the control of infectious diseases. All of these issues will be dealt with in the presentations to follow.

Dr. Nils Daulaire of the U.S. Agency for International Development will talk about health and population policies. Then I will recount the bizarre intellectual history of debates about population issues. Third, you will hear from Dr. Thomas Homer-Dixon on the links among population, environment, and human ingenuity. And finally, Dr. Hania Zlotnik of the United Nations will speak on the powerful forces of international migration. It is striking to me that the four members of this panel represent a kind of North American free-trade area: two Americans, one Canadian, and one Mexican national.

Global Health, Population Growth, and United States Policy

NILS M.P. DAULAIRE[a]

Chief Health Policy Advisor, U.S. Agency for International Development, Washington, D.C., USA

We are here to consider the ethical and social issues arising out of advances in the biomedical sciences. Our conference organizers have put together a masterful progression, from the *micro* to the *macro*—from molecular genetics, to cellular neurology, to systems of domestic health-care delivery, and finally to considerations on a global scale.

How many powers of ten have we traversed?

The common theme running through all these presentations has been our responsibility as health-care professionals to use the exponentially increasing powers of biomedical knowledge and analysis for human good.

Vice President Gore in his address repeatedly stressed the ethical and moral framework that must underlie any serious consideration of policy. That issue is starkly highlighted when we confront the question of global population growth, a growth in human numbers from two billion to nearly six billion in the space of his lifetime, when it took the 10 thousand human generations before him to reach two billion. I will leave projections into the future, and their implications for global well-being, to the presenters who follow me.

I will focus instead on the issues of today and the very near future: the realities faced by a majority of the world's people; the potential contributions of the biomedical sciences to deal with these problems; and our ethical and moral responsibilities both as physicians and as citizens of the world's most powerful and affluent society. Let me describe how these considerations underlie United States policy on global health and population.

I start with a fundamental teaching we learn as physicians: *primum non nocere*—first, do no harm. Are advances in the biomedical sciences over the past century responsible for the explosive growth in human numbers that threatens to swamp the earth's carrying capacity? Have we done harm?

This question has been widely debated and thoroughly analyzed, and the answer is a strong but qualified *no*: health care as we traditionally define it has had an effect on overall population growth only at the margins. Without question, population growth has come through increasing survivorship in the context of continued high birth rates, but the largest contributors to this improved survival have derived from increasing economic productivity and trade, from increasing food production and distribution, and from broad public-health measures such as improved sanitation and immunization programs. Individual, curative health care directed at a specific illness in the individual has played only a very small role in this trend.

---

[a]Present address: President and Chief Executive Officer, Global Health Council, 20 Palmer Court, White River Junction, Vermont 05001.

So if we are not responsible for the current state of affairs, do we have any responsibility at all?

Again, as physicians we are taught that it is our obligation to turn our knowledge to the benefit of those who need it and can benefit from it. And in this sense, our current and potential contribution is vast. In my role as a policy-maker at the U.S. Agency for International Development, I have been asked whether the goals of stabilizing global population and of improving health are not in fact contradictory. I firmly believe that they are not, and that we can deal with them using a consistent ethical and moral approach.

I would like to share a personal experience that helps to illustrate some of the fundamental issues underlying this question:

When I had finished my medical school training, but before I started my internship, I had the good fortune to be able to work for several months in a rural clinic in Bangladesh. Given the scarcity of their resources, I was treated as a full-fledged doctor and had a wide range of clinical responsibilities. My favorite was obstetrics.

As a medical student I had delivered several dozen babies and found those to be the happiest and most positive of my clinical experiences. You start with one patient in pain and distress and end with two persons who are happy and healthy.

In my third week on duty call in Bangladesh, I was summoned to our crude operating theater to see a woman in labor. The patient was a 19-year-old mother of two experiencing her third pregnancy. She had been brought to the clinic on an oxcart by her husband, a trip that had taken them five hours from their remote village. After an uneventful pregnancy she had begun labor six days earlier; had been attended at home, as is the custom in most of the developing world; and for the past two days had been increasingly febrile and exhausted, with no movement from the baby. As is generally the case in much of the developing world, her husband did not bring her to the clinic until traditional approaches had been exhausted and he was afraid she was going to die.

A rapid assessment required only the most primitive and fundamental sense organ —the odor of anaerobically putrefying flesh filled the operating theater. The patient was unconscious, with a high fever, shallow and rapid respirations, and a thready pulse of over 150. It required little clinical acumen to know that this woman had suffered an obstructed labor, that her baby had died in the process and was decomposing, and that she herself was severely septic as a consequence.

I quickly prepped her for an emergency delivery, but within a minute of getting her on the table she suffered a grand mal seizure, and her respirations and pulse ceased. Efforts at resuscitation were unsuccessful, and a few minutes later I had to inform her husband that she had died before I could deliver her baby. He was calm in the face of this news, but he told me he could not take her home for burial unless the baby was extracted, and so for the next hour I undertook this task, piece by piece. In the process, I discovered that the young woman's uterus had ruptured during labor and that the child had died in her peritoneal cavity, spreading infection everywhere.

With my grizzly task finally done, I returned to the husband. He was waiting outside with his two young children, both girls—one barely 15 months old, the other three years old—and with the younger sister of the woman who had died; she was perhaps 14 years old.

The husband's first question to me was "Was it a boy child?" I told him that as far as I could tell it was not. He shook his head and said that in that case it was probably just as well—his wife could only have given him more girl children.

The story of her short life, as I pieced it together from her husband and sister, was typical for much of the developing world today, as it would have been typical here in the Upper Valley when Dartmouth Medical School was founded 200 years ago. Never schooled, married at 14, pregnant for the first time at 15, her husband eager for a male child, she had worn herself out before she reached the age of 20. I asked her sister whether she had considered family planning, which was available through the clinic where I worked. Her sister, shyly, said that she knew her sister did not want to be pregnant again, but that these things were in the hands of God and of her husband. There was nothing she could have done to prevent it.

But the story doesn't end there. Eight weeks later, the younger of the two daughters was brought back to the clinic. She had been thin when I saw her before, but now she was totally wasted and wrinkled. She was brought by the wife's younger sister, who said that the father had already made arrangements for a new marriage, and that without a mother to care for her, the child had been fed only thin gruel since the mother's death. The little girl had had persistent diarrhea for the past month and by the time she came to the clinic was severely dehydrated.

Again, biomedical science had limited impact. I had had her on an IV for less than an hour before she died.

As we are taught to do in our medical training through clinico-pathological conferences and grand rounds, I tried to piece together the underlying causes of these two linked deaths, and what interventions might have resulted in different outcomes.

The hard facts of the case forced me to recognize that at the foundation of these deaths lay the status and condition of women and girls in Bangladesh. Had the mother been given the opportunity for even a basic education so that she could read and write, and thereby have some idea of what options might be available in her life and some idea of how to seek out these options; had her marriage and first pregnancy taken place at a later age; had either of these two victims been more highly valued in their society—the outcome for both her and her daughter would in all likelihood have been different.

If she had had access to family planning services and contraceptives in a way that she could understand and use, she might well have avoided the unintended pregnancy that killed her, and she might have delayed the prior pregnancy that left her second daughter so frail and vulnerable.

If even rudimentary maternal and child health services had been available, her high-risk situation—her third pregnancy within three years, all before the age of 19 —could have been identified and closer follow-up instituted. Even rudimentary links between the village setting and adequate clinical services might have taken note of her obstructed labor and gotten her to a place where a safe delivery could have been carried out before she became severely septic.

As for her daughter, again the underlying cause of her death was the closely spaced pregnancies that did not allow for a sufficient period of breast-feeding and a mother who was nutritionally depleted. Ironically, family planning could have saved this young child's life. Poverty and inadequate food kept her nutritional state marginal until she lost her mother, at which point her lack of reserves turned her lack of care into a terminal condition. Poor sanitation and widespread contamination of food and water made her a ready candidate for infectious diarrhea. And again, the poor linkage between village and clinical services meant that she did not get clinical care when it might have affected her outcome.

This small pair of personal tragedies is not unique. In fact, it illustrates the most widespread set of health issues in the world.

Let me put this in context. We sit today on the crest of the largest human wave in history. The number of children born in this generation will not only be the largest number ever yet born; if projections are correct, they will be the largest generation there will ever be. So what we do now has tremendous downstream potential.

Every year, nearly 140 million children are born—today alone almost 400,000. Surveys from around the world show that as many as 40% of these pregnancies are unintended and not desired by the women who bear them. And this is in addition to the estimated 50 million unwanted pregnancies a year that are terminated by abortion, most of them in situations where abortion is both illegal and extremely unsafe, and where women put their lives at risk through a considered decision that they do not want to carry this pregnancy to term. Whatever one's moral views on abortion, this is a public-health crisis that we as health professionals must address.

Most of this could be prevented. Surveys show that between 100 million and 150 million couples around the world would like to limit or space their families, but do not yet have access to reliable family planning services. This is despite the fact that biomedical science has provided us with increasingly effective contraceptives, with diminishing side effects, that are currently being used by nearly 300 million couples around the world.

Could we not do better?

As with the woman I described to you, pregnancies—particularly early, multiple, and closely spaced pregnancies—pose the highest health risk these women will face throughout their lifetimes. In the United States, 12 of every 100,000 women who become pregnant will die as a consequence, a figure we find unacceptable, and which we look to reduce. In the poorest countries of the developing world, that risk is 60 times higher—a level of 700 or more maternal deaths for every 100,000 births. Combine these high risks with the large number of pregnancies per woman, and in places I have worked over the past two decades one of every dozen women entering marriage will not survive the consequence of her own fertility.

This year, 580,000 women will die as a direct consequence of pregnancy and childbirth; today alone, over 1,500.

And what about their children? The highest risk period in life is infancy and early childhood. This year, more than 12 million children under the age of five will die, almost 35,000 today. Most of these deaths are due to diarrhea, pneumonia, and malaria, infectious diseases readily treated with our modern biomedical technology. But too often that technology is unavailable where it is most needed. Of course, underlying many of these deaths is weakened resistance due to chronic malnutrition, which lies coiled like a serpent at the heart of poverty.

You certainly do not need to be a physician to recognize that sex is the ultimate cause of pregnancy, both intended and unintended. Over the past few decades we have seen the emergence of an enormous new threat due to sex: HIV and AIDS.

Let me underline how we must view HIV in the developing world differently from HIV in the U.S. First, because the principal mode of transmission of this disease is different: approximately 85% of infections in the developing world are transmitted through heterosexual intercourse, while that accounts for a minority of transmission in the West. HIV/AIDS is, in most of the world, a classic sexually transmitted disease.

As it spreads its reach, this year nearly six million people will become infected; more than 16,000 today. Who is the typical person who will be infected with HIV this year? She will be a young woman in sub-Saharan Africa or Asia, in her twenties, married, with several children, who has throughout her entire life had sexual relations with only one person: her husband. She has not made so-called lifestyle choices, and yet she—and her children—will nonetheless be the principal victims. By the year 2010, more than 40 million of these children will have lost one or both parents, creating the largest cohort of orphans in history. The impact on individuals and on their societies will be enormous.

The recent good news in the U.S. concerning effective treatment of infected patients is a hollow promise in the developing world, where the drug costs of treating a single patient would deplete the entire annual health budget of most medium-sized towns. Of the nearly six million people infected this year in Africa and Asia, virtually all will die of AIDS within the next decade. Expensive drugs and complex therapeutic regimens, no matter how effective in our own context, will do nothing to help these people. So the second major difference in contrast to the U.S. is the recognition that the only practical way to deal with this epidemic in the developing world is through preventive strategies, both behavioral, and—of critical importance from the biomedical standpoint—through the development of a vaccine that can be used effectively and affordably in the developing world. The new AIDS Vaccine Initiative offers the first glimmer of hope in this area.

I have described some enormous challenges, challenges that can truly be termed *macro*. For years their very scope has caused people to throw up their hands at the hopelessness of the task.

But we have the means to deal with these challenges, and much of the contribution can and should come from the biomedical sciences.

For 20 years I have seen the positive side of the sad story I have shared with you:

- A growing recognition on the part of young couples around the world of the value to themselves of smaller families.

- Increasing commitment and capacity on the part of health services for active outreach to communities.

- Locally tailored strategies for reaching even those far from hospitals and clinics.

- The development of appropriate technological solutions—often low-tech rather than high-tech—for the challenging conditions in which biomedical solutions have to be applied.

- Testing and validation of approaches to diagnosis and care of major diseases that recognize the fact that it is not doctors but rather health workers with limited education and training who are most often there when they are needed.

- Health education that informs and empowers mothers to improve their children's and their own health.

- The discovery of new health-care approaches that have dramatically reduced mortality, such as supplementation of children's diets with high-dose vitamin A capsules—shown to reduce child mortality by one-quarter.

- The growing involvement of the indigenous private sector in meeting some of these needs, such as pharmacies in the remotest corners of the world that now have begun to sell basic contraceptives and essential, low-cost pharmaceuticals.

- And, perhaps most fundamentally, seeing the growing value of girl children, and of the importance of education to their lives.

On the basis of the statistics I have shared with you and of my two decades of experience in the developing world, it was clear to me when I joined the U.S. Agency for International Development in 1993 that there was an ethically and morally compelling case for a coherent set of policy principles and that these principles could in fact be practically carried out in the real world.

Subsequently, we have put these policy principles in place in our foreign assistance programs under five basic tenets:

(1) That no woman should have to become pregnant unless she wishes to bear a child.

(2) That no woman should be put at risk of death as a consequence of pregnancy.

(3) That no family should have to face the needless death of a young child.

(4) That no person should have her or his life placed at risk as a consequence of responsible sexual activity.

(5) And that no person, and particularly no woman, should enter adulthood without the basic educational skills that will enable her to become a part of our global society.

Vice President Gore mentioned the importance of the 1994 Cairo Conference—the International Conference on Population and Development—in helping to make this into a global consensus. His leadership played an important role in that conference's successful outcome, and I was privileged to serve in the capacity of principal U.S. negotiator on the health aspects of that Program of Action.

The tenets I have cited have now been globally accepted, under the broad categories of reproductive health, child health, and basic education.

Let me stress what is categorically rejected in such a set of principles: the idea that we, the affluent societies of the North, must somehow act to control the population growth of the poor societies of the South. Or that governments should have the authority to control through coercive means population growth within their countries.

Population control—even "for their own good"—is not an ethically and morally acceptable concept, especially for physicians whose first responsibility is to the well-being of their individual patients. Yet I have heard the term used repeatedly and erroneously as a synonym for voluntary family planning, or as a sobriquet to tarnish all our efforts used by those who oppose family planning altogether. I urge you to consider its implications and strike this phrase from your lexicon.

There is solid evidence that building programs based on the five positive ethical principles I have described, in the context of a clear strategy to reduce poverty and hunger, leads to declines in both birth and death rates. In Bangladesh, for example, where I began my own journey 21 years ago, the average family size at that time was nearly six and a half children, and one of every seven children born did not survive to its fifth birthday. Today, after two decades of concerted international efforts to make available basic maternal and child health services, including a wide variety of contraceptives to meet differing needs, the average family size has dropped to fewer than three and a half and is continuing to drop, and child mortality has been cut nearly in half. This achievement has bettered the lives of millions of poor Bangladeshis, and has been a consequence of their own choices and decisions supported by basic health services.

Even in Africa, long considered to be entrenched in the ideal of large families, we are now seeing dramatic declines in fertility rates in places like Kenya, where concerted attention has been paid to developing services that meet people's needs, not those that tell them what they should do.

What are our ethical and moral imperatives as biomedical professionals in the face of these challenges?

We heard yesterday from Professor Edelman about the incredible individuality of the human being. This has profound implications. It means that we must deal with the four billion human beings living in the developing world not as an amorphous, interchangeable mass, but as individuals, each with unique potential and inherent value. But as physicians we already know this. The fact that they are far away, or out of sight, does not lessen their human importance.

Because of that, we must consider the implications of biomedical developments not just from the standpoint of what is possible scientifically, but from the standpoint of what can improve the lives of these people.

We cannot ignore their poverty, or the fact that the average health-care expenditure by the governments of the developing world generally is less than two dollars per person per year. We risk using our magician's wand to increase the distance between the medical haves and have nots, rather than lifting the latter to levels that will allow them a solid basis for their lives.

So our biomedical solutions must be affordable, if not today then in the foreseeable future:

- Contraceptives that increase the ability of women and their partners to choose when and if they become pregnant, that have minimal side effects, and that cannot be imposed against their wishes.

- Answers to the highest pregnancy risks—hemorrhage, obstructed labor, infection—which do not require high-tech medical centers and which can be made available through paraprofessionals found where the people are.

- Inexpensive vaccines and pharmaceuticals for children that protect them from the principal infectious disease risks they face, available in a form that can stand up to heat and humidity, transportation and storage, and administration by health personnel with very limited training and skills.

- Vaccines and other preventive technologies and approaches targeted on HIV transmission that can be widely and effectively applied in the poorest communities of the world.

We are on the crest of the largest generation in human history. It is fortuitous that we are also on the verge of decoding the human genome, of deepening our understanding of the human mind, and of appreciating in a concrete fashion the unique potential of each human being. While two billion of our fellow humans live in deep poverty, they do not live in hopelessness. There are fewer hungry people today than there were two decades ago, the lowest proportion of the world's population ever living in poverty, and remarkable signs of economic growth and vitality from all regions of the world.

Now is the time to welcome them in: to share the full benefits of our scientific knowledge, and to all share with each other the benefits of our diverse and unique human ingenuity.

Science and Polemics on Population

MICHAEL S. TEITELBAUM

Program Officer, Alfred P. Sloan Foundation, New York, New York 10111-0242, USA

An alternative title for this presentation could be "Visions of Progress, Specters of Apocalypse" because those characterizations have been often applied to discussions of population trends. Different writers have described population growth, on the one hand, as the very engine of human ascent, leading to a state that transcends all other life forms, and, on the other hand, as a fatal flaw of the human species, leading to its self-destruction. We have been buffeted by extreme visions—from the gloomy images of the Reverend Thomas Malthus and some modern environmentalists to the enthusiastic pronatalism of early utopians, old-line Marxists, and modern-day supply-siders of the New Right: excess and dearth, vigor and decay, boom and bust. Within the past half-century alone, American polemics on this subject have gone full circle, a complete 360 degrees. Opinions have lurched from alarms about "race suicide" in the 1930s, to the "population bomb" fears of the 1970s, and most recently to anxiety about an alleged "birth dearth."

Given such extreme images of despair and euphoria about human population growth, many of us might be surprised to learn that there is, in fact, a substantial consensus—a scientific consensus of a far more moderate character—as to the underlying effects. Let me give you a very quick tour of the subject.

At the dawn of the industrial revolution in the 18th century, there were about 770 million human beings living on Earth. As of 1997, the estimated population has reached nearly 5.9 billion. The pattern was one of only gradual increase in the early part of that period, followed by an acceleration in growth during the time since World War II. This was an acceleration so dramatic as to have produced a virtual discontinuity with all past human history. The truth is that the bulk of all human demographic growth since the emergence of the species has occurred within the lifetime of everyone here.

One way to illustrate the exceptional nature of this recent period is to look at the spans between successive billions of living human beings. It took millions of years of human existence to reach the first billion; by happenstance, this occurred at about the time this medical school was being founded in 1797. It took over a century more to reach the second billion; another 33 years to reach the third billion; about 14 more years for the fourth billion; and 13 years for the fifth billion. The six-billion landmark should be reached in roughly a 12-year interval, about a year from now [1998]. And there has been a similar trajectory for the U.S. population. In 1797, there were about five million Americans. In 1997, there are about 268 million. The primary cause of this increase has been a remarkable acceleration in mortality control, sanitation, and public health.

Sometime in the late 1960s, about two decades after the onset of that post-war acceleration in population growth, there was what could be described as a global point of demographic inflection. As Dr. Daulaire has said, most demographers and other analysts believe that this point of inflection will prove to have been an all-time peak in annual increase for the species—about 2% for the world as a whole. Over the ensuing decades this global rate of increase has drifted very slowly downward. Currently it appears to be about 1.5%. As Dr. Daulaire noted, this decline did not result from an increase in mortality but rather from sustained declines in fertility. Nonetheless, the decline in the global population growth *rate*—while it is significant, because it represents a reversal of a very long-term trend of accelerating rates of population growth—has not been of sufficient size to reverse the trend of absolute, *numerical* population growth. The annual increment in the world population continues to rise owing to the momentum of population growth, which lasts for 30 to 50 years after fertility declines take place.

From the perspective of science, or demographic analysis, there is substantial agreement about the broad outlines of population change. It is in the interpretation where there is disagreement, and that's mainly what I intend to talk about—the human significance of these issues. This subject encompasses an intellectual tradition that is breathtaking in its sweep and diversity. It stretches from Plato through medieval theology and encompasses all the major intellectual and political themes since the 18th century—the views of the mercantilists, physiocrats, classical economists, Malthusians, Marxians, and more recently, supply-siders and libertarians of the New Right. Then, superimposed upon these intellectual and political traditions (and perhaps important to the level of energy with which those positions have been espoused) have been differing religious views as to the acceptability of various human techniques of fertility regulation. For example, Mother Teresa, who just died, was a strong opponent of what she considered to be artificial contraception and, of course, abortion.

Although I must oversimplify some of these positions here, you will see that four general points stand out. The first is that recent debates have, in substantial measure, repeated and recapitulated arguments that go back 200 years. Second, perspectives on demographic change have been deeply entwined with leading political, economic, scientific, and religious theories of the period. Third, the intellectual history of the subject is littered with mistakes and misunderstandings; with the animosities and personal quirks of the protagonists; with extraordinarily strange bedfellows—people who would not otherwise speak to one another agree on these kinds of issues; with ironic zigs and zags; and with political and religious dogma encrusted upon everything. And fourth, many vocal advocates of the most recent period seem blissfully unaware of past debates; in some cases, they are quite unaware of similarities between positions they are strenuously arguing now, and those drawn from ideological perspectives that they despise.

I mentioned that theorizing about population goes back at least to Plato. Plato advocated an optimum population size of 5,040 citizens, with that size to be maintained by conscious birth control. But let us skip past that period, since Plato's prescription was never embraced by anyone, to my knowledge.

The modern debate begins with the mercantilists. These thinkers dominated European economic and political thought from the 16th to the 18th century. The mercantilists viewed people as the basic resource of the state, of the monarchy —a position that should not be surprising, since they lived in the aftermath of the demographic disaster of the Black Death, but before the emergence of steam power. People then were seen primarily as producers rather than as consumers, and people, particularly men, were critical determinants of military power. In the words of

Frederick the Great: "The number of the people makes the wealth of states." This view, combined with the centralizing tendencies of these monarchists, was used to justify state interventions aimed at increasing fertility, and at discouraging the departure of subjects by prohibiting out-migration.

Mercantilist thinking ultimately gave way to two streams of thought based on profoundly different world views: that of the 18th-century utopians and that of the physiocrats and classical economists. The utopians are a very interesting group of thinkers who included among their number the father, Daniel, of the Reverend Thomas Robert Malthus. They embraced the population optimism of the mercantilists, but within a very different set of ideas about human progress and perfectibility. Like the mercantilists, utopians believed that population size was the principal factor determining the amount of resources. But the utopians saw a perfected humankind as requiring no coercive institutions such as police, law, property, or family. Moreover, they advocated a society in which the resources produced by the population's labor would be held in common by all persons. Hence progress was consistent with any level of population.

Meanwhile, the physiocrats favored an approach they termed *laissez faire.* They were strongly opposed to state interventions, such as those of the mercantilists. Moreover, the physiocrats saw economic surplus as attributable to land rather than to labor, as the mercantilists maintained. Hence for the physiocrats, growth in the number of workers could not increase national wealth; only growth in usable land could. For both of these reasons they opposed pronatalism, or promotion of higher fertility, by the monarchies of the day. And physiocrats such as François Quesney argued that human multiplication should not be encouraged to a size beyond what could be sustained without widespread poverty.

In a way, these physiocrats were the first scientists of population. They made, for the first time, extensive use of pioneering data and analyses that had just been developed and that for the first time made possible quantitative assessment of population size and rates of growth and mortality.

The classical economists, such as Adam Smith and David Ricardo, were heavily influenced by these physiocrats. Land was one of three factors of production for the classical economists, but unlike the other two, labor and capital, land was of fixed supply. Thus, they said, there would inevitably be decreasing returns to inputs of labor and capital, and hence limits on the scale of both food production and industrial activity. They shared with the physiocrats a belief in the optimal role of free markets —*laissez-faire* versus state intervention.

The truth is that none of the classical economists anticipated the Industrial Revolution, which was incipient as they were writing. The sweeping technological advances of this revolution would transfer economic activity from the land to raw materials such as coal, and would increase the agricultural productivity of the land, lower mortality, and ultimately lower fertility, not by marriage deferment but by conscious fertility regulation within marriage. None of them anticipated these powerful trends that were clearly under way.

One of the leading classical economists was Thomas Malthus, son of the utopian Daniel. He was a close friend of Ricardo's and eventually became the central figure in the population debate of the 19th and 20th centuries. His first venture in this field was a hastily written polemic published in 1798 and entitled "An Essay on the Principle of Population as it Affects the Future Improvement of Society, with Remarks on the Speculations of Mr. Godwin, Monsieur Condorcet, and other Writers." (The "other writers" included his father.) For Malthus, human welfare could not be furthered if the fundamental biological capacity for population growth was not subjected to conscious restraint. It was a polemic, this first essay. His position was easy to misrepresent, and his equally polemical critics misrepresented it with gusto. And there the matter might have rested, as another polemical footnote to intellectual history, had the criticisms he received not provoked Malthus to undertake a more careful and deliberate study, based on data. He had hypothesized in his essay that a country with plentiful land (remember, land was seen as the source of prosperity) relative to its population would experience rapid population growth unrestrained by high mortality. And so he sought data in the land-rich country of the period, the United States. On the basis of the sparse data he had, he estimated that this population, which was then small, was doubling itself in less than 25 years. Surprisingly, since the data were poor, that turns out to have been pretty close to the truth. Malthus argued that in settings lacking the United States' unusual richness of natural resources, a rapid population increase would be constrained by what he termed the "positive checks" of sickly seasons, epidemics, pestilence, and plague. Unless, he added, "prudential restraints" were practiced. What did he recommend? The prudential restraint he advocated was drawn from the experiences of Western Europe, which had a pattern of very late marriage. He termed this "moral restraint." He was also aware of other potential preventive checks and alluded to them—promiscuity, prostitution, homosexuality, birth control, and abortion. But he forcefully rejected these checks, which, as an Anglican curate, he considered to be immoral vices:

> Promiscuous intercourse, unnatural passions, violations of the marriage bed, and improper arts to conceal the consequences of irregular connections, are preventive checks that clearly come under the head of vice.[1]

And again:

> I have never adverted to the checks suggested by Condorcet without the most marked disapprobation. Indeed, I should always particularly reprobate any artificial and unnatural modes of checking population, both on account of their immorality, and their tendency to remove a necessary stimulus to industry.[2]

For Malthus, no humane society could ignore the imperative of moral restraint. The alternatives, he said, were the terrible checks of war, famine, and epidemic. He acknowledged that existing welfare, poor laws, and charity were well-intentioned, but he said they might well be counterproductive, because they would increase rather than decrease suffering if they caused their recipients to increase their fertility.

These were provocative arguments, and they led to denunciations of Malthus from all sides. Progressives portrayed him as a reactionary, though the fact is that Malthus was a radical in many ways. He favored then-radical ideas such as free medical assistance for the poor and universal education. And he supported democratic institutions in the context of a great reaction against the French Revolution among the European establishment of which he was a prominent member. Meanwhile, the conservative religious bloc accused him, an Anglican cleric, of blasphemy—despite his traditional opposition to the practices of contraception and abortion. Finally, he was vilified, mostly after his death, by Marx and his followers.

But Malthus did have a major impact on the English Poor Laws, on the ideas of the classical economists, and even on evolutionary biologists. For example, Charles

Darwin referred to Malthus's theorizing as instrumental in his development of the theory of natural selection.

There were followers of Malthus and, as is often the case, his followers deviated significantly from his views. These "neo-Malthusians" accepted his main arguments about the links between high fertility and poverty. However, they rejected his prescription of delayed marriage and his opposition to birth control. Rather than using these arguments from Malthus in support of conservative ideas, the neo-Malthusians, prominent among whom were Charles Bradlaw and Annie Besant, were political and religious radicals. They described themselves as free-thinkers, and saw birth control as an important way to diminish the social inequality experienced by the lower classes. For their efforts, they incurred the wrath of the British political and religious establishment. They were both actually tried, convicted, and jailed for publication of "obscene" materials, specifically, a 40-year-old American text about birth control.

I alluded earlier to a harsh attack made upon Malthus by Karl Marx in the 1860s and 1870s, long after Malthus's death. This attack led to one of the greatest and most persistent ironies in the two-century-old debate about population and resources. Let me give you an idea of the language used by Marx about Malthus:

> Parson Malthus [was] contemptible, [a] plagiarist [and] sycophant of the ruling classes [who spread this] sin against science, [this] vile and infamous doctrine, this repulsive blasphemy against man and nature.[3]

For Marx, the resource limits emphasized by Malthus would arise only under capitalism:

> Every special historical mode of production has its own special laws of population, historically valid within its limits alone. An abstract law of population exists for plants and animals alone, and only in so far as man has not interfered with them.[4]

Almost all that Marx ever said about population is embodied in these two sentences. He never had much to say in a positive sense. Basically, he simply attacked the Malthusians. He also did not seem to think very highly of "parsons." According to Marx:

> [M]ost of the population-theory teachers are Protestant parsons …—Parson Wallace, Parson Townsend, Parson Malthus and his pupil, the arch-Parson Thomas Chalmers, to say nothing of the lesser reverend scribblers in this line.[5]

However, in contrast to other Protestant clergymen, who, Marx said, "generally contribute to the increase of population to a really unbecoming extent," Malthus "had taken the monastic vow of celibacy."[6] The fact that Marx calls Malthus a monastic, celibate priest suggests that he knew little about the person he was attacking, who was, in fact, a married father of three.

In general, these anti-Malthusian views of Marx's were continued and extended by the Marxians who followed him. But there were exceptions. The prominent German Marxist theorist Karl Kautsky did break with this tradition, saying that there was no conflict between Marxism and Malthusian reasoning:

> The sterile rejection of population theory, at least on the part of socialism, is definitely out of place, for the two are not in principle incompatible …. Only a transformation of society can extirpate the misery and vice that today damn nine-tenths of the world to a lamentable existence; but only a regulation of population growth by the most moral means possible, probably the use of contraceptives, can forestall the recurrence of this evil.[7]

Kautsky was put under tremendous pressure by Engels for this apostasy, and eventually he recanted 30 years later.

So by the time of the Russian Revolution, the anti-Malthusian position was well established as Marxian orthodoxy. It now seems rather bizarre, but early in the revolutionary period, in 1921, Lenin promulgated an order legalizing abortion in the Soviet Union as the "right of the woman to control her own body." Yet Lenin opposed contraception as shabby Malthusianism. Apparently Lenin was unaware that Malthus too had opposed contraception. Later, Stalin adopted a pronatalist set of policies as a stimulant to economic progress—which began to sound a bit like the mercantilists. And in the 1930s, these pronatalist policies of Stalin's turned coercive. In parallel with similar measures in Nazi Germany, the Stalinist government banned abortion in the 1930s, even though under Lenin abortion had been seen as a woman's basic human right. To the extent that traditional Marxism-Leninism still exists, its proponents continue to view abortion as a women's rights issue, while contraception continues to be suspect as "Malthusian," thereby perpetuating a century-old mistake.

It was only in the world's largest Marxist-Leninist state, the People's Republic of China, that a new challenge arose to this position. In the 1980s, Chinese leaders began to argue that the very future of socialism in China would depend on draconian state action to bring about sharp declines in fertility. They adopted policies to affect the age of early sexual activity and marriage (the Malthusian notion of moral restraint) and also to affect fertility within marriage by limiting births via contraception (the neo-Malthusian idea) and via abortion (the Leninist idea). So the Chinese put all three together, if you will. In the embrace of Malthusian and neo-Malthusian perspectives, one could hardly imagine a more complete reversal of the traditional Marxist-Leninist stance than what happened in China in the 1980s.

Ironically, there is still another zig and zag to all of this, because just as Marxist-Leninist thinking was being turned on its head by the Chinese, right-wing thinking in the West was moving dramatically toward the old-line Marxist tradition. This was especially true of the New Right, the libertarian thinkers who emerged into visibility in the 1980s. During the Reagan Administration, such arguments, emanating largely from the Heritage Foundation and the Cato Institute, led to a sharp revision in traditional U.S. policy. In 1984, the Reagan White House produced the following statement for the 1984 World Population Conference in Mexico City:

> First and most important, population growth is, of itself, a neutral phenomenon. It is not necessarily good or ill. It becomes an asset or a problem only in conjunction with other factors, such as economic policy, social constraints, need for manpower, and so on.
>
> The population boom [in developing countries] was a challenge; it need not have been a crisis .... [I]t coincided with two negative factors which, together, hindered families and nations in adapting to their changing circumstances.
>
> The first of these factors was governmental control of economies .... One of the consequences of this "economic statism" was that it disrupted the natural mechanism for slowing population growth in problem areas .... That pattern might be well under way in many nations where population growth is today a problem, if counter-productive government policies had not disrupted economic incentives, rewards and advancement. In this regard, localized crises of population growth are, in part, evidence of too much government control and planning, rather than too little.
>
> The second factor that turned the population boom into a crisis was ... an outbreak of anti-intellectualism which attacked science, technology and the very concept of material progress.[8]

This statement's basic argument is that population growth is "neutral," that everything depends on the economic system. Countries with "statist" economic systems will have problems; those with "free markets" will not.

In this revisionist, conservative ideology, precisely as in old-line Marxist writings, population surplus can occur only under incorrect economic policies. Of course, the correct policies of the New Right differ from those promoted by the Old Left. But the structure of the argument is exactly the same. For both, population surplus is only apparent; in reality, it occurs only because the economic system is defective. The correct economic system will both eliminate poverty and generate automatic mechanisms by which fertility will be regulated. Of course the defect for the Marxists is capitalism, and the correct system is socialism; and the defect for the New Right is socialism or economic-statism, and the correct system is free-market capitalism. But the structure of the argument is identical—a similarity about which the New Right's anti-Communist proponents presumably are only murkily aware.

The policies that followed this Reagan Administration analysis were among the first to be reversed by President Clinton. But the debate is still continuing.

Let me try to summarize this convoluted history. The mercantilists saw population as wealth and advocated state intervention to increase both population and wealth. The free-market physiocrats saw land as wealth and rejected the mercantilist interventions. The utopians embraced the optimism about population of the mercantilists, but advocated equitable distribution of resources. The classical economists saw decreasing agricultural returns to labor and capital and advocated free markets. (They anticipated some more recent thinking, by the way; Adam Smith wrote that with free markets, population would automatically regulate itself.) The Malthusians rejected the population optimism of the utopians, but opposed "unnatural" interventions such as contraception. The neo-Malthusians accepted the population pessimism of the Malthusians, but advocated voluntary contraception (they also, by the way, opposed abortion). The Marxist-Leninists embraced the population optimism of the utopians, attacked the Malthusians and the neo-Malthusians, and opposed contraception but embraced abortion. The Chinese Marxists rejected the population optimism of their Marxist-Leninist colleagues and embraced strong state intervention to promote both Malthusian and neo-Malthusian restraint, using both contraception *and* abortion. And finally, the American New Right embraces the population optimism of the utopians, the mercantilists, and the traditional Marxist-Leninists, while it rejects the economic-statism of the Marxist-Leninists and the mercantilists. The New Right shares with traditional Marxists the notion that population size is self-regulating, along with vigorous criticism of Malthus's attribution of poverty to excessive population growth.

So here we have a history that is replete with misunderstanding, bizarre zig-zags, personal animus, passionate rhetoric, and extraordinarily strange ideological bedfellows. This is so even though there is a strong scientific consensus about the demographic facts of the situation. That leads me to quote Edward R. Murrow: "Anyone who isn't confused, doesn't understand the situation."

Historians of the future will be fascinated by the emergence in the late 20th century of an ideology based upon an unlikely amalgam of mercantilism, Marxism, and libertarianism. If nothing else, recent developments prove that whatever scientific research may show, the conclusions of ideologues about population and resource issues are almost impossible to predict.

Let me close with an admonition to these ideologues from Mark Twain, who, as usual, had the best advice: "Get your facts first, and then you can distort them as much as you please."

REFERENCES

1. Quoted by COALE, A.J. "T.R. Malthus and the population trends of his day and ours." Ninth Encyclopedia Britannica Lecture, University of Edinburgh, November 1, 1978.
2. Op. cit.
3. MEEK, R.L., Ed. 1954. Marx and Engels on Malthus. International Publishers. New York.
4. MARX, K. Capital. Vol. 1. p. 693.
5. PETERSEN, W. 1964. The Politics of Population. Doubleday and Co. Garden City, NY.
6. Op. cit.
7. KAUTSKY, K. 1880. The Influence of Population Increase on Social Progress. Boch and Hasback. Vienna. pp. 166-192.
8. United States Policy Statement at the United Nations International Conference on Population and Development. Mexico City. 1984.

Population, Environment, and Ingenuity

THOMAS HOMER-DIXON

Director, Peace and Conflict Studies Program, University of Toronto, University College, Toronto, Ontario M5S 1A1, Canada

I'm going to talk about some of the social consequences of population growth and the natural resource scarcities that sometimes arise from that growth. Most importantly, I'm going to talk about how societies respond to these stresses—demographic stresses and natural resource stresses—and whether they can respond well or not so well.

The previous presentations have set mine up very nicely; you'll see some resonance between those points and what I have to say. I am going to focus on the role of ideas, or what I call ingenuity, in the social adaptation processes that some societies carry out in response to severe population and ecological stresses. I will build a simple theory of social adaptation that is keyed to three core notions: ingenuity requirement, ingenuity supply, and the ingenuity gap between rising requirement and supply.

My argument is that in many cases population and resource stresses increase the *requirement* for ingenuity, while at the same time restricting the *supply* of ingenuity in response to that rising requirement. This leads to what I would call an ingenuity gap—a gap between rising requirements and static or declining supplies of ingenuity. Persistent and serious ingenuity gaps, I would argue, lead to various kinds of social pathologies, including increased poverty, institutional collapse, and ultimately, perhaps, civil violence of various kinds, including rebellion, insurgency, and ethnic violence.

These ideas are derived from work I've done with others over the last seven years on how various kinds of "environmental scarcities" can contribute to civil violence, or violence within society, such as insurgency, rebellion, coups d'état, and ethnic clashes. By environmental scarcity, I mean scarcities of renewable resources: principally croplands, fresh water supplies, forest resources, and fish stocks. Those are the main resources that we've examined. And we've looked principally at developing countries in our research, on the assumption that developing countries would be affected first and worst by the social crises arising from scarcities of such environmental resources. These projects—there have been about four of them all told—have involved around 100 researchers and advisors on four continents, and we have focused in detail on 15 case studies, including the links between water scarcity in the Jordan River Basin and in the Gaza Strip in the Middle East and the chronic Palestinian unrest in that area, a story that's not often told. We have studied how land scarcity in Bangladesh, partly caused by rapid population growth, has contributed to large-scale migrations to certain areas in India such as the states of Assam and Tripura, which in turn have contributed to quite violent ethnic clashes between the incoming migrants and people already in those receiving regions. We have looked at local conflicts over forest resources in Indonesia and at cropland and forest scarcities and their contribution to the Zapatista rebellion in Chiapas, Mexico, in 1994 and 1995.

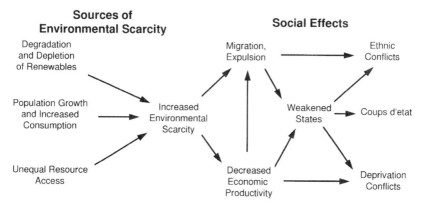

FIGURE 1. Some sources and consequences of environmental scarcity.

Examining all these cases has allowed us to derive a general model for some of the linkages between environmental scarcity and conflict.

FIGURE 1 shows a very simple model of three sources of environmental scarcity: degradation and depletion of renewables, population growth and increased resource consumption, and unequal resource access. The first source of scarcity—degradation and depletion of renewable resources such as cropland, forest supplies, or water supplies—can be thought of as a shrinking of the resource pie, a drop in the supply of the resource. The second—population growth and increased per-capita resource consumption—constitutes an increased demand for the resource. In other words, as population grows, a static quantity of land is divided into smaller and smaller portions for each individual. This is what we call demand-induced scarcity, that is, scarcity that arises from increased demand for the resource. And the third common source of scarcity, something we see in all of the cases we examine, is unequal resource access, wherein some groups or individuals get a disproportionately large slice of the resource pie, while others get too small a slice to meet their subsistence needs.

Our research shows that these three sources of scarcity interact in various ways to produce environmental scarcity. And increased environmental scarcity contributes to various social effects: migrations; decreased economic productivity; weakened social institutions, in particular governments; and, ultimately in some circumstances, various kinds of conflict—ethnic conflicts, coups d'état, and deprivation conflicts, such as insurgency or rebellion. This sort of conflict is diffuse, chronic, and subnational—it is *within* countries, not among countries. It is the kind of subnational conflict that we have seen in places such as Rwanda and Somalia and that our conventional military institutions have the most difficulty containing.

But such conflict does not happen in all societies affected by severe environmental scarcity. In fact, just seeing this model by itself can be a little misleading, because it suggests that there are almost deterministic linkages from scarcity on one side of the diagram across to conflict on the other. But when you do your research, you find that there are many societies where environmental scarcity is severe and where cropland and water supplies are not widely available and yet there is not severe social dislocation, not severe poverty, and, ultimately, not serious conflict. Some societies adjust well and some don't. Whether they adjust well or not is determined by what we call *contextual factors*. Imagine that this diagram is, in a sense, embedded in a sea of other variables that influence the strength or weakness of each arrow in the diagram. This diagram should not be interpreted as representing an inevitable or deterministic model.

One of the arrows is particularly important and has received a great deal of attention, and that is the one between increased environmental scarcity and decreased economic productivity. What is the relationship between scarcity of resources, perhaps induced by population growth, and the production of wealth in a society? Is this link tight or loose? And what are the contextual factors, the particular political, economic, social, institutional, and cultural characteristics of a given society that influence the strength of this link? The debate over that particular question has tended to divide into three camps in recent years, as Michael Teitelbaum has explained. I''ll now give you my own account of the contemporary debate, and you will see a lot of resonance between our points of view.

I would divide the contemporary debate into roughly three camps. The central question is whether increasing resource scarcity limits economic development. The neo-Malthusians answer that question *yes*; they feel that human development is constrained by strict physical limits. The neoclassical economists answer the question *no*; they believe that with the right economic institutions, especially markets, humans can increase their prosperity indefinitely. The third camp is what I call the "distributional" view, and members of this camp would say the question is secondary—what really matters is the social distribution of resources.

This debate, however, is largely sterile. In the United States, for example, although there is vigorous discussion between the protagonists—in particular between the neo-Malthusians such as Paul Ehrlich and neoclassicists such as Julian Simon—they merely go back and forth, lobbing shells, and ultimately nothing seems to be achieved.

We have attempted in our work to move beyond this tripartite and often bipartite debate and take the discussion to a new level. I start by accepting that the neoclassical economists have something important to say. Human beings often exhibit extraordinary ingenuity and creativity in response to the problems they face, especially in the context of markets and market mechanisms. We must not underestimate the power of new ideas to change our world. That was Joseph Goldstein's point yesterday in his introductory remarks to this conference. But what determines the need for and the flow of these new ideas? It turns out that economists have not much to say about that question. In addressing it myself, I began with the concept of ingenuity. By that I mean something quite specific. Ingenuity by my definition consists of ideas applied to solve practical social and technical problems. There are two kinds of ingenuity: social ingenuity and technical ingenuity. Technical ingenuity is what we normally think of when we think of ingenuity. We think of new technologies that address resource scarcities, such as new hybrid grains that can grow in eroded or nutrient-depleted soils. We think of water and fuel conservation technologies, such as stoves that can be used in a village hut to cook food and that consume a lot less fuel.

The other kind of ingenuity is what I call social ingenuity. This is ingenuity in the form of new and reformed institutions and social arrangements within a society. These institutions include clear and enforced property rights, efficient markets that get the right prices for scarce resources, or competent bureaucracies and government agencies. To refer to some of the things that Nils Daulaire talked about in his presentation, social ingenuity can take the form of hospitals, rural clinics, and family-planning extension services in the countryside. Social ingenuity can also take the form of uncorrupt police and judicial systems, of financial agencies that can deliver capital when and where the entrepreneurs who are trying to respond to scarcity need it.

The important thing about this particular model is that the social ingenuity is a prerequisite to technical ingenuity. You need the foundation of institutions, clear property rights, sufficient markets, and uncorrupt police and judicial systems to enforce contracts in order to provide the right incentives for technological entrepreneurs to respond effectively to resource scarcities. In fact, it turns out that the institutional arrangement of a society is probably much more important in determining its adaptability to resource scarcity than the technologies that the society can deploy. That is surprising, because we often think that the best way to respond to resource scarcity is through various kinds of technological fixes. But I would say that institutional responses are often much more powerful, and in any case have to precede the technological response.

It turns out that economists now recognize that something like ingenuity is a central contributor to economic growth in all societies. That idea has been captured by a new subfield in economics called new economic growth theory, or sometimes endogenous growth theory. This field has been pioneered by Paul Romer at Stanford. He asks what the sources of economic growth are. The traditional neoclassical answer focuses on inputs of labor and capital and in some cases on resources such as land and minerals. By "capital," economists mean principally physical capital in the form of factories and physical plants. But in the late 1950s, the economist Robert Solow, who eventually won a Nobel prize for his work, showed that a portion of economic growth cannot by explained by the input of labor and capital. He did a cross-national analysis of many economies, looking at their growth rates and their inputs of labor and capital, and he found in every case that a significant proportion of economic growth could not be accounted for by labor and capital. This "Solow residual," as it came to be known, has caused real problems for neoclassical economists and for traditional growth theory. Solow suggested that it could be accounted for by new technologies within the economy. Others have suggested other things that could account for the Solow residual, and Paul Romer, in particular, has focused on what he calls ideas. I'm persuaded by Paul Romer's argument that ideas are the factor that explains the Solow residual and that ultimately explains a good portion of economic growth and of a society's capacity to produce wealth.

Paul Romer's argument is persuasive, but here I will read just one pithy and succinct sentence he wrote that is particularly important: "Ideas are the instructions that allow us to combine resources in arrangements that are ever more valuable." I find that quite an extraordinary statement. If ideas are important, how can we think about their role in an economy? This is where I've taken Paul Romer's work and the work of other endogenous growth theorists and have focused on two variables—the requirement for ingenuity and the supply of ingenuity. For the rest of my talk, I'm going to discuss briefly the factors that influence both requirement and supply.

On the requirement side, my thesis is very simple—I suggest that worsening environmental scarcities in many parts of the world will drive up the requirement for ingenuity in those regions. About half the world's population depends on local renewable resources for their day-to-day well-being. It's very easy for us to forget this fact in the industrial and postindustrial economy we live within, a society where it's often possible to get to a McDonald's in four minutes. But we have to remember that half the world's population depends upon local water supplies, local fuel supplies, local cropland, and local fish stocks for their day-to-day livelihood and well-being. In fact 60% of the world's population, about four billion people, depends upon traditional fuels such as wood, charcoal, straw, or cow dung, for at least a portion of its cooking and heating energy requirement. Many regions and billions of people around this planet are now affected by multiple scarcities of land, water, forests, and fish. Again, that is something that is relatively easy for those of us in advanced industrial societies to forget. And many of these scarcities are increasing. They are also exhibiting what specialists call "nonlinear effects." In other words, these are complex ecological systems that the societies are embedded in, and constant human pressure on those systems causes them to shift their dynamic suddenly and in unexpected ways. For instance, as forests are gradually removed from a region, you might get a sudden and unexpected result—a so-called "nonlinear shift"— in rainfall patterns due to a change in the hydrological cycles between the land and the atmosphere that produce rainfall. Or you might get nonlinear shifts in the availability of wildlife or in the prevalence of crop pests.

On a global level, human-induced flows of material and energy now rival those of nature around the planet. Yet in the next 25 years, population growth and increased per-capita consumption of renewable resources will double this material and energy throughput. We can therefore assume that current scarcities of renewables will become much worse in some regions in the world, though they're already severe in some areas, especially South Asia, the Sahelian region of Africa, the interior of China, Central America, and the Caribbean. These multiple, faster-paced, and often nonlinear environmental problems increase the complexity, urgency, and unpredictability of the decision-making environment in which problems must be solved. The societies that confront these environmental scarcities are going to have a very large requirement for ingenuity, for sophisticated markets, for sophisticated financial agencies and health facilities, for systems of incentives, and for proactive bureaucracies to allow the societies to respond effectively to scarcity.

So just to summarize my point here, I argue that increased environmental scarcities in some regions of the world will increase the requirement for both new technologies and new forms of institutions and reformed institutions in response to those scarcities.

Now we can turn to the supply side of the problem. When I speak of the supply of ingenuity, I don't mean just the generation of ideas in research laboratories and government think tanks, but also the delivery and implementation of that ingenuity in the real world. Out in rural areas, or in government agencies and institutions or in nongovernmental organizations, supplied or delivered ingenuity is ingenuity that is actually implemented. Optimists such as neoclassical economists often assume that supply responds more or less automatically to demand—that the supply of new ideas in an economy reacts to changes in demand for those new ideas. In terms that economists would use, the supply of ingenuity is infinitely elastic. Or in the vernacular, which the rest of us would use, necessity is the mother of invention. Often these optimists are right—necessity *is* the mother of invention—but not always.

There are four reasons why the optimists may not be right, four factors that can limit the supply of ingenuity— market failure, social friction, capital availability, and constraints on science.

Let's look first at market failure. The key point here is that to have an optimal ingenuity response in an economy—to get the right flow of ingenuity in response to scarcities of land, or water, or energy supplies—you have to have accurate price signals that reflect the scarcity of that resource. If you get inaccurate price signals, you're not going to get the kind of entrepreneurial response that you need to deal with the scarcity problem.

But there are two problems that can inhibit the generation of accurate price signals. The first is that many of the resources we're talking about, such as hydrological cycles and high-seas fisheries, are essentially dynamic; they move around. It's very hard to divide them up into salable and tradable units or to establish property rights for them, so it's hard to establish clear prices for those resources. As a result, dynamic resources tend to be underpriced. The second market-related problem is something economists call negative externalities. These are costs borne by individuals who are not participating directly in the market transactions for scarce resources or the goods and services produced by those resources. So, for example, there might be downstream damage resulting from the consumption or extraction of a resource, as when a logging company takes timber off a hillside in the Philippines, which produces serious erosion that plugs up irrigation systems and hydroelectric reservoirs. But the people who are affected severely by these downstream costs are not participating in setting the prices for the resource, and so the price of the timber does not accurately reflect all the costs that its extraction and consumption entail. So both the dynamic nature of these renewable resources and negative externalities mean that you get inaccurate price signals that do not reflect accurately resource scarcities, and so you get an inadequate supply of ingenuity in response to such resource scarcities. Many economies, in fact just about all economies around the world, are riddled with these kinds of market failures.

The second factor that may limit the supply of ingenuity is what I call social friction. The focus here is on the activity of narrow coalitions, often elite groups, that seek to redistribute resources in their favor. Scarcities of resources can stimulate very aggressive, self-interested behavior on the part of these narrow interest groups, and this can block institutional reform and the flow of social ingenuity in response to resource scarcity.

In Haiti, for example, a country that was entirely forested when the Europeans discovered it in the 15th century, there has been very serious deforestation. Now, only about 4% of its forests remain, and these forests are disappearing at a rate of about 2% a year. This is an economy that depends heavily on fuelwood, especially the rural economy, and a good portion of the urban economy, and the increased scarcity of fuelwood has, of course, driven up fuelwood prices. But the fuelwood and charcoal market is largely controlled by elite groups within Haiti, especially remnants of Papa Doc's *Ton-Ton Macoutes*, basically the paramilitary thugs that he used to control society. These elite groups do not have any interest in seeing the price of charcoal and fuelwood come down, so they often send out thugs to reforestation programs and have them rip up the seedlings in order to sustain the price of fuelwood. Here, scarcity is not stimulating invention, at least not a societally optimal form of invention, but instead is stimulating behavior that blocks the ingenuity that would allow reforestation to take place and the scarcity to be resolved, or at least reduced to a certain extent.

Another example is South Africa. Here, the apartheid system pushed millions of blacks into Bantustans, or tribal homelands, that were often located on some of the worst lands in the region. These blacks, when they were dumped into the Bantustans, were often victims of predatory local governments and chieftains. And because of the lack of capital and lack of local knowledge, the damage to land and forests and water supplies in those Bantustans, such as Transkei, Ciskei, Bophuthatswana, and Venda, was absolutely extraordinary—some of the worst land degradation I've ever seen. As apartheid has collapsed, we've seen the movement of millions of people out of those homelands into cities such as Durban, Johannesburg, Pretoria, and Cape-town, where they live in squatter settlements. And in the cities, these blacks have again relied upon local environmental resources—local streams, local fuelwood supplies, and, in many cases, patches of land beside their huts to grow supplemental food supplies. Those resources are in extremely short supply, and local warlords, especially in the vicinity of Durban, have mobilized their followers in order to seize resources from neighboring groups, often of a different ethnic identity. The result of all this competition has been the collapse of local institutions that regulated the flow of people into these communities and their use of local resources. So once again, we see social friction, a situation where environmental scarcity has stimulated predatory behavior that has interfered with the flow of ingenuity.

The third factor that influences the supply of ingenuity is capital availability. The supply of ingenuity depends on an adequate supply of financial and human capital. Financial capital—money—is important for funding of schools and universities and research laboratories and for greasing the wheels of institutional reform. Let's face it, in a lot of societies it's necessary for political and institutional leaders to have access to capital to buy off potential political opponents as they're trying to reform institutions. And human capital in the form of skilled people is, of course, essential for ingenuity supply. Societies that are facing acute resource scarcities need engineers, scientists, and trained civil servants to respond to those scarcities effectively. Yet many countries facing severe environmental scarcities are very poor and are hemorrhaging human capital—educated people—often to rich countries. For example, between 1985 and 1990, Africa lost 60,000 mid- and senior-level managers. In 1980, sub-Saharan Africa had only 45 scientists and engineers involved in research and development for every million people, compared to almost 3,000 for developed countries. Societies suffering from severe shortages of financial and human capital are going to be able to supply less ingenuity in response to their resource problems.

The fourth and final factor is what I call constraints on science. The presentations that we have heard at this symposium leave one awed by the power of science and technology and by the progress made in recent decades, and no one should underestimate that progress. But we must remember that there are limits to the progress of science and to its ability to solve all the problems we face. Because of their particular relevance to this conference, I'm going to talk briefly about three of these limits.

The first is cognitive limits. Many problems of environmental scarcity and its social consequences involve unimaginably complicated systems that are probably too complex and chaotic to be managed effectively by even the best human minds. The renowned entomologist E.O. Wilson at Harvard has suggested that managing even a relatively simple ecosystem is a bit like trying to unscramble an egg with two spoons.

The tool that we're trying to apply to the problem is too crude and ultimately incapable of doing the job. I think that this is true for many of the problems in poor societies around the world. And cognitive limits are going to be more severe for those poor societies that have inadequate human capital, because the few people who remain are utterly overwhelmed. Kenya, for example, in 1992 had only three Ph.D.-level hydrologists in a country that faces critical water shortages, and they were chronically overwhelmed with work.

A second constraint on science is the increased cost of science as it progresses. The cost of scientific instruments and of training personnel tends to rise as science delves deeper into nature. Many environmental problems that developing countries face will demand quite advanced science, such as molecular biology. And yet the cost of science today is leaving behind poor countries who often cannot afford adequate supplies of even the most basic equipment, such as pipettes and petri dishes, or of even the most important scientific journals.

A third constraint on science is the time lags inherent in scientific progress. Science is cumulative. Scientific knowledge is built in layers, and the theoretical foundation for practical engineering progress can take many years to lay down. The pace of scientific advancement cannot be easily forced, yet the pace of environmental scarcity worldwide is rising. Problems are happening faster, over larger areas, and there is a risk that the scientific solutions to address these problems will arrive too late to be of much help.

So to conclude, if the requirement for ingenuity rises sharply, while the supply of ingenuity falls or remains static, then we can expect a society to face an ingenuity gap—an inability to adapt to its resource scarcities. This is liable to contribute to various kinds of social turmoil, migrations, increased poverty, and, perhaps ultimately, violence, as we've seen in some of the cases we've examined over the last seven years.

There are two important implications that I would like to leave you with. The first is that it is not useful or accurate to speak strictly of physical limits to population growth and to human prosperity, as neo-Malthusians tend to. Instead, we should say that the limits our societies face are a function of the interaction in a given society between the society's physical environment and the ingenuity that it is able to bring to bear on that environment. Rather than speaking of limits, it is better to say that some societies are trapped in a race between a rising ingenuity requirement and their ability to supply ingenuity in response to that rising requirement. Some crucial countries around the world, what are often called pivotal states, such as China and India, are caught in such a race.

The second important implication is that some societies and some subgroups within societies will win this race. Therefore, there are reasons for optimism. On the other hand, others are going to lose, with the result that we will see an increase in the differential between the powerful and the weak, between the wealthy and the poor, between those groups that have access to resources and those that have much less access to resources. We are going to see a widening of the already huge power and wealth gulfs among and within societies. These differentials are not conducive to long-term social and political stability. If numerous ingenuity gaps appear, particularly in pivotal states such as India and China, the spillover effects to rich countries such as Canada and the United States may be severe.

We are now living cheek-by-jowl on an extremely crowded planet, and we cannot isolate ourselves economically and politically from problems on the other side of the world. Ultimately, if ingenuity gaps appear in many societies around the world, the overall prospect for humanity will not be nearly as bright as the optimists seem to suggest.

Population Growth and International Migration at the End of the 20th Century

HANIA ZLOTNIK

Chief, Mortality and Migration Section, United Nations Population Division, 2 United Nations Plaza, New York, New York 10017, USA

As a demographer, I see the world in terms of three very important processes—fertility, mortality, and migration. The first two, fertility and mortality, of course affect everyone, but migration does not necessarily affect every person in the world and is left to the side by many demographers. But that is the aspect of the topic that I have been asked to cover.

About 15 years ago I was an expert on fertility and mortality, topics that have a biological basis for existence: Everyone has to be born and everyone has to die, facts that set a biological limit on what can happen. But with migration there are no laws; anything is possible. It is complicated to analyze the topic and especially to make a connection between migration and the issues involved in caring for the health of a population. The only simple relationship I can think of is that of the United States, which has one of the world's highest immigration intakes, has had special programs to admit nurses because of a shortage of nursing professionals, at the same time as it has put barriers on the immigration of medical doctors trained in other countries because of a surplus of physicians. But, except for this aside, in this presentation I will be talking about complex relationships between fertility, mortality, and migration.

Demographers make a strict distinction between internal and international migration, and I would note that internal migration, which occurs *within* countries, is not well studied except in a few, mostly developed countries. Rough estimates of internal migration worldwide show that between 1990 and 1995 perhaps as many as half a billion—500 million—people moved from one place to another within a country. And that does not even include people moving within the same city, but only those moving between different political or administrative divisions of a country. During the same period, our best estimates of international migration show that in net terms something like 15 million people moved across international borders. In other words, on a global scale, international migration represents only a tiny fraction of population mobility. Yet it is that aspect of mobility that attracts the most attention because, as Dr. Homer-Dixon implied, international migration is the product of economic and political events that make a difference for the societies that send and that receive migrants. Therefore, a lot of attention is placed on international migration, while internal migration is often ignored.

As of January 1, 1990, something like 120 million people worldwide could be classified as international migrants. The year 1990 is special because it marked some key events in world politics, most notably the disintegration of the Soviet Union. That is a seminal event in terms of international migration, because from one day to the next, at the point when the new Commonwealth of Independent States came into being, many people who had been internal migrants suddenly became international migrants. This created a major discontinuity in the statistics, with as many as 20 million migrants being added to the statistics literally overnight. All the estimates I will show you don't yet reflect that change because they refer to a date before the breakup to the former U.S.S.R. The same thing happened, on a smaller scale, in the former Yugoslavia, where population movements have resulted from the internal conflict that has wracked the countries that emerged from the disintegration of the larger state.

Demographers have spent much time studying the fact that the growth rate of the world's population has been declining. But that decline has varied considerably depending on whether we are looking at *developed* or *developing* countries. In fact, developed countries showed a sharp decline in population growth starting almost a century ago. As a result, their populations are now growing very slowly. In contrast, developing countries saw their population growth rate increase drastically after 1950, especially as a result of the widespread use of antibiotics and of epidemiologic interventions that improved public health. More effective insecticides and better nutrition, for example, lowered mortality and thus raised the rate of population growth. Only during the late 1960s did fertility start declining in developing countries. Therefore, there is now a large gap between the developed and developing countries' rates of population growth.

These trends in the rates of population growth lead to the possibility that there may be, at some time in the future, an actual decline of the population in developed countries. In view of this possibility, demographers have posited that it is likely that people in developing countries will move to developed countries, because there will be a need there for more people to do the jobs that the developed countries' populations don't want. Essentially, this model says that there will be a population vacuum in the developed world that is going to be filled by the excess population of developing countries. This view can be interpreted as meaning that the higher a developing country's population growth rate, the higher the tendency for that country to be a source of international migrants.

But anyone who actually looks at the data, despite their lack of accuracy, can see that this simplistic model is not quite true. I must admit here that our data *are* distorted: we don't have good information about international migration in most countries of the world. However, I can still explain the problems with the interpretation I just described. Let me start by describing the relationship between international migration and population growth. The way we demographers view the world is that we count all the people in a given population at a certain time, denoted by $P1$, and we compare that to the number of people at a previous time, let's say $P0$. In the intervening period, there will have been some births, say B, and some deaths, D; the births have to be added to the population, and the deaths subtracted from the population. That is, $P1 = P0 + B - D$. In addition, if the population is open, as the populations of many countries are, then you would also have some more people being added due to immigration (say, I) and some being subtracted because they have left as emigrants (say, E). Consequently, $P1 = P0 + B - D + I - E$. So there are two ways of adding to a population—the excess of births over deaths $(B - D)$ and the excess of immigrants over emigrants $(I - E)$. Then, if we consider the elements of change in the population over the period by looking at the following equation: $(P1 - P0) = (B - D) + (I - E)$, we find that the growth in population is equal to what we call natural increase, which is births minus deaths, and what we call net migration, which is the difference between the number of immigrants and the number of emigrants. Now, if we divide both sides of this last equation by the size of the population at the midpoint of the period, we get a new version of the same equation, which now looks like this: $r = ni + nmi$—that is, the growth rate of a population (r) is equal to the rate of natural increase (ni) plus the net migration rate (nmi).

Let me intrude here with several caveats. First, you may be surprised to learn that despite all the advances made by the populations of the world, and the scientists of the world, we don't have good population counts for all countries of the world at exactly the same time. Censuses are carried out periodically in most countries, but at any point in time at least 40% of the countries of the world just don't have a recent census. For instance, in the case of the country with the world's largest population, China, a census was conducted in the 1950s but then there was no other source of demographic information for the whole country until the 1980s. That is, for 30 years, demographers were essentially "inventing" population trends in a country that accounted for between one-fourth and one-fifth of the whole population of the world. Today we *do* know a lot about China, but now there are many other countries for which we have relatively little information. So there are gaps in our information base that can produce errors.

Another important thing to keep in mind is that all the components allowing us to calculate population growth have not been measured with equal accuracy. Not only do we lack data for some of these components, but in addition the data are sometimes measured with varying accuracy. Deaths are not recorded as completely as births, or the existing population is not counted as completely as other components of change. Furthermore, for many countries, the estimates of net migration are rather weak and you have to take that into account in interpreting the information that I will present. Even the United States, despite being the world's major destination for immigrants, does a very poor job of collecting migration statistics: what the U.S. Immigration and Naturalization Service (INS) measures is inadequate in comparison to what we would like to see measured. Essentially, the INS collects information mainly about people receiving green cards—that is, people who have been given permission to stay in the country forever. But there are many ways in which people can come into the United States and stay without having a green card—and I don't mean only those who enter the country illegally, but many people who are admitted legally under different permits; those people are essentially not included in the statistics you see commonly cited in the press. What we would need is someone standing at every entry point of every country, counting everyone who comes in and everyone who goes out. But if you try to imagine doing that, even for this room, you'll see how difficult it would be to do it with accuracy. The United States used to do some counting of border-crossers in the 1920s; back then, it was reported that between Mexico and the United States there were something like 20 million entries every year. And that was in the 1920s, with poor and inefficient transport systems. Nowadays, the number of persons crossing the Mexico–United States border is in the billions. So most countries, with the exception of islands, don't use that method of counting. Be that as it may, the intrinsic deficiencies in migration statistics is another element of inaccuracy to bear in mind.

And lastly, let me note that the division of the world into just two camps, developing and developed, is somewhat artificial.

TABLE 1. Five-number summaries of the distribution of countries according to different indicators of net international migration (1960–1995)

	Lower extreme	Lower quartile	Median	Upper quartile	Upper extreme
Net number of migrants (000)	−6,733	−453	−44	126	19,837
Net migration rate (percentage)	−1.9	−0.2	−0.1	0.1	3.4
Net migration rate as percentage of natural increase	−71.2	−11.1	−2.6	4.2	646

So with all these caveats, let me show you the estimates of net migration—in terms of both raw numbers and rates—for as many countries in the world as possible. According to the United Nations' Population Division, that set includes 164 countries, not counting the successor states of the former Soviet Union and Yugoslavia, which would bring the total to 183. I have considered information for a relatively lengthy period, from 1960 to 1995, in order to lend stability to the estimates presented. TABLE 1 shows the five-number summaries of the distribution of countries according to the net number of migrants they had over the period 1960–1995 (see the first row in the table). Over those 35 years, the lower extreme—that is, the country that lost the most people through international migration—was Mexico, with a net number of emigrants amounting to 6.7 million. At the other extreme, the country that gained the largest number of migrants was the United States, which absorbed 19.8 million people. Now let us focus on the central portion in this distribution of countries according to their net number of migrants (the part between the lower and upper quartiles). According to TABLE 1, over the period 1965–1990, half of the countries of the world experienced a net migration that varied between a loss of at most 453,000 persons and a gain of at most 126,000 persons. For most countries, numbers of such magnitude over a 35-year period represent very small gains or losses annually. In terms of the average net migration rates over the 1960–1995 period, the distribution shown in the second row of TABLE 1 indicates that for at least half of the countries of the world, net migration rates have been very low, varying between − 0.2% and 0.1%. And even for the other half of the countries in the world, net migration has generally not made a major contribution to population growth. Countries recording relatively large values in the net migration rate tend to have small populations so that, although the number of migrants they send or receive is small, these migrants represent important losses or gains in relative terms. Thus, the country with the highest net migration rate (3.4% per year) is the United Arab Emirates, and the one with the lowest is Samoa (−1.9% annually), both of which have populations of less than 4 million.

The next thing we can do is relate net migration to natural increase by calculating net migration as a percentage of natural increase, so as to assess its relative importance (see the third row in TABLE 1). For some countries, net migration represents a huge percentage of natural increase. That is the case of Germany, for example, where net migration is 646% as large as natural increase (that is, six and half times as large). This is because the population of Germany grew very slowly from 1960 to 1995. With a natural increase of only 0.04%, migration had a very significant impact on its growth. At the other end of the distribution, Hungary saw its natural increase reduced by 71% by net emigration. But again, the emigration experienced was small

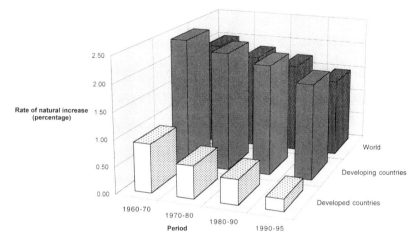

FIGURE 1. Rate of natural increase for the world and developed and developing countries, 1960–1995.

in relative terms, since natural increase was also a low 0.12% annually. Very few countries show these low values for natural increase and, consequently, net migration generally represents a low or at most moderate percentage of natural increase. Thus, for half of the countries of the world, net migration contributes to a reduction in natural increase of at most 11% or to an increase of at most 4%.

Now let me give you an overview of trends in natural increase for the world—data that are especially interesting in relation to some of the earlier talks. FIGURE 1 shows natural increase all by itself—not including net migration—for the world as a whole, as well as for developed and developing countries, and illustrates the difference between the way the populations of developed and developing countries have been growing since 1960. At the high end, a rate of natural increase of 2.4% per year implies that the population doubles about every 30 years. That is where developing countries were in the 1960s and 1970s. But then what we call a demographic transition kicked in, and fertility started a steady decline worldwide, especially in developing countries (as illustrated by the middle row of bars in FIGURE 1). That has been the good news about population dynamics. But even so, when you compare the rates of natural increase for developing countries and those for developed countries, you see how much there still is to be achieved. In developing countries, the rate of natural increase has declined to 1.8% per year in the 1990s, but in developed countries it is close to zero, at about 0.2% annually. This fact underlies many of the contentious issues arising between developed and developing countries today.

Let me also show you how these figures vary by region, because there are some significant variations in regional rates of natural increase. FIGURE 2 shows that falling at the high end, at about 3% annual growth, is Africa, which had very high rates of natural increase in the 1960s. And Africa was not only late in coming to a decline, but there was even an upturn in its rate of natural increase in the 1970s and 1980s. However, the most recent estimates and projections by the United Nations show that

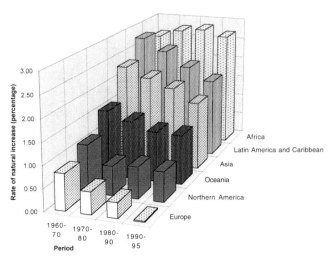

FIGURE 2. Rate of natural population increase for the major world regions, 1960–1995.

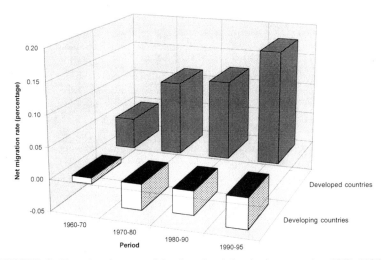

FIGURE 3. Net migration rate of developed and developing countries, 1960–1995.

Africa is finally seeing its rate of natural increase decline. In Latin America and Asia the transition has been more consistent; there, natural increase started at a lower level and has gone down quite a bit. However, I should point out that much of the decline in Asia is driven by China, where the reduction in fertility has been extremely rapid since 1980. There are also some variations among developed countries. Canada and the United States, for example, are still growing at a higher rate than Europe. Europe in the 1990s is almost not growing at all. The projections are that Europe will have a negative rate of natural increase in the future if current trends continue. Some people worry that populations there may actually decrease, in the absence of international migration.

Now let us return to the subject of migration. Since there is no way yet to emigrate to Mars or Jupiter, the net migration total for developing countries must balance out the net migration total for developed countries; in other words, all the people being lost by developing countries are being gained by developed countries. But because the total population of the world's developing countries is much greater than the total population of developed countries, the *rates* of migration are not the same. The proportionate loss in developing countries is smaller than the proportionate gain in developed countries (FIG. 3). FIGURE 3 also shows that there has been a sharp increase in the gain of developed countries since the 1960s. So developed countries see themselves as gaining too many people, people who were not necessarily invited in, from developing countries—and that view has been driving the migration debate recently.

What does this tell us about the relationship between population growth and migration? FIGURE 4 shows a plot of natural increase on the horizontal axis and net migration on the vertical axis; each dot represents one of the 164 countries of the world in 1990, and you can see that the scatter is quite wide. There is indeed a slight negative relationship between the rate of natural increase and net migration; the higher the rate of natural increase, the more likely a country is to have net emigration. However, that emigration will not necessarily be to developed countries; it could be to other developing countries. And statistically, the relationship is not strong enough to explain most of the variation in the points plotted in FIGURE 4.

Now let's look at the same sort of plot, but using only developing countries (FIG. 5). Actually, I eliminated from this plot only the market-economy, Western countries, which most of you would probably take to mean developed countries, but which do not include the Eastern bloc countries of Europe that used to be considered

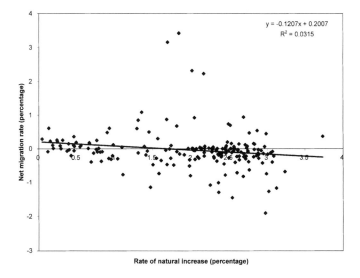

FIGURE 4. Net migration related to natural increase, all countries, 1960–1995.

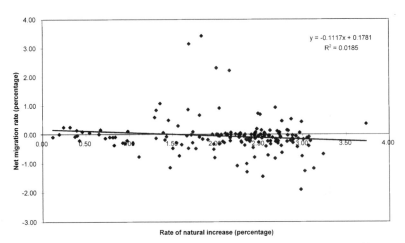

FIGURE 5. Net migration related to natural increase, excluding Western bloc countries, 1960–1995.

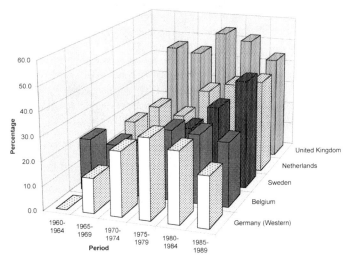

FIGURE 6. Percentage of migrants to selected European countries originating in developing countries.

developed and that now form a group of their own. So the plot in FIGURE 5 includes the developing countries plus the former Eastern bloc countries, now called "countries with economies in transition." Again, the relationship between natural increase and net migration is slightly negative, though even weaker than when the developed countries were included. So these data show that the relationship between population growth and international migration is not as simple as one might expect. High natural increase does not necessarily lead to high emigration. High natural increase is not even strongly correlated with high emigration.

Another interesting way of looking at the issue is to examine the experience of a few specific developed countries, to see how many migrants from developing countries they have received over the 1960–1994 period. FIGURE 6 shows the proportion of migrants from developing countries received by the United Kingdom, the Netherlands, Sweden, Belgium, and Germany. From reading the newspapers, you might imagine that Germany, for example, is being "invaded" by people from developing countries. But as FIGURE 6 shows, Germany has received a fairly low percentage of migrants from developing countries. Its highest percentage from developing countries was about 25% in 1975–1979, and it has come down to about 10% in the 1990s. On average, over the whole period, only about 22% of migrants to Germany were from developing countries. Of course, immigrants from developing countries *are* quite obvious in Germany: the Turks, for example, are a small but visible minority. It is important to keep in mind that their numbers are not large in relative terms, however. The United Kingdom, on the other hand, may not be a country that people identify as a major receiver of migrants from developing countries. However, nearly half of the migrants received from 1960 to 1994, 45% to be exact, were from developing countries; that is one of the highest proportions in Europe (and certainly the highest among the countries shown in FIGURE 6). Although the United Kingdom experienced negative net migration during the period—that is, more people left than entered over some years—of its inflow, almost half was from developing countries. All the other countries in FIGURE 6 received only about 25% of their incoming migrants from developing countries.

Now let us look at the traditional receivers of immigrants—Australia, Canada, and the United States. FIGURE 7 shows that in all three countries, especially in Canada and the United States, the proportion of migrants originating in developing countries has been growing steadily. For the United States, it is now almost the entire flow of migrants—up to 88%. But the United States has always been an extreme case

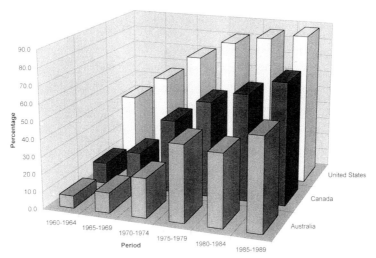

FIGURE 7. Percentage of immigrants to the traditional countries of immigration originating in developing countries.

compared to other major receiving countries in the developed world. In Canada, the proportion of immigrants originating in developing countries is 50%, and in Australia it is 30%. That is, the United States is not representative of what is happening in most developed countries. The sense that all developed countries are being "flooded" by migrants from the developing world is not validated by the statistics that the developed countries gather.

Let us consider again the data from the eight developed countries examined so far, which represent most of the main receivers of migrants. FIGURE 8 shows a line representing the total migrant gain by those countries over the period 1960–1970 according to region of origin. The bars represent the natural increase in each region of origin during that period. The line indicates that in the 1960s, most of the migrants going *to* the developed world (that is, to the eight countries whose data were presented in previous figures) also came *from* the developed world (that is, from other market-economy Western countries). It was during the late 1960s and early 1970s, when the rules regarding restrictions on the admission of migrants from developing countries changed in most of the receiving countries, that the number of migrants from developing countries began to increase. But until that time, there were relatively few migrants from developing countries to the developed world because of barriers to their entry. The only exception was migration between Latin America and the United States, which was not subject to major restrictions. As FIGURE 8 shows, most of the migrants to the eight countries considered originated either in developed countries, Latin America, or Eastern bloc countries (denoted as "Europe in transition"). Comparing the migrant intake originating in each region with the region's rate of natural increase depicted in FIGURE 8, it appears that there is a low correlation—or even a negative correlation—between a region's rate of natural increase and its level of emigration to the developed world. In fact, FIGURE 8 suggests that the lower the rate of

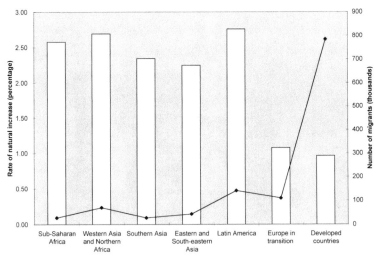

FIGURE 8. Relation between natural increase and number of migrants to selected developed countries by region of origin, 1960–1970.

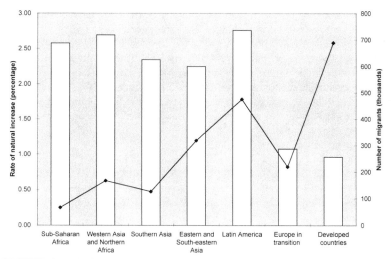

FIGURE 9. Relation between natural increase in 1960–1970 and the number of migrants to selected developed countries by region of origin in 1980–1989.

natural increase of a region, the *more* likely it was to be a source of migrants for the eight developed countries considered.

One might argue that we need to consider the fact that children born in developing countries now won't be looking for jobs in developed countries for another 20 years. So let us consider the lagging effect of natural increase: let us compare the natural increase from the 1960s with the migration level of the 1980s, the period when the children born in the 1960s would have started looking for jobs. This modification changes the migration pattern by region of origin, as shown in FIGURE 9. Now there are considerable numbers of migrants originating in eastern and southeastern Asia and in Latin America. The numbers originating in Eastern bloc countries (Europe in transition) have also increased in comparison with the 1960s. But still there is not a positive correlation between natural increase and emigration. This result stems from the fact that countries in Europe are still receiving large numbers of migrants from other European countries and not as many, in relative terms, from the developing world. So this is one more piece of evidence validating my point that people from developing countries are not exactly "invading" the developed world.

Yet where opportunities for migration exist, people from developing countries are taking advantage of them to move to developed countries. But the data show that those flows are not out of control. It is important to keep these facts in mind when you hear assessments of migration and the imbalance of population growth between developed and developing nations. The truth is that migration, especially international migration, is a very costly undertaking. I'm sure that you have all read in the newspapers how people have to pay thousands of dollars to be smuggled into the United States. They also have to pay the same amount of money, or a lot of money by developing-country standards, to migrate legally. Most people in developing countries don't earn the kinds of salaries that would allow them to move. If they move at all, it is mostly within their own countries, not to the developed world. The developed world is still unreachable for the vast majority of them.

Looking to the future, is migration to the developed world going to increase? Probably yes, because an imbalance does exist. And it is not only an imbalance in terms of demographics, it is an imbalance in economic terms. There are several worrisome aspects to the fact that many countries are being left behind because of structural barriers to economic development or because of a lack of ingenuity to change their social systems and to adapt to resource scarcities. Consequently, more pressures for migration will exist in the future, and they will have to be accommodated. But an immense flow of people is not likely.

Once again, in this respect, the United States is likely to have a special role to play. Like Canada and Australia, the United States is essentially a country built by immigration, and that is unlikely to change in the near future. So the geneticists who spoke yesterday will probably have an interesting time analyzing the genes of the United States' population, because they incorporate a mixture of many peoples!

Let me also add, on a more serious note, that there has been much talk about how migrants import not only their genes, but also their diseases. Especially with respect to the transmission of HIV, there have been many theories about its being imported from elsewhere. But I must point out, and I think the medical community knows this very well, that you don't need to be a migrant to be an importer of disease—you only need to travel. There is an enormous amount of travel today: only a few hours are needed to be halfway round the world and transmit one's viruses to whoever is around. Disease transmission is not a problem exclusively tied to migration—it is a problem related to population mobility in general.

To conclude, perhaps it is pertinent to tell you what I say when people ask, as they often do when they hear that I am chief of something called the Mortality and Migration Section of the United Nations, "Why those two topics—mortality and migration—together?" In fact, it is just a quirk of fate. But sometimes I will answer, "Well, you have two choices for leaving a population. It's up to you to choose which one." I guess, since one of the panelists in this symposium has noted that California has given us the option of whether to die (or to migrate—to outer space perhaps), this might be the sort of answer a Californian might give!

REFERENCES

1. UNITED NATIONS. 1999. World Popluation Prospects: The 1996 Revision. United Nations Publications, Sales No. E.98. XIII. 5. New York.
2. ZLOTNIK, H. 1991. South-to-North migration since 1960: the view from the North. Pop. Bull. U.N. **31/32:** 17–37.
3. ZLOTNIK, H. 1994. International migration: causes and effects. *In* Beyond the Number. Laurie Ann Mazur, Ed.: 359–377. Island Press. Washington, D.C.
4. ZLOTNIK, H. 1998. International migration 1965–1996: An overview. Pop. Devel. Rev. **24**(3): 429–468.

Commentary on the World Population Session

RONALD M. GREEN

Cohen Professor for the Study of Ethics and Human Values and Director, Ethics Institute, Dartmouth College, Hanover, New Hampshire 03755, USA

To many Americans, it seems obvious that the world faces a population problem. Popular literature of the past several decades, including best-sellers like Paul Ehrlich's *The Population Bomb* and the Club of Rome's *The Limits to Growth,* have driven this concept into our minds. The facts supporting this conviction also seem evident. They include the unprecedented rise in human numbers. As several contributors to this symposium have noted, growth has become exponential. It took tens of thousands of years for the world's population to reach one billion people; it will take only 12 years to add the billion that will bring the human population to six billion in 1999. Equally obvious is the association between human suffering and high growth rates or high absolute levels of population. Around the world, high population density and high growth rates seem to go hand in hand with underdevelopment, unemployment, famine, disease, and war. The problems of Bangladesh, Sudan, and Ethiopia are notorious examples.

Simple mathematics supports these observations and conclusions. In any situation of fixed resources, a growing population must lead to a declining share of resources per person. As per-capita well-being declines, at some point it finally descends beneath a welfare floor, and widespread suffering ensues. It may be possible for a period of time to evade the logic of this fatal equation by increasing resources in proportion to growing numbers. This is what we have done so far to sustain current massive population levels. By bringing technology and stored energy resources to bear, we have greatly increased each individual's ability to produce the necessities of life. In some regions, increased productivity has even outpaced the effects of population growth. But in a fixed global environment, mathematical logic must ultimately prevail. Eventually, some critical factors in production show themselves to be fixed. In the 1970s, attention initially focused on the declining supplies of fossil fuels that we used to increase productivity. More recently, attention has turned to the limited ability of the earth's environment to absorb the stresses placed on it by our previous technological "fixes." The phenomenon of global warming, emphasized by Vice President Al Gore in his address to this gathering, now alerts us to the frightening toll that ever-larger population levels may be taking.

If people are the problem, then reducing the numbers of people must be the remedy. Massive social evils invite a "demographic" solution. In policy terms, this thinking leads naturally to an emphasis on population control measures. Delivery of birth-control information and devices, advertising campaigns that encourage people to reduce family size, and the use of incentives—including, perhaps, the threat of coercion as a desperate last resort—all make sense when social problems are perceived this way. This logic reached a high point in India during the early 1970s, when the government of Indira Ghandi implemented forced sterilization programs as a response to the nation's perceived population problem.

The implications for medical professionals of this mode of thinking are interesting. Physicians' most important skills are at best irrelevant, and at worst pernicious. Individual curative medicine plays very little role in alleviating the problems caused by population growth. Each life saved only increases the denominator of the fatal equation. Even more harmful are massive public health interventions—improved water and sanitation, mass inoculation programs, and efforts to eradicate agricultural pests or disease-bearing insects. Within the logic of population growth as an inevitably malign force, these public health measures only increase vulnerable populations to unsustainable higher levels. Catastrophe is deferred and accentuated, not avoided.

If all this seems self-evident, it is not. In his address, Vice President Gore drew on the wisdom of Yogi Berra to remind us that "what gets us into trouble is not what we don't know, [but] what we know for sure but just ain't so." The remarks by each of the contributors to this section also call into question any narrow emphasis on demographic explanations of perceived social problems. Each presenter tried to place population growth in perspective and to offer information that might counter irrational and panicked responses. Some of this information also has the effect of validating the role of medical professionals in helping us respond to population-related social problems.

Michael Teitelbaum, program officer for the Alfred P. Sloan Foundation, and Thomas Homer-Dixon, director of the Peace and Conflict Studies Program of the University of Toronto, developed the long traditions of theorizing among philosophers, ethicists, economists, and social scientists about the causes of population growth and the appropriate responses to it. Teitelbaum traced what he called the "intellectual history of zigs and zags" that marks this question and its answers. Although the tradition of reflection began with Plato's proposal for compulsory population control in his utopian state, the most heated debates occurred in the early 19th century with the work of Thomas Robert Malthus. Human population growth, Malthus argued, necessarily outpaces any possible growth in food supplies. While food production increases arithmetically, population growth increases geometrically, or exponentially. These facts, Malthus argued, explained the misery that was apparent among England's rural poor. It followed that no charitable efforts, no welfare schemes or poor laws, could ameliorate the plight of the poor. Although Malthus's Christian moral beliefs prevented him from advocating artificial methods of birth control, he found some glimmer of hope in the prospect of delayed marriage and sexual continence. Later neo-Malthusians like Charles Bradlaugh and Annie Besant abandoned Malthus's opposition to artificial birth control, but they shared his view that unchecked population growth is the major cause of poverty and social distress.

This essentially demographic explanation of social misery was dramatically challenged by Karl Marx and later communist and socialist thinkers. In Marx's view, poverty and hunger result not from the high birth rates of the poor, but from the unjust workings of the capitalist economic system. "Parson Malthus," as Marx derisively called him, was merely an apologist for this system. The aim of his writings on population, Marx asserted, was to blame the poor for their condition, to divert attention from the social and economic causes of poverty, and to stifle efforts at change or reform. Many later socialist and communist theorists followed Marx's lead. Reacting against Malthusianism in all its forms, they emphasized the capacity of society, through technological innovation and social reforms, to accommodate limitlessly expanding populations. This pro-growth population ideology was often obscured by socialist and communist regimes' commitment to the provision of contraception and abortion services, policies that were an extension of their advocacy of women's rights. In the Soviet Union and Eastern Europe, decades of war, social turmoil, and economic hardship also lowered fertility rates and allowed governments the luxury of this pronatalist ideology. Only in China did Marxist theory confront the reality of a burgeoning population growth that taxed the ability of the economic system to keep up with it. Still, it was only in the 1980s that the Chinese communist regime abandoned what had been a fundamental tenet of Marxist belief and inaugurated a deliberate population policy.

Remarkably, just as Marxist thinking was reversing itself, some thinkers adhering to a more conservative free-market economic position, which had previously championed Malthusianism, were moving closer to the Marxist view. Organizations like the Heritage Foundation and the Cato Institute began to argue that population growth is neutral and that everything depends on the economy. Allowed to function on its own, the free market can solve all problems of resource scarcity. The real problems, these theorists maintained, are statist central planning and controls. Although the conclusions of this argument are anticommunist, Teitelbaum observed, its structure is similar to that of Marx: not demographic factors but faulty economic systems are the principal cause of overpopulation and human misery. To further compound the ironical nature of this debate, the Roman Catholic Church adopted a position broadly similar to that of the early Marxists. According to current authoritative Church teaching, the solution to the observable social dislocation and suffering associated with underdevelopment is not birth limitation but social justice. Recent papal documents denounce birth control and abortion as part of the "culture of death." The Church-approved response to the population problem is increased international sharing of resources and technology.

Viewed against the background of these debates, the perspective offered by Homer-Dixon stands within the broader Malthusian tradition. Research by his Toronto-based Peace and Conflict Studies Program suggests that fixed physical resources (such as land and water) are not, as Malthus believed, the limiting factors in a society's ability to respond to rising population. Rather, the critical considerations are human technological and social ingenuity. The former encompasses such things as the development of highly productive new seeds; the latter includes everything from more open markets to reduced police corruption. Nevertheless, even with this theoretical adjustment, the logic of Malthus's fatal equation remains in force. Population increases exponentially, while at some point ingenuity can only progress arithmetically. Incessant population growth will eventually challenge the ability of even human ingenuity to cope with population-induced stress.

Homer-Dixon's position and research highlight the continuing force of the Malthusian view. Nevertheless, criticisms of this view also continue to be voiced. Although few modern students of demography dispute the inevitability of limits in one form or another or favor uncontrolled population growth, the exclusively demographic focus of Malthusian perspectives has been widely criticized. In particular, the role of high fertility as a leading independent variable in social distress has been questioned. Without abandoning the awareness that population growth can exacerbate social problems, theorists have emphasized the prior role of social, cultural, and economic factors in inducing large families. At the level of both theory and practice, a view combining elements of both sides of the traditional debate has emerged. Like Malthus and his intellectual descendants, those who hold this view accept the fact that demographic factors may worsen social problems. They also acknowledge that unceasing human growth is impossible. Nevertheless, they have a very different understanding of why high fertility and poverty are associated. They emphasize how poverty and underdevelopment cause high fertility, rather than the other way around. They also offer different solutions to the problem. Although family planning programs are valuable, they cannot be isolated from major efforts directed at social reform, economic development, the emancipation of women, and the provision of a full range of basic medical services.

In his address, Vice President Gore voiced the key insight here. Recent U.S. policy, he observed, has been shaped by the wisdom that "the most powerful contraceptive is the confidence that one's children will survive." In poor countries, he noted, large families have traditionally been people's insurance against illness and old age. High mortality rates for children promote large family size because they undermine parents' confidence that their children will reach maturity. This remains true even when public-health measures or improved nutrition have substantially reduced aggregate mortality rates. Where good primary health care is lacking, parents can still lose some or all of their children to disease and trauma. Realizing this, they continue to have large families. In an environment of reduced overall mortality, these individual decisions by parents to sustain traditional family size are the driving force for rapid population growth.

Contributing to this situation is the low status of women in many underdeveloped societies. In the absence of educational or economic opportunities, women's prestige and security depend on the number of their surviving children. Large families and the burden of dependency further anchor women to traditional roles, and the cycle of poverty, high fertility, female dependency, and high fertility continues.

By itself, the provision of birth-control devices or information is not effective in terminating this vicious cycle. Without fundamental social change, appeals for reduced family size fall on deaf ears. Compulsory birth control or sterilization measures, when separated from other positive social programs, come to be viewed as oppressive and are evaded as much as possible. Without balanced efforts to enhance the choices facing families, social pressures to reduce fertility can even lead to a backlash.

One key to breaking the vicious cycle are programs that improve economic opportunities, particularly educational and economic initiatives that create opportunities for women. Not only do these provide alternatives to early marriage and frequent childbearing, but they also enhance women's self-esteem and increase their value as something other than mothers. Access to basic health care and programs for maternal and child health are also essential. Apart from increasing parents' confidence that their children will survive to adulthood, they provide an excellent context for the provision of family planning information and materials. In various ways, family-focused primary health care contributes to the empowerment of women, which is a crucial factor in breaking the cycle of poverty and high fertility.

For all these reasons, medical professionals, far from being unwitting contributors to the population problem, are crucial actors in helping us implement a balanced response to it. They play a role not only in developing the programs for basic health care and maternal and child health that are at the center of the issue, but also in educating the public and political leaders to ways of responsibly addressing demographic problems. The remarks by Nils Daulaire, chief health policy advisor to the U.S. Agency for International Development, provided many important illustrations of this point. Informed by his own experience as a primary-care physician in Bangladesh, Daulaire has played a role in moving U.S. policy away from the narrow emphasis on the provision of birth control that marked our efforts at least until the 1994 Cairo Conference. That older policy had set the U.S. at odds with many socialist bloc and Third World nations as well as the Roman Catholic Church. At Cairo, however, the U.S. forged a new alliance with women's movements from around the world and with others who stressed economic and social development as the primary response to underdevelopment. This new policy, as Daulaire reported, rests on a series of basic tenets, among them that no woman should have to become pregnant unless she wishes to bear a child; that no family should have to face the needless death of a young child; and that no woman should enter adulthood without the basic educational skills that will enable her to become a part of our global society.

Despite this progress in conceptualizing and addressing population-related problems, old ways of thinking die hard. Throughout human intellectual history, narrowly demographic explanations of observable distress stand alongside eugenic or racist theories as monuments to the human instinct to find simple answers to complex questions. The closing remarks at this session of the symposium by Hania Zlotnik, chief of the Mortality and Migration Section of the United Nations, provided a different reminder of the continuing allure of demographic explanations for social evils and of the need to counter with facts seemingly "self-evident truths" in this area.

As Zlotnik made clear, many developed nations have lowered population growth rates, and, in the case of some European and Eastern European nations, populations are actually failing to replace themselves. Although she did not develop the point, the dynamic of negative population growth rates also invites demographically based explanations of social problems. This was seen earlier in this century when low birth rates among the middle and upper classes in many Western European nations were viewed with alarm as a leading indicator and cause of social decline.

In our day, lower birth rates in developed countries and continuing high fertility rates in many less-developed countries contribute to the belief that developing nations are exporting their high fertility to developed nations through massive movements of legal and illegal migrants. The fact that immigrant communities usually occupy lower rungs on the economic ladder and often evidence social problems associated with that position only reinforces the popular perception that immigration is the major cause of social and economic turmoil.

These beliefs have been common in the United States, where liberal, post-1965 immigration policies and our proximity to Mexico account for the fact that a very high percentage (80%) of our immigrants come from developing countries. However, as Ms. Zlotnik made clear, the U.S. is an outlier in this respect. On a global basis, international migrations account for a relatively small part of the movements of populations, most of which take place within nation-states as people seek improved economic opportunities.

Ms. Zlotnik acknowledged that despite their relative unimportance in absolute terms, migrations from poor countries with high growth rates remain a contentious issue. Demographic trends also suggest that the issue will not soon go away. While developing nations have recently begun to reduce fertility rates, they remain high. In addition, the negative growth rates of some developed countries will create a demand in the developed world for laborers from poorer countries, with all the problems of cultural assimilation this involves. Nevertheless, she emphasized that amidst these flows of human beings and the resulting social controversies, it is important to remain grounded in facts and to resist the allure of simplistic explanations. For example, it is a mistake to blame epidemics such as the spread of HIV on immigrants. Disease transmission of this sort results primarily from the greatly increased international travel that is mostly engaged in by the affluent citizens of developed nations.

Issues of world population growth do not form part of the standard curriculum of medical education. Nevertheless, as the contributors to this session made clear in various ways, the medical profession has an important role to play in shaping our response to population dynamics. Medical educators and physicians can develop the programs of health care and the research initiatives needed by people around the world as they seek to improve opportunities and choices for themselves and their families. Physicians, by understanding and communicating the complex ways in which high fertility relates to social distress, can be voices of reason in an arena so often charged with emotion and prejudice. Michael Teitelbaum introduced this section by observing that its inclusion in the Bicentennial Symposium was another example of the "exceptionalism" that has so often characterized Dartmouth Medical School. Certainly, the decision to give this topic consideration among the most important issues facing medical education in the next century is a sign of Dartmouth's commitment to pioneering new content and methods of medical education.

Closing Session:
The Future—Through the Looking Glass

Medicine, Liberal Learning, and the Pursuit of Wisdom

S. MARSH TENNEY

Nathan Smith Professor of Physiology Emeritus and Former Dean, Dartmouth Medical School, Hanover, New Hampshire 03755, USA

I am pleased to welcome you to the final session of this symposium, "The Future: Through the Looking Glass." In 1960, a symposium was held at Dartmouth Medical School entitled "Great Issues of Conscience in Modern Medicine." This symposium, titled "Great Issues for Medicine in the 21st Century," has included all of the topics that were on the agenda 37 years ago, plus one additional topic—that of health-care systems and finances. Let us hope that the next symposium is not titled "Still Greater Issues in Medicine."

I addressed the opening ceremony of the 1960 symposium, and I am honored that the program committee for this symposium has asked me to make a few introductory remarks for this final session.[1]

The profession of medicine occupies a special place in society, and its practitioners play a unique role in our lives. A physician is likely to be our first and our last human contact in life. In life's passing, decisions and actions with consequences that may determine survival or death will often depend on a doctor's competence. Small wonder that society has great expectations of the profession. The physician must be kind and caring, knowledgeable and skillful. But above all else, there should be manifest that attribute of character called wisdom. It is a pity that it cannot be taught.

The theme of this session focuses on the future, but I am going to look back. In fact, it will be a parochial view. In the next few minutes, I will examine an aspect of a few prominent early persons in the history of Dartmouth Medical School and of the Medical School as a part of Dartmouth College. The aspect I have in mind, one more apparent in the past than in the present, is a more undifferentiated manner of thinking—one that led to greater cohesion in institutional function and a wider scope of individual practice. It influenced the outlook of both lay and medical populations in a way that was at once reciprocal and connective. My purpose is not to remind ourselves that there are lessons to be learned from history, but to reflect on those attributes of some persons and places worthy of emulation.

First, there was a man and his idea. The story of Nathan Smith and the founding of Dartmouth Medical School has been retold many times,[a] but few have commented on the character of this revered physician and teacher, especially upon the principles that guided him in his professional work. First, it is clear that Smith, early on, sensed the inadequacy of the apprentice system of training that he had learned by, but it was all that was available in northern New England at the time. As a practitioner with apprentices under his own supervision, he became increasingly concerned about their limited exposure to emerging medical science. This was a strong motive for his petition to the president and trustees of Dartmouth College to establish a medical school. It would make accessible a formal medical education in a region devoid of any such opportunity. The only three possibilities in this country at the time were at the University of Pennsylvania in Philadelphia, at King's College (later Columbia University) in New York, and at Harvard University in Cambridge, all impossibly far removed for northwoods New England boys.

The College's acceptance of Smith's request, one year after his first course of lectures, included the awesome academic title "Professor of Anatomy and Surgery, of the Theory and Practice of Physic, of Materia Medica and Botany, and of Chemistry." The story goes that this title caused Oliver Wendell Holmes, who joined the Dartmouth medical faculty some years later, to deliver a much-quoted quip that Smith didn't occupy a chair at Dartmouth, but a whole settee. It was not unusual in the early medical schools of this country for a professor to teach many subjects, but Smith's case was unique, and he carried this load for several years without help except from his former student Lyman Spalding, who assisted in anatomy.

On top of his classroom obligations, Smith maintained an active practice, and his clinical skills were widely sought as his reputation continued to grow. Furthermore, in carrying out his clinical duties, Smith was forced to travel long distances on horseback. Medical students routinely accompanied him to learn at the bedside. There is ample evidence that Nathan Smith was conscientious in everything he undertook, and especially in the care of patients; he was thoughtful of their personal as well as their medical problems.

The stature of Smith's character is clarified by examining the development of his personal philosophy of medicine, especially therapeutics. The theories of William Cullen and Benjamin Rush dominated medical thinking at the time. Their views were set forth with uncompromising dogmatism, and they advocated vigorous therapies, especially praising the value of repeated purging and blood-letting. Smith was inclined to be conservative, but, more important, he relied on his own experience to assess what was good and what was bad. He presented the teachings of Cullen and Rush in his lectures but then refuted them by citing case histories from his own extensive practice. In short, he was following that old maxim: sound judgment comes from experience, although experience often comes from bad judgment. Simply put, Nathan Smith was a practitioner of common sense, or, in more exalted terms, a man who had acquired the capacity to judge rightly in matters of life and conduct, which is the definition of wisdom.

Smith did not have much formal education and he made no pretense of being a learned man, but he always introduced his lectures with a historical review of the subject at hand. He frequently referred to Hippocrates, whose views he found generally acceptable—especially his counsel that treatments should aim to assist nature in the healing process and his caution that the physician should take no action that

---

[a]The first truly full-scale biography of Nathan Smith was published shortly after the Bicentennial Symposium, as another of the School's anniversary observances. Titled *Improve, Perfect, & Perpetuate: Dr. Nathan Smith and Early American Medical Education,* it was written by Oliver S. Hayward, M.D., and Constance E. Putnam and published by University Press of New England (Hanover, N.H., 1998).

might harm the patient. Ancient learning and a critical attitude of mind, ever on the alert for sources of error, led Smith to sound conclusions.

Medical knowledge is deeply rooted in science, but good medical practice still requires much that lies outside the domain of science. There are those who feel that the growth of one has been at the expense of the other—that science and technology have left no room for the human factor in medicine. That simple explanation seems unlikely; I suspect there are a great many widespread social factors at work, and everyone can construct a growing list of everyday transactions with no human involvement at all. The movement toward depersonalization is facilitated by technology, but there has also occurred a subtle change in attitude, an aspect of mind that accepts a categorical separation in the branches of learning, encouraging an intellectual split where once a natural fusion was taken for granted.

Let us look at the first aphorism of Hippocrates (and let us also note in passing that the first edition in modern times of the *Aphorisms of Hippocrates* was published by François Rabelais, a physician at Montpellier who was, of course, better known for his literary masterpiece *Gargantua et Pantagruel):*

> Life is short, the art long, opportunity fleeting, experience treacherous, judgment difficult.

It is on the first phrase—"Life is short, the *art* long"—that I want to focus, and, within it, on the word "art," which is the word the translator has chosen to convey the meaning of the original Greek, *techne.* "Techne" is the root of many words in today's vocabulary, like technology and technique, but in ancient Greece its meaning was much more inclusive and was by no means restricted to the category of matters we call technical. It could mean either art or science, but any distinction between the two was blurred. Skill, as a result of knowledge, was implied, but the clear separation of meaning that we now understand was not apparent in the classical mind. A derivative, possibly, is found in the long tradition of the medical profession to roam freely in the arts and sciences.

In fact, when I consulted my copy of Pickering's Greek lexicon regarding the word *techne,* I found in the preface an acknowledgment of the contribution of sections B to O by Professor Daniel Oliver of Dartmouth Medical School. Oliver was appointed here in 1822, the first full-time member of the faculty—that is, the first to have no medical practice on the side; he held titles in Physiology, Physic, Materia Medica, and Botany, and he was also Professor of Moral and Intellectual Philosophy in the College. Like Oliver Wendell Holmes, who was appointed Professor of Anatomy and Physiology here in 1838, Daniel Oliver could claim professional legitimacy as a humanist as well as a scientist. One can be sure that the teachings of both men, in whatever department, prepared their students for the work of life, which is a goal of the liberal arts. And as was the case with Smith, the personal example these men provided was at least as important as what they taught.

In the contemporary university structure, a Faculty of Arts and Sciences is routine, but it is unusual to find individuals qualified in both divisions. Also, today's medical faculties sometimes teach on the undergraduate level, and medical students are encouraged to take courses on the college level, but the general phenomenon of college students attending medical school courses has become relatively rare. By contrast, records from the early history of Dartmouth Medical School reveal that almost half of the students enrolled in medical courses were from the College, and it is clear that their ambitions were not to train for a career in medicine. They apparently saw medicine as one of the "liberating arts." And during the revitalization of Dartmouth Medical School (DMS) in the late 1950s, a strong scientific base was introduced on the premise that science need not be illiberal. One finds that Daniel Webster was just such a student at DMS. Based on his experience with medical subject matter, he was moved to deliver a commencement discourse on the chemical theories of Lavoisier. President Freedman has already told you of the remarkable prayer offered by President Wheelock after he had attended a lecture by Nathan Smith. This singular example of a college president, so inspired as to thank the Almighty for a lesson in anatomy and chemistry, would have achieved immortality in the annals of medical history if Wheelock had concluded the prayer: "... and we thank Thee for this medical school."

The interesting fact is that medicine, viewed as a systematic body of knowledge, was once considered a worthy subject for some study by any well-educated person. Thomas Jefferson, for example, listed medicine along with philosophy, music, and architecture as fields in which he read widely. And at his newly created university in Charlottesville, he recruited the famous London physician Robley Dunglison to join the faculty long before he contemplated founding a medical school.

This symposium has been devoted to a forward look into the 21st century, but in these past few minutes I have cast a backward look at this place and some of its people with the purpose of identifying a few features that were once more apparent than they are now. The public today is critical of the medical profession for being uncaring, cold, technique-oriented, and indifferent to human beings. All science and no humanity, in other words. The growing popularity of "alternative medicine" and the alarming tendency to reject science are no solution to the problem. Medical progress will depend on more, not less, science, and medical students must understand the principles on which the profession rests. Possibly the compartmentalization of a once more homogeneous body of knowledge has led to compartmentalized thinking. "Either/or" has become the didactic rule, instead of "and."

The proper conjunction of art *and* science is the reliable road to wisdom. There may be some merit in the stratagem introduced by many medical educators of including courses in literature in the medical curriculum, apparently to titrate the impersonal logic of science. But what would have a far greater impact is contact with teachers and physicians whose character exemplified both scientific and humanistic virtues. Of course, reading great literature enriches our lives; educated individuals read for pleasure. And it cannot be denied that both medical students and doctors enrich their lives by this means. But it should be acknowledged that the coin has another face. Everyone, not just doctors, should have some knowledge of how the human body works and of those principles that govern healthy life, and some insight into its dislocations and perturbations that we call disease.

It is ironic that not so long ago it was commonplace for students in the liberal arts to attend medical lectures, but that now, when television presents a disease-of-the-day and a health-conscious public is confused by a blizzard of recommendations and warnings based on uninformed opinions, a valuable custom once prevalent has nearly vanished. We urge that there be a responsible citizenry, one informed about the laws of our country, but there is no such sentiment for being informed about the workings of the body we inhabit. A once more open academic society, one that fostered a community of ideas, has given way to a separation and sacrifice of intellectual scope.

In as many ways as possible, I hope that the academic component of medicine will be brought back into a more integral relationship with the university. The Faculty of Medicine is the historic base for studies of human biology. Medicine, which strives to improve the health and welfare of mankind, resonates sympathetically with the humanities' goal of fostering human interests and ideals. Physicians and humanists share a common faith in man and a devotion to human well-being. There still exists a synergistic bond, but it needs to return to its former strength.

Finally, we return to Nathan Smith, a physician and teacher who combined art and science in his practice, a man whose knowledge was shaped by experience, a man of character justly known as wise. It has been said that an institution is the lengthened shadow of one man. For Dartmouth Medical School, Nathan Smith stands tallest.

NOTE

1. I would like to make a point here of recognizing Heinz Valtin, a professor emeritus of physiology at Dartmouth Medical School, an internationally known authority on renal physiology, and the chair of the Bicentennial Symposium Planning Committee. And personally, I would like to note my nearly 40 years of collegiality and close friendship with him at Dartmouth, and, in fact, even further back at the University of Rochester, where we were also colleagues. I treasure our friendship and admire his professionalsim. The ability that he displayed in leading the Symposium Planning Committee, an effort to which he devoted his full energy for three years, is evident in these proceedings. I would like to convey to him the gratitude of the faculty and of the audience on behalf of President Freedman and Dean Wallace.

The Conflict between the Science and the Art of Clinical Practice in the Next Millennium

SIR DAVID WEATHERALL

Regius Professor of Medicine, University of Oxford, and the Institute of Molecular Medicine, John Radcliffe Hospital, Headington, Oxford OX3 9DU, United Kingdom

It is a great honor for somebody from the old world to congratulate you on the magnificent achievements of the last 200 years and to extend every good wish for the next several hundred. You may have noticed that I phrased those remarks with exquisite care—I said "honor," not "pleasure." That's no insult to your fine medical school. It is simply that having studied the psychopathology of public speaking for many years, I realize now that anybody who gets up in a situation like this and says it's a pleasure is either a liar, intoxicated, or senile. And in the ancient university where I work, usually a neat mix of all three.

I suspect that the difficult topic I was invited to address here is the result of *Science and the Quiet Art,*[1] a book that I wrote a few years ago at the request of Lewis Thomas and the Commonwealth Fund. My brief was to try to analyze the role of the biomedical sciences in medical practice, both in the past and in the future. In trying to tackle this complex issue, it was necessary to touch briefly along the way on the conflict between the practice of clinical science and the art of handling sick people; this seemed particularly relevant at a time when the basic medical sciences are engaged in the reductionist pastime of stripping individuals down to their last DNA building block and when there is increasing public disillusionment with high-technology medicine and the biological sciences.

There are several reasons why the discrepancy, whether real or apparent, between the scientific basis of medicine and its day-to-day practice remains an important issue. It still tends to polarize the staff of our major teaching centers into academic physicians, who try to combine their clinical practice with research, and "proper doctors," who devote all their time to clinical care. But more importantly, there is a growing fear that as our approach to disease becomes increasingly reductionist, it will have a dehumanizing effect on medical care. What, it is asked, will medicine look like in a few years' time, when disease is being defined at the level of sick molecules and cells and the activities of doctors are being driven largely by the pressures of a marketplace economy? And these fears are only part of a broader public concern about modern medicine and biology. Is it right to be tinkering with our genes, the very essence of life itself? Will these tensions tend to drive biomedical scientists and those who practice medicine even further apart?

Undoubtedly these questions will raise considerable problems and challenges for the medical educators of the future. In addition, they may pose increasing difficulties for clinical investigation, which, as discussed elsewhere in this symposium, is going through a particularly difficult period. But is it inevitable that the tensions between the science and the practice of medicine will worsen in the future? To address these problems, we must look first to the past and see how they have arisen. A better understanding of their origins and of how they have been perpetuated, together with a more holistic view of disease set in its broader biological perspective, offers the hope of avoiding some of these difficulties in the future.

Although it is difficult to define the moment at which "scientific medicine" came of age, many historians find it convenient to date it to the 1628 publication of the account by William Harvey (1578–1657) of the circulation of blood. This view was eloquently summarized by William Osler in his Harveian Oration to the Royal College of Physicians of London in 1906:

> But at last came the age of the hand—the thinking, devising, planning hand; the hand as an instrument of the mind, now re-introduced into the world in a modest little monograph of 72 pages, from which we may date the beginning of experimental medicine.

The divide between the science and the practice of medicine can already be seen in the remarkable period of scientific endeavor that followed Harvey's insights. In the mid-17th century a group of physician-scientists, some of whom were founding members of the Royal Society, met regularly in Oxford to discuss various aspects of natural philosophy and to describe their experiments. They included Thomas Willis (1621–1675), Richard Lower (1631–1691), and the philosopher and physician John Locke (1632–1704). When Thomas Willis returned to Oxford after the civil war, he was accompanied by Thomas Sydenham (1624–1689), another great physician who was to have a major influence on medical practice, though in a different way from his Oxford contemporaries. Sydenham, who has been called the English Hippocrates, had an enormous influence on medical practice and his ghost still walks the wards of many teaching hospitals—and not just in Great Britain. He was extremely skeptical of academic activities and stated that it was better to send a man to Oxford to learn shoemaking than to practice medicine. He disliked the pretensions of doctors who believed that their scientific research was more important than their day-to-day practice, and he taught that medicine could only be learned by observation at the bedside. He emphasized the primacy of the doctor-patient relationship, stressed the acquisition of knowledge and skills by apprenticeship and contact with patients, was suspicious of theory and of the value of laboratory research, and looked upon good doctoring as a pragmatic art. "Anatomy, botany, nonsense," said Sydenham, "go to the bedside—there only will you learn disease." This attitude permeated the medical scene thereafter, and to some extent still does today. When the great pharmacologist Henry Dale arrived at St. Bartholomew's Hospital as a medical student in 1900, his chief, Samuel Gee, told him that he could forget all the physiology he had learned in Cambridge, since medicine was not a science but merely an empirical art.[2,3]

While the polarization between medical academics and medical practitioners may not be important in itself, these attitudes have had a deleterious effect on the practice of medicine over the centuries, not in the least in the medical profession's apparent reliance on dogma and disregard for scientific evidence. The medical historian William Bynum has addressed the difficult problem of why historical partnerships between science and medicine, knowledge and practice, have never been straightforward.[4] He has traced a tradition of medical practice, based on admiration for Sydenham and his views, which is still a major force in our teaching hospitals. It reflects a view of medicine as an individualistic art, founded on systematic bedside observations and skills, together with a deep suspicion of theory and laboratory research. But he does not see it as naively antiscientific or dogmatic. In part, he suggests, it may result from the different attitudes of mind required of the producers of medical knowledge and of those who dispense it. One of the founders of clinical science in England, Sir Thomas Lewis, summarized these qualities as follows:

> Self confidence is by general consent one of the essentials to the practice of medicine, for it breeds confidence, faith, and hope. Diffidence, by equally general consent, is an essential quality of investigation, for it breeds inquiry. Here then are the chief characteristics, each necessary in its own sphere, each unsuited to the other.

In the second half of the 20th century, as clinical practice has become more and more reliant on the fruits of basic science and technology, the demarcation between the producers and dispensers has become less marked. And with the recent rediscovery of evidence-based medicine, first popularized by Pierre Charles Alexandre Louis (1787–1872) and the Paris school, many practitioners have relied less on dogma. Yet during the latter half of this century, other tensions between the basic biomedical sciences and medical practitioners have arisen.

Over the last 20 years, there has been a change in the emphasis of medical research. Rather than concentrate their efforts on patients or diseased organs, scientists are now focusing their attention on pathology at the level of cells and molecules. While many of those who have been most successful in this new type of biomedical research have had some knowledge of the foibles of clinical medicine, many have not. The latter, in their enthusiasm for the remarkable potential molecular biology holds for a better understanding of disease mechanisms, have made claims that are often premature and naive. This kind of thinking is exemplified by the distinguished molecular biologist Leroy Hood in an article entitled "Biology and Medicine in the 21st Century,"[5] in which he writes:

> The diagnosis of disease-predisposing genes will alter the basic practice of medicine in the 21st century. Perhaps in 20 years it will be possible to take DNA from newborns and analyze 50 or more genes for the allelic forms that can predispose the infant to many common diseases—cardiovascular, cancer, autoimmune, or metabolic. For each defective gene there will be therapeutic regimes that will circumvent the limitations of the defective gene. Thus medicine will move from a reactive mode (curing patients already sick) to a preventative mode (keeping people well). Preventative medicine should enable most individuals to live a normal, healthy, and intellectually alert life without disease.

It is claims like these, or the predictions for the early successes of gene therapy in the early 1980s, that have tended to produce a further divide between practicing clinicians and biological scientists. Hardly a day goes by without the announcement of yet another "gene" for a particular disease, usually associated with a footnote that this new discovery will have a major beneficial effect for clinical practice in the near future. And yet time goes by and these benefits do not seem to materialize. Hence there is a growing suspicion among practicing doctors that all this hype is, and will continue to be, irrelevant to their day-to-day activities; Sydenham was right all along!

In short, current tensions between the science and the practice of medicine seem to stem from the exaggerated hopes and claims of the remarkable developments in molecular biology of recent years, together with the fear that this increasingly reductionist approach to biomedical research will simply exaggerate the dehumanizing effect of modern high-technology medicine. But neither of these problems is insoluble. If the medical sciences and medical practice are willing to recognize the complexities of sick human beings, this should breed more humility on the part of our biomedical research community and, at the same time, a better understanding of the problems that will face them on the part of our doctors of the future. If, at the same time, we can somehow convey the message that the study of disease at the level of molecules and cells does not necessarily mean that medical practice will take a more reductionist approach to patients, it may still be possible to temper these conflicts in the future.

In his remarkable book *This is Biology, the Study of the Living World*,[6] Ernst Mayr discusses the thorny problems of how the life sciences are structured and how their important questions are defined. After describing the efforts of innumerable committees to clarify this problem he comes up with the refreshingly simple answer. There are only three big questions, he says: "what," "how," and "why." The "what" questions deal with descriptions of things as they are. While the term "descriptive biology" has a somewhat pejorative ring about it, it is the vital base upon which the more complex questions can be explored. The "how" and "why" questions can be addressed under two main headings. First, there are the proximal causes—that is, how things actually work. These encompass such disciplines as physiology, cell biology, and molecular biology. Second, there are the ultimate causes. How did things get like they are and why are they as they are? These require the application of such disciplines as evolutionary biology, transmission genetics, ecology, and ethology.

This approach to the definition of the central questions of biology can be equally well applied to the problems of diseases and patients. How does the simplest disease state—that is, one due to a single defective gene—fare when approached in this way? Since I have been studying genetic anemias due to single defective genes for the last 30 years, I thought it would be interesting to see how far we had advanced towards a genuine understanding of the biology of what should be one of the less complicated problems in modern medicine.

The thalassemias, hereditary disorders of hemoglobin, are the commonest monogenic diseases in man.[7] Over a period of about 20 years, after their first description in 1925, their clinical heterogeneity together with their widespread occurrence in many populations of the world was described in detail; by the early 1950s, the "what" questions of their descriptive biology had been adequately answered. In the 1960s, it was possible to start to answer some of the questions relating to their proximal causes—first their cell biology and later their molecular pathology. Indeed, the tools of molecular and cell biology have enabled us not only to understand how the primary mutations of the ß-globin genes are manifest in abnormalities of the function and development of red cell precursors and their progeny, but also provided some genuine understanding about how the action of a limited number of other genes can modify the phenotypes of these single gene disorders.

What of the ultimate causes of these diseases? In recent years, it has been possible to obtain unequivocal evidence that their remarkably high frequency in many populations is the result of the protection of heterozygotes against severe forms of malaria. In fact, the most recent work in this field suggests that children with these diseases may be protected from other infections, possibly as a secondary effect stemming from the fact that malaria is such a debilitating disease in populations in which it is holoendemic. Thus we are beginning to see how these single gene disorders can have a profound effect on the pattern of the health of populations in which they are common, and we are starting to obtain some information about evolutionary biology and transmission genetics.

Work of this kind has also begun to provide insights about the remarkable differences in individual response to a wide range of other infections that are very common in children with these blood diseases. During the relatively short period—that is, in evolutionary terms—in which human races have been exposed to malaria, it is not just the hemoglobin disorders that have been selected by heterozygote resistance. Many other polymorphisms, including those of the HLA-DR system and a variety of cytokines, have also been selected. Because this has also happened over a short evolutionary time, every population has a different set of polymorphisms, just as they have different sets of thalassemia mutations. Hence in every population in which thalassemias are found, there is a different background of genetic susceptibility to infection.

It is also apparent that ecological factors play a major role in modifying the phenotype of children with the same type of genetic disease. The environment in which they live has—through factors such as nutrition, patterns of infection, availability of health care, and many others—a major effect on their reaction to the disease. And it is increasingly clear that ethological factors are of importance. Different societies have widely varying approaches to genetic illness, and individual religious groups have an equally broad spectrum of attitudes to how these conditions should be viewed and handled; there is also a remarkable variation in individual patients' approaches to their disease, much of it depending on cultural and family factors.

In short, a simple, single gene disorder has to be viewed in an individual patient as something that reflects layer upon layer of increasing complexity. If we apply this approach to the study of the common killers of Western society, things get infinitely more complex. Here we are not dealing with diseases with a single cause—that is, a mutant gene or an infectious organism; instead, heart disease, stroke, and cancer reflect the interaction of many different genes with a wide variety of environmental factors together with the ill-understood biological changes of aging. Anybody who believes that a simple genetic test at birth will be able to predict the age of onset of a heart attack or of diabetes in middle life should think again. It may be that in the long-term future, when the interplay among our thousands of genes, the environment, and the effects of aging are better understood, this may be possible. But the very complexity of these interactions suggests that this will not be feasible in the near future.

This is not to decry this kind of research. Along the way, as we understand the action of the genes that make us more or less susceptible to our common killers, much valuable information will be obtained, not in the least for the pharmaceutical industry. And as we come to grips with the complexities of cancer, or the actions of the nervous system at the cellular and molecular level, similar benefits will arise.

It is important, therefore, that the multiple layers of biological complexity as outlined by Mayr are emphasized in the future—not only as we develop new approaches to medical education but also as a constant reminder to biomedical science that it needs to take a more humble view of some of the problems that it is tackling, regardless of the remarkable new technology that it has at its fingertips.

So what of the future? The divide between the science and the practice of medicine remains, as it always has been, based on mistrust largely stemming from lack of communication and understanding between investigator and practitioner. Both need to think more carefully about the nature of their skills. Medical researchers need to constantly remind themselves about the extreme complexity of the biology of sick people. Similarly, practitioners educated to an increasingly sophisticated level about the biology of disease also have to come to grips with this problem. Having tried, with limited success, to bridge both camps for many years, when writing *Science and the Quiet Art* I tried to summarize the position as follows:

> The principal problem for those who educate our doctors of the future is how, on the one hand, to encourage a lifelong attitude of critical, scientific thinking to the management of illness and, on the other, to recognize that moment when the scientific approach, because of ignorance, has reached its limits and must be replaced by sympathetic empiricism. Because of the dichotomy between the self-confidence required at the bedside and self-critical uncertainty essential in the research laboratory, it may be difficult to achieve this balance. Can one person ever combine the two qualities? Possibly not, but this is the goal to which medicine must aspire.

Several important issues must be emphasized in the education of biomedical scientists and those who wish to become practicing clinicians in the future. First, the study of disease at the cellular and molecular level, while it is reductionist, does not necessarily mean that medicine will become more dehumanizing and less holistic. On the contrary, it could well have the opposite effect. Since World War II, medical practice has become split into more and more watertight specialties, not always to the benefit of the patient. As medical research has moved to the molecular and cellular level, this has had the effect of breaking down these barriers; medical scientists from a wide variety of different clinical disciplines are now using exactly the same tools to study disease. This attitude can and should spread to clinical practice. With our increasing aged populations, fewer and fewer patients are being encountered who have disease involving only one system. Our teaching hospitals of the future will have to revive the central role of the generalist just as, when the Human Genome Project is complete, the next generation of biologists will have to take a more holistic view and, using biomathematical approaches that have not yet even been dreamed of, try to put the human organism back together and see how it works as a whole.

Another message from the DNA era, and one that also has to be emphasized in medical education, is that the study of human genes tells us that everybody is unique. This simple observation seems to be lost on those who decry our reductionist approach to medical research, and it is one that cannot be overemphasized by medical educators.

But the central issue to be understood by the doctors of the future is the complexity of the biology of disease and of sick people. This can best be taught by using simple examples of the kind that were described earlier. Thus although much of medical education will have to remain rooted in the "what" questions of pathology, the "hows" and "whys" and their complexities must not be underemphasized. If the medical students of the future, together with biomedical scientists, fully appreciate and accept these complexities for what they are, both should achieve a level of humility that will tend to reduce the stresses and strains between the investigators and practitioners. It will also help to emphasize for our students the vital importance of the old skills of communication and of clinical method that, given the multifaceted problems of sick people, will probably always be required, whatever the sophisticated technology of the diagnostic laboratory has to offer. Finally, viewing the future in this way should underline the increasing importance of the "middleman," that is, the clinical investigator, in drawing together the worlds of medical research and practice.

REFERENCES

1. WEATHERALL, D.J. 1995. Science and the Quiet Art. W.W. Norton & Company. New York; and Oxford University Press. Oxford.
2. BOOTH, C.C. 1989. Clinical research. *In* Historical Perspectives on the Role of the MRC. J. Austoker and L. Bryder, Eds. :205–241. Oxford University Press. Oxford.
3. BOOTH, C.C. 1993. History of science in medicine. *In* Science in Medicine: How Far has it Advanced? G. Teeling-Smith and C. Roberts, Eds.: 11–22. Office of Health Economics. London.
4. BYNUM, W. 1993. Historical background: medicine as dogma. *In* Science in Medicine: How Far has it Advanced? G. Teeling-Smith and C. Roberts, Eds. 1–10. Office of Health Economics. London.
5. HOOD, L. 1992. Biology and medicine in the twenty-first century. *In* The Code of Codes. D.J. Kevles and L. Hood, Eds.: 136–163. Harvard University Press. Cambridge, Mass. .
6. MAYR, E. 1997. This is Biology, The Science of the Living World. Harvard University Press. Cambridge, MA.
7. WEATHERALL, D.J. Historical perspectives. *In* The Thalassaemia Syndromes, 4th ed. D.J. Weatherall and J.B. Clegg, Eds. Blackwell. Oxford. In press.

The Making of a Physician-Scientist: 2000[a]

MICHAEL S. BROWN

Distinguished Professor of Biomedical Sciences, University of Texas Southwestern Medical Center at Dallas, Dallas, Texas 75235-9046, USA

It is an honor to be here, and especially to be the last speaker in a long but exciting symposium. I was reminded of an experience that a friend of mine had a couple of years ago when he spoke at a Gordon Conference, right here in New Hampshire. At the last session of the last day, when he got up to give his talk, my friend looked out at the audience and saw only one person. "Nevertheless," he thought to himself, "I might as well give the talk anyway." So he gave his whole talk, and the man in the audience applauded, and my friend went down and shook his hand and said, "Well, sir, I don't know you, but I guess you must be very interested in this topic and I'm really glad you came." And the man said, "Interested in this topic? Hell, no, I'm the next speaker." So at least more than the next speaker showed up this morning, and I am grateful.

We have celebrated 200 years of history by discussing the problems of the present and the promise of the future. And as Dartmouth enters its third century, it is appropriate that we close this symposium with a discussion of the problems that will confront medical education over the next hundred years. I will focus on one of those problems: the need to educate a new breed of physician-scientists to perform patient-oriented clinical research.

You have just heard a magnificent example from Professor Weatherall of how a clever, creative physician with a deep interest in a particular disease can use modern technologies to define the molecular nature of that disease and, by extension, to learn important lessons about other diseases. The problem is we are not producing enough David Weatheralls—not enough physician-scientists—to take advantage of the enormous technological breakthroughs that the basic scientists are giving us. In particular, we are not producing enough individuals who conduct patient-oriented research.

By patient-oriented research, I mean research that requires, and is stimulated by, direct contact between a scientist and a patient. It is not the same as disease-oriented research, even though both are directed toward the eradication of disease. Disease-oriented research may use patient material such as DNA or cultured cells, but it does not use the whole patient. It can be performed by Ph.D.'s as well as M.D.'s, and it does not require a medical background. But patient-oriented research must be performed by physicians who observe, analyze, and manage individual patients. As a rule of thumb, if the investigator shakes hands with patients in the course of the research, that scientist is performing patient-oriented research. Disease-oriented research is now flourishing as never before, but patient-oriented research is falling further and further behind.

[a]This presentation was adapted from Goldstein, J.L. & M.S. Brown. 1997. The clinical investigator: bewitched, bothered, and bewildered—but still beloved. *Journal of Clinical Investigation* **99**: 2803–2812.

Joseph Goldstein began this symposium by telling us about three revolutions in his lifetime: burgers, chips, and genes. All three represent great technological advances. Burgers and chips revolutionized our lives, but genes have not. While 1,300 biotechnology companies have been formed, they have so far produced only 17 products. Some of these products are helpful, but none has brought about a therapeutic revolution on the order of penicillin or aspirin. Genetics has given us the names of the defective genes in cystic fibrosis and Huntington's disease and breast cancer, but it hasn't given us cures for them. I believe that most of the ethical controversy about genetics would disappear tomorrow if we could treat these diseases as well as we can diagnose them.

The really great therapeutic successes of medicine have come in the fight against microbes that invade our bodies from the outside. We have conquered polio and tuberculosis and pneumonia, but we have made barely a dent in diseases that are caused by internal problems like mutant genes. (David Weatherall's example of thalassemia is quite the exception to this rule.) To conquer the chronic degenerative diseases like Huntington's, Parkinson's, Alzheimer's, cancer, diabetes, and heart attacks, we need a new kind of physician-scientist, one who is trained both in medicine and in science and who brings the same creativity to the bedside that the basic scientist brings to the laboratory.

The failure to cure disease is particularly tragic, because basic scientists have given us unprecedented tools. We have learned a whole new way to discover drugs. First, we clone human genes that produce enzymes, hormones, receptors, or ion channels. Then we use these genes to produce the products in a test tube. Through combinatorial chemistry—a totally new mechanism of chemical synthesis—we produce millions of new chemicals, and then we use robots to test each one of these millions of chemicals for their ability to inhibit the cloned products. And we end up with biological modifiers of unprecedented power and specificity. The process is extremely efficient. One large drug company claims a 95% success rate when searching for inhibitors of any enzyme.

But just as this technology should be leading to treatments for disease, we have hit a roadblock. We create chemicals that do wondrous things in test tubes, but when we test them in people they don't work. Sixteen of the last 17 clinical trials by biotechnology firms have failed. The big companies do not do much better. What's wrong? Why haven't the basic scientists cured more diseases?

I believe the answer lies in the widening gap between basic scientists and clinical practitioners. All of the advances that I have mentioned were made by scientists who do fundamental laboratory research. They can inhibit any enzyme, but who tells them which enzyme to inhibit? Who exposes the Achilles heel of common diseases? For this task, physician-scientists are needed—rare individuals who practice medicine on a daily basis, who understand the complexities of disease, and who, at the same time, are versed in the tools of scientists. Basic scientists can design the weapon and they can load it with ammunition, but only the physician-scientist can aim it.

Let me give you a few examples. The only reason that we recognize Huntington's disease, Parkinson's disease, and Alzheimer's disease is because three doctors named Huntington, Parkinson, and Alzheimer discovered them. Alois Alzheimer is a good example. He was a physician practicing in Germany at the turn of the century. At that time nearly all patients with dementia were thought to suffer from syphilis.

In 1907, Alzheimer described a single patient, a woman who died from progressive dementia. He performed a postmortem examination and used a technological breakthrough of his time, a new histochemical stain that had just been developed. With this stain he saw plaques and tangles that are now recognized as the hallmarks of Alzheimer's disease. With his one patient, Alzheimer separated his disease from syphilis and directed scientists to the pathologic plaques, which eventually led to all the progress that has been made in understanding this disease.

The arena of drug discovery contains many examples of accomplishments by creative physicians. Let me mention just one: the discovery of cortisone, the first anti-inflammatory steroid. The story begins with Philip Hench, a rheumatologist at the Mayo Clinic. In 1929, he observed that his patients with rheumatoid arthritis often improved during pregnancy. He thought that pregnancy must induce the production of some internal anti-inflammatory hormone. In the 1930s, he began to collaborate with a chemist, Edward Kendall, also at the Mayo Clinic, who was isolating steroids from the adrenal glands of cows. Hench administered these steroids to his patients, and after 20 years of trial and error he found one that had a remarkable effect. He gave this steroid to a woman who had been bedridden for months with severe, crippling rheumatoid arthritis, and within 24 hours she rose from her bed and walked the halls of the Mayo Clinic. That chemical was cortisone. Hench's discovery marked a major milestone in the treatment of inflammatory disease. His work paved the way for the later discovery of nonsteroidal anti-inflammatory drugs such as ibuprofen, which are in widespread use today. So the next time you take an Advil or Motrin for a headache, give thanks to Dr. Philip Hench.

But before you think that all of this is ancient history, let me provide two contemporary examples. In 1981, an astute physician named Michael Gottlieb at UCLA noticed three homosexual men who entered the hospital with a rare infection called pneumocystis pneumonia that only strikes people whose immune systems are weak. Working with a basic immunologist at UCLA, Gottlieb used a brand new reagent to show that the homosexual men had a deficiency of helper T-cells. Gottlieb's 1981 paper was the first description of AIDS.

And in the 1980s, Barry Marshall, a young physician-in-training in Australia, isolated a bacterium called *Helicobacter pylori* from the stomachs of patients with ulcers. He made the audacious suggestion that ulcer disease is not caused by acid as everyone then thought, including me, a trained gastroenterologist, but rather by *Helicobacter.* This work was greeted with extreme skepticism, but Marshall went on to show that the disease could be cured by treatment with antibiotics. Today, ulcer disease is almost always cured by antibiotics, and surgery is almost never performed for this condition—a direct result of Dr. Marshall's discovery.

Now let me give you an example of patient-oriented research that I am *not* talking about: drug trials, at least as they are practiced today. The usual story is that a company develops a drug and after minimal testing on animals, the drug is given to patients; the physicians are told exactly how to administer the drug—the schedule and the dose; and they are told what parameters to measure. Unfortunately, the drug usually doesn't work and is discarded. Of course we need physicians to conduct these trials. But I do not consider this type of work to be creative patient-oriented research. Physicians should be telling the drug companies what drugs to develop, not the other way around. You have heard that war is too important to be left to the generals; like-

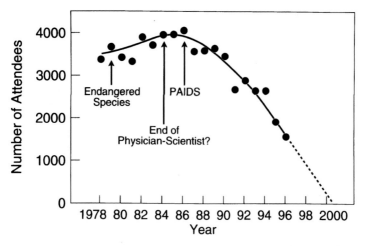

FIGURE 1. Declining attendance at the annual joint meetings of three societies devoted to patient-oriented research: American Society for Clinical Investigation (ASCI), Association of American Physicians (AAP), and American Federation for Medical Research (AFMR). The arrows indicate landmark publications on this topic: by James Wyngaarden in 1979; Gordon Gill in 1984; and Joseph Goldstein in 1986. PAIDS = Paralyzed Academic Investigator's Disease Syndrome.

wise, drug development is too important to be left to the drug companies. We need creative physicians at the beginning to help design drugs and to figure out how best to use them.

But, tragically, just when the need for physician-scientists is greatest, the supply is shrinking. This problem was first pointed out by James Wyngaarden, a former director of the National Institutes of Health. In 1979, Wyngaarden published a paper entitled "The Clinical Investigator as an Endangered Species." He pointed out the sharp decline in the number of NIH grants awarded to physicians who were doing clinical research. Over the succeeding 20 years, that trend has continued and has gotten much worse. Last year, only 20% of research grants from the National Institutes of Health went to M.D.'s.

The trend is reflected in another way, too, in the decline of learned societies devoted to clinical research. FIGURE 1 shows the annual attendance at the joint meeting of three societies for clinical research. For nearly a century, these meetings were the arena in which the most exciting clinical research was shared. In fact, Hench's discovery of cortisone was first presented at this meeting, in 1949. As you can see, the attendance since about 1986 has been declining in a linear fashion. If the decline continues at this rate, the attendance will hit zero early in the 21st century.

The decline in physician-scientists is manifest not only by a drop in grants and attendance at meetings, it is apparent in the composition of every clinical academic department in this country. In their glory days, these departments were as described by Professor Weatherall. Apparently his unit in Oxford maintains this tradition, but most of our departments do not. These departments used to contain a mixture of pure physicians, physician-scientists, and even a few basic scientists, all united in their quest to understand and treat human disease. Now these departments are split. An enormous gap separates those who practice medicine from those who practice science. Rarely do they attend the same conferences and barely do they communicate. As a result of this isolation, most scientists have left clinical departments, including those who hold the M.D. degree.

I should point out, by the way, that many of the symposium speakers who dealt with advances in genetics and neuroscience were M.D.'s who, by and large, do not see patients: Goldstein, Collins, Rakic, and Edelman, for example, are all M.D.'s. They went to medical school and got their M.D. but then left clinical practice. We need to find a way to keep people with that kind of imagination involved with patients.

Why are so many talented scientists leaving the clinic? The causes are clear. Clinical departments face tremendous pressures to provide revenue from clinical services. Academic medical centers compete with private hospitals and health maintenance organizations. Their economic survival depends on caring efficiently for large numbers of patients, leaving little room for research, which is costly, distracting, inefficient, and usually irrelevant to the outcome for a particular patient. Clinical research is also made difficult by the stringent attendance policies of managed care and federal health insurance programs. They demand the constant physical presence of a physician and they prohibit the practice that used to allow academic physicians to supervise patients through residents, thereby freeing time for research.

Not only are physician-scientists being pushed out of clinical pursuits, but they are also being pulled into full-time research. The pace of basic science has increased as a result of technological breakthroughs that produce renewable reagents. These reagents include cloned genes, proteins, and monoclonal antibodies. To the scientist, the rapid dissemination of research tools is good news and bad news. The good news is that you can do lots of experiments. The bad news is that your competitors can also do lots of experiments. This threat increases the pressure to work intensely to stay ahead of the pack, and this competition renders the dual research/clinical career increasingly difficult to follow.

There is yet another reason for the growing split between medicine and science, a problem that both Dr. Tenney and Dr. Weatherall addressed earlier. I consider it to be the most profound problem and one that may be impossible to correct: physicians and scientists have to approach their tasks differently; they simply must think in different ways.

A physician's job is to diagnose and treat disease. Here, the most precious attributes are knowledge, skill, and the ability to act decisively. The physician must know all that can be known about the human body, how each cell works, how cells work together to produce organs, and how organs work together to produce a human being. Physicians must know how diseases disrupt this organization, but they need more than knowledge. They need skills. Physicians must develop their senses so that they can size up a patient with their hands, eyes, and noses, and, most importantly, their ears. Physicians must also be ready to act. There isn't time to look things up in books. Sick patients need action now, and when doctors see 50 patients a day, they must be able to recognize diseases quickly and intervene decisively. This task can be accomplished only if physicians have precise knowledge and buoyant self-confi-

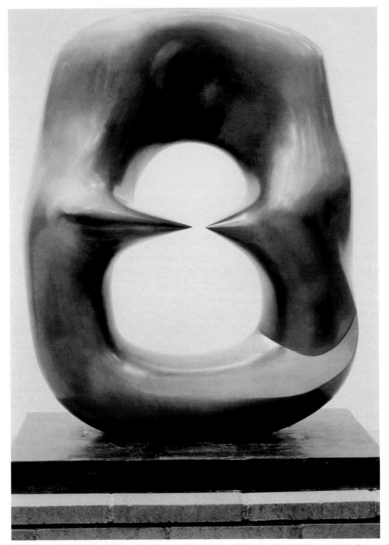

FIGURE 2. Reclining Nude. Sculpture by Henry Moore. © C. Herscovici, Brussels/ Artists Rights Society (ARS), New York.

dence. Physicians must trust the information they gather with their own senses and they must be ready to act.

How does the scientist differ from the physician? The physician knows all there is to know, while the scientist knows all that is *not* known. The scientist sees the gaps in our knowledge. This fundamental difference is illustrated by FIGURE 2, which shows a typical sculpture by the great artist Henry Moore. These great masses of bronze surround large areas of air. The physician sees the masses of bronze, the solid facts that establish the statue. The scientist sees the spaces between the masses. The scientist's job is to discover the invisible architecture that unites the bronze and makes it into a unified structure. To be a scientist, one must learn to think like a scientist. One must learn to appreciate the quality of facts. One must be a tough critic and always be doubting. One must have limitless imagination and curiosity. One must ask *why* something happens, not just *what* happens. One must think hypothetically: "What would happen if the truth were exactly the opposite of what we now believe?"

Medicine and science require complementary thought processes; the processes that work for one are devastating for the other. Many individuals have the type of mind that lends itself to medicine. They can absorb a mass of facts, relate them all, quickly assess problems, and act decisively. These people make great physicians. Others have minds preoccupied with questions. They don't want to practice what's known, they're absorbed with the unknown. These people make excellent scientists. But there are rare individuals whose brains can somehow handle both, who can work with patients decisively using skills that are based solidly on current art, yet who can also work in the lab to *advance* the current art.

Unfortunately, I believe the way we now produce physician-scientists is inadequate to the task. The most popular programs are those leading to the dual M.D./Ph.D. degree. I direct such a program in Dallas, where I have 96 mouths to feed. Our students spend eight to nine years in medical school in order to obtain both the M.D. and the Ph.D. But even though I direct an M.D./Ph.D. program, I believe this prototype to be inadequate. The nation has 125 medical schools, 30 of which offer M.D./Ph.D. programs. Last spring, 15,000 students received M.D. degrees in this country, but only 180 received M.D./Ph.D. degrees in NIH-sponsored programs—roughly one out of 100. Let me put the number in perspective. There are 1,300 biotechnology companies. If there were a competitive, NFL-style draft for newly graduated M.D./Ph.D.'s, it would take seven years before each company could hire even one. And not a single M.D./Ph.D. would be left over to join an academic faculty. Clearly the M.D./Ph.D. programs cannot meet the need for physician-scientists. These programs have other flaws as well, about which I will say more.

So how can medical schools correct the shortage of physician-scientists? Here I'm going to be a little controversial. For the sake of argument, I propose two steps: (1) I think we need special education programs directed specifically at training physician-scientists; and (2) we need protected positions on the faculty for those engaged in patient-oriented research.

Let us consider the educational aspects first. We must recognize that the process that produces inquisitive physician-scientists is different from the one that produces accomplished medical practitioners. Our students have been telling us this for years. Every medical school in the country has been cutting back on the amount of science taught to medical students in order to increase the time students spend with patients. This move, I believe, is both understandable and appropriate. Students who plan to practice medicine must learn how to care for sick people. Of course, they must learn scientific facts and principles as well, but not necessarily the process by which these facts or principles were obtained. By and large, the experimental details are irrelevant and the students reject them—and I believe they are right.

The problem is quite different for those interested in clinical research. To the scientist, experimental detail is everything. Prospective medical scientists must learn

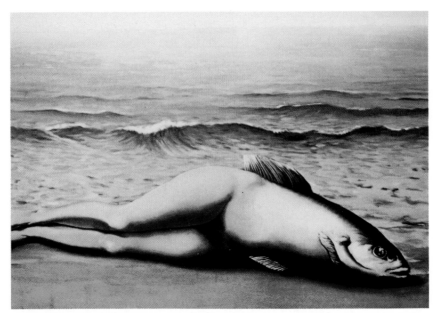

FIGURE 3. *L'Inventive collective* [The collective invention]. René Magritte. © 1997. C. Herscovici, Brussels/Artists'Rights Society (ARS), New York.

the powers and limits of experimental methods. More important, they must be shown the frontier of knowledge. They must be guided by faculty to this frontier and they must be encouraged to use their imaginations to cross that frontier.

The educational aims of the practitioner and the scientist have diverged sufficiently so that a single curriculum can no longer satisfy both. I believe we must offer separate medical school courses to students with separate interests. The separation will help the future practitioners by allowing them to focus their scientific exposure on the relevant facts and principles, freeing up more time for patient care and humanistic pursuits. Prospective scientists, after learning the problems of medical science in the classroom, will then work in the laboratory for at least two to three years in order to absorb the thought processes of science. They would then work with patients during the final two years of medical school and in their residencies.

Although these programs will be separate, in my view they are equal. Both curricula will produce trained professionals who will serve society in separate but equally important roles. Just for the sake of argument, I would propose that perhaps one-third of all medical schools might offer such a dual program but that the majority of schools would continue in the present fashion. In those schools that offer the program, I imagine that perhaps one-third of the students would enroll in the medical scientist program. Overall, therefore, about 10% of our graduates would receive the medical scientist degree, for a total of about 1,500 annually. This output would be enough to supply the biotechnology companies, the drug companies, and the medical schools with trained, young, imaginative medical scientists.

The program I am describing would differ sharply from today's M.D./Ph.D. programs. The most important difference would be the focus of the educational process. Currently, M.D./Ph.D. students take the same medical school courses as do other medical students, but they interrupt the standard medical curriculum in the middle by enrolling in a standard graduate school science program for four to five years. The total length of the program averages eight to nine years, which is much too long. These people are elderly by the time they ever get to set up their own laboratory.

Moreover, the two parts of the program are totally disconnected. Medical school courses don't teach the scientific basis of medicine (at least not adequately), and the graduate school work is usually irrelevant to medical problems. The M.D./Ph.D. ends up something like the chimeric creature in FIGURE 3 painted by René Magritte. You saw many other examples of his work in Joseph Goldstein's presentation. When we published an article on this topic recently, the *Journal of Clinical Investigation* put this painting on their cover with the quote "The Physician–Scientist: All Washed Up." The point is that, like this chimeric creature, the physician-scientist is often divided into two halves. Young students going through an M.D./Ph.D. program are subjected to two totally different types of educational processes, and, as a result, many of them, like this reverse mermaid, are at home neither on land nor at sea, neither in the laboratory nor at the bedside. Frequently, basic scientists will tell M.D./Ph.D. students that clinical practice is boring and nonintellectual, and physicians will tell them that rat doctors know nothing about medicine. No wonder that less than 10% of M.D./Ph.D. graduates end up in patient-oriented research.

The medical scientist program that I propose avoids these pitfalls. The medical scientist will have a medical school curriculum that focuses on the scientific frontier and a research curriculum that focuses on approaches and thought patterns that relate to that frontier. Clinical training will also be targeted toward the inquisitive side, as opposed to the acquisitive side, of medicine.

But of course there is no point in training patient-oriented researchers if there is no place for them to work. So the second part of my proposal is for research-oriented medical schools to establish endowed faculty positions to support patient-oriented researchers in clinical departments. The purpose is to free them from the need to generate their salaries through clinical practice. We have evolved a system in this country where faculty in clinical departments are supported almost entirely by fees that are charged for clinical services by that faculty. Only small amounts of money are available to support salaries for members of clinical departments who are not generating sufficient money from patient care. By providing the endowed positions that I propose, faculty members doing patient-oriented research will have the freedom to select patients because they are relevant to their research program, not because they generate a profit for the department.

Let me urge you not to misunderstand my point: I am not saying that medical schools should abandon community obligations and surrender to the desires of selfish scientists. Medical schools should continue to serve their patients and communities as before. I am simply asking that certain schools set aside a portion of their faculty resources to support the training and practice of patient-oriented researchers.

In conclusion, let me again state how honored I am to be included in the celebration of the 200th anniversary of Dartmouth Medical School. Right now, I don't expect to be around for Dartmouth's 300th anniversary; but if we could turn out a Barry Marshall or a Philip Hench interested in the field of geriatrics, who knows?

I wish to add one more thought. On behalf of Joseph Goldstein and myself and all of the invited speakers at this symposium, I want to express our sincere thanks to Professor Heinz Valtin for the three years of work that went into planning this symposium. He and his colleagues on the Dartmouth faculty spent a huge amount of time selecting the fields that would be covered, picking the speakers who would address those issues, making all the logistic arrangements, and handling about a million-trillion other details that are necessary to put on such a well-integrated and organized symposium. I think we all owe Heinz Valtin a major debt of thanks.

Closing Remarks

HEINZ VALTIN

*Vail and Hampers Professor Emeritus, Dartmouth Medical School, and Chair,
Bicentennial Symposium Planning Committee, Hanover,
New Hampshire 03755-3836, USA*

Now it is time for *me* to express heartfelt thanks. On behalf of Dartmouth Medical
School, of Dartmouth College, of the Symposium Planning Committee, and of you,
the audience, I extend our most sincere thanks to all our distinguished speakers, especially to Drs. Goldstein and Brown, who agreed to chair this event, and to the generous donors who supported it. We are confident that the thoughts expressed here
will stimulate much continuing discourse.

And now, having just given thanks on behalf of the audience, I would like to turn
the tables and thank you, the audience, for your active participation in this
symposium.

It would take far too long to credit here the many persons who contributed their
time, imagination, and energy to the success of this symposium. You know who you
are and though I do not name each of you here, please know that my thank-you to
you as a group comes from the heart. There is, however, one person whom I would
like to single out, and that is Barbara Blough. Her official title during these past three
years has been vice chair of the Bicentennial Symposium Planning Committee, but
there has been absolutely nothing assistant or subordinate in the role that she has
played; rather, she has been a full partner in these endeavors, contributing her initiative and extraordinarily good judgment to the planning of this event. Barbara, thank
you!

Now let me introduce Dr. Christopher Longcope and Dr. David Longcope, who
are two direct descendants of Nathan Smith, the founder of Dartmouth Medical
School. Dr. Christopher Longcope is the great-great-great-grandson of our founder,
and his son David is therefore the great-great-great-great-grandson of Nathan Smith.
They represent the sixth and seventh generations since Nathan Smith and are members of an unbroken line of physicians since Smith.

From the moment three years ago when we started planning Dartmouth Medical
School's bicentennial year, we have wanted this symposium to be the centerpiece. In
our invitations to the prospective participants, we said that we were seeking an international gathering of world-renowned scientists, scholars, and public-policy leaders
who would try to grapple with the critical issues facing the biomedical community
in the years ahead. Now, having experienced these three days, I think we can all
agree that our intent became reality.

Appropriately, this symposium has continued a tradition begun at Dartmouth
Medical School by its founder. Nathan Smith was passionately committed to a scientific approach to medicine. At the same time, however, both Dr. Smith and Dartmouth Medical School have always recognized the importance of the humanities to
our pursuits. Thus, Dartmouth Medical School continues to follow the path set by
Nathan Smith with a curriculum that stresses the interrelatedness between excellent

science and empathetic patient care, and it is not by accident that this symposium has focused on that interrelatedness.

It is noteworthy that while the speakers have identified major problems, many of them have, at the same time, conveyed the message that biomedical scientists stand ready and willing—in fact, eager—to accept the challenges; and by and large, they have expressed conviction that, given enough time, we can solve the problems.

It is on this note of optimism that I would like to close these proceedings. We have full confidence in the future of biomedicine. Our motivation to understand natural phenomena and our fascination with discovery will continue to drive biomedical research even if the newly gained knowledge raises profound and unanticipated questions. We express confidence that as new facts and capabilities raise novel ethical and social issues, means will be found to deal with these problems.

Thus, as we close this symposium, we salute the young people in this audience as well as future generations of physicians and teacher-scientists, who will deal with the great issues for medicine in the 21st century.

Symposium Participants

[Illustrations by Robert Gosselin, M.D., Ph.D., the Irene Heinz Given Professor of Pharmacology Emeritus at Dartmouth Medical School.]

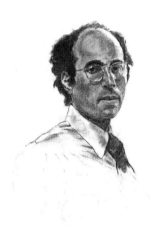

RICHARD AXEL, M.D., a professor of pathology at Columbia University, is a Howard Hughes Medical Institute Investigator and holds Columbia's Higgins Professorship in Biochemistry and Molecular Biophysics. Dr. Axel's major research interest is the application of molecular genetics to problems of neurobiology. His recent work has focused on the molecular biology of perception, particularly the sense of smell. This sense, he has written, has as its basis the largest gene family thus far identified in mammals, which "perhaps reflects the significance of this sensory system for the survival and reproduction of most mammalian species." His recent awards include the John Jay Award, the Science Pour L'Art Award, the Unilever Science Award (shared with Dr. Linda Buck), and the Rosenspiel Award (shared with Dr. Buck and Dr. James Hudspeth). Dr. Axel is a 1967 graduate of Columbia and received his M.D. from the Johns Hopkins University School of Medicine in 1970.

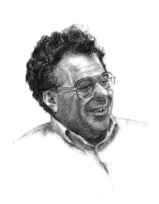

DAVID BOTSTEIN, PH.D., is a professor of genetics and chair of the Department of Genetics at Stanford University School of Medicine. Dr. Botstein's work has centered on the use of genetic methods to understand biological functions. In the early 1970s, he devised novel genetic methods for studying the actin and tubulin cytoskeletons and developed the use of localized random mutagenesis technologies to understand protein structure and function relationships. His theoretical contribution to linkage mapping of the human genome began, with collaborators, with the suggestion that the restriction fragment length polymorphisms could be used to produce a linkage map of the human genome and to map the genes that cause disease in humans. Dr. Botstein, who received an A.B. from Harvard in 1963 and a Ph.D. from the University of Michigan in 1967, was elected to the National Academy of Sciences in 1981 and to the Institute of Medicine in 1993. Among his awards are the Eli Lilly Award in Microbiology, the Genetics Society of America Medal, and the Allen Award of the American Society of Human Genetics. He currently serves on the Advisory Council of the National Human Genome Research Institute and is the author of *The Dynamic Genome* (1992).

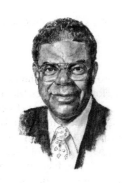

LONNIE R. BRISTOW, M.D., served as president of the American Medical Association from June 1995 to June 1996. A member of the AMA's board of trustees from 1985 to 1997, Dr. Bristow had earlier served as chair of the Section on Internal Medicine of the California Medical Association and as president of the American Society of Internal Medicine. In 1977, Dr. Bristow was elected to membership in the Institute of Medicine of the National Academy of Sciences. He is a graduate of the City College of New York and received his M.D. degree from the New York University College of Medicine in 1957. He has written and lectured extensively on medical science as well as on socioeconomic and ethical issues in medicine. He was appointed by President Clinton to chair the board of regents of the Uniformed Services University of the Health Sciences, and he has served on the Institute of Medicine's Committee on the Effects of Medical Professional Liability on the Delivery of Maternal and Child Health Care, on the Federal Interagency Committee on Smoking and Health, on the Centers for Disease Control's HIV Prevention Advisory Committee, and on the 1989 Quadrennial Advisory Council on Social Security. In addition, he was one of two public representatives in the settlement talks between tobacco companies and a group of state attorneys general.

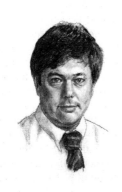

MICHAEL S. BROWN, M.D., was awarded the 1985 Nobel Prize in Medicine or Physiology with his colleague Joseph L. Goldstein for their work in identifying the process by which receptors on human cells trap and absorb bloodstream particles that contain cholesterol. The discovery led to a new understanding of how excessive levels of fatty cholesterol accumulate to clog human arteries and cause strokes and heart attacks. Dr. Brown earned both his bachelor's degree and his M.D. from the University of Pennsylvania, and did postdoctoral training in biochemistry at the National Institutes of Health. His work focused on gastroenterology, specifically the role of enzymes in controlling the chemistry of the digestive system, before he became a research fellow at the University of Texas Southwestern Medical School in Dallas; there, he and Dr. Goldstein began a collaborative study of the cells of victims of familial hypercholesterolemia (inherited high blood cholesterol), looking for genetic abnormalities. The Nobel committee's citation said, "Michael S. Brown and Joseph L. Goldstein have through their discoveries revolutionized our knowledge about the regulation of cholesterol metabolism and the treatment of diseases caused by abnormally elevated cholesterol in the blood." Currently, Dr. Brown holds a Regental Professorship at the University of Texas and is a Distinguished Professor of

Biomedical Sciences at UT Southwestern Medical Center. In addition, he is director of UT Southwestern's Jonsson Center for Molecular Genetics.

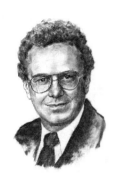

DANIEL J. CALLAHAN, Ph.D., cofounder of the Hastings Center and its president from 1969 to 1996, is now director of the Center's international programs and a senior associate for health policy. Dr. Callahan received a B.A. from Yale, an M.A. from Georgetown University, and a Ph.D. in philosophy from Harvard; in addition, he holds honorary degrees from several institutions. He is the author or editor of 33 books, including *What Kind of Life: The Limits of Medical Progress* (1990); *Setting Limits: Medical Goals in an Aging Society* (1987); *Ethics in Hard Times* (1982); and, with his wife, Sidney, *Abortion: Understanding Differences* (1984). A noted and frequently quoted authority on medical ethics, Dr. Callahan is an elected member of the Institute of Medicine of the National Academy of Sciences, a Fellow of the American Association for the Advancement of Science, a member of the Director's Advisory Council at the Centers for Disease Control, and a former member of the Advisory Council of the Office of Scientific Integrity of the U.S. Department of Health and Human Services. He won the 1996 Freedom and Scientific Responsibility Award of the American Association for the Advancement of Science.

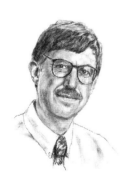

FRANCIS S. COLLINS, M.D., Ph.D., is a physician-geneticist and the director of the National Human Genome Research Institute, which is engaged in a 15-year project to map and sequence all of the human DNA by the year 2005. Collins received an undergraduate degree in chemistry at the University of Virginia and a doctorate in physical chemistry at Yale, before becoming interested in molecular biology and genetics and entering medical school at the University of North Carolina. After his residency in internal medicine at Chapel Hill, Dr. Collins returned to Yale for a fellowship in human genetics and then went on to a faculty position at the University of Michigan, where he worked on methods of crossing large stretches of DNA to identify genes responsible for specific diseases. This approach, positional cloning, allowed Dr. Collins and colleagues to identify the gene for cystic fibrosis in 1989, the gene for neurofibromatosis in 1990, and the gene for Huntington's disease in 1993. A scientist who combines passions for religion, motorcycles, and the practice of medicine, Dr. Collins has won dozens of awards, including the Susan G. Komen Breast Cancer Foundation National Award for Scientific Distinction for his work in searching for the genetic causes of both inherited and randomly arising breast cancer. He is a member of the National Academy of Sciences.

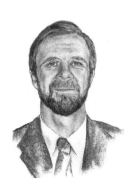

NILS M.P. DAULAIRE, M.D., M.P.H., was at the time of the Bicentennial Symposium the deputy assistant administrator for policy and chief health policy advisor at the U.S. Agency for International Development; since 1998, he has been the president and CEO of the Global Health Council. In his former position, he was responsible for policy development and oversight of all of USAID's sustainable development programs in health, population, food security, women's empowerment, girls' and women's education, basic education, poverty alleviation, and the environment. He previously served as director of the International Center for the Prevention and Treatment of Major Childhood Diseases and as director of the international health division of the John Snow Public Health Group. A graduate of Harvard College, Harvard Medical School, and the Johns Hopkins School of Hygiene and Public Health, Dr. Daulaire has devoted two decades to field work in international public health, principally in southern Asia and sub-Saharan Africa. He has been a member of the faculty at Dartmouth's and Harvard's medical schools and has published widely in international journals. In his post at USAID, he was the Clinton administration's most senior appointed official devoted to international health and population issues in the developing world. In addition to English, Dr. Daulaire speaks, in order of fluency, Norwegian, French, German, Nepali, Spanish, Swedish, Danish, Bangla, and Bambara.

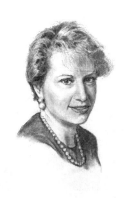

SUSAN G. DENTZER, a 1977 graduate of Dartmouth College, was at the time of the Bicentennial Symposium an economics writer and contributing editor for *U.S. News & World Report*, where for more than 10 years she specialized in political and economic issues, particularly health-care policy and the economics of the Medicare program. Currently, she is a correspondent on PBS's *NewsHour with Jim Lehrer,* and before her stint at *U.S. News & World Report* she was a senior writer at *Newsweek*. Dentzer is also currently a member of Dartmouth's Board of Trustees and is the recipient of an honorary master of arts degree from Dartmouth, as well as the College's Presidential Medal for Achievement. While a Nieman Fellow at Harvard in 1986-87, she studied health economics, management psychology, and other disciplines; she also held a fellowship in the Japan Society's U.S.-Japan Leadership Program in 1991 and has since then pursued an interest in U.S.-Japanese economic relations and the effects of the aging Japanese population. Dentzer has been a frequent guest on such television programs as *Nightline, The McLaughlin Group,* and *Washington Week in Review* and a commentator on Public Radio International's business news show, *Marketplace.*

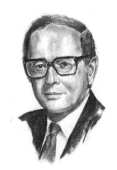

GERALD M. EDELMAN, M.D., Ph.D., the Nobel Laureate in Medicine or Physiology in 1972, is president of the Neurosciences Research Foundation, Inc., and director of the Neurosciences Institute, as well as the chairman of neurobiology at the Scripps Research Institute. He earned his B.S. from Ursinus College, an M.D. from the University of Pennsylvania, and a Ph.D. from the Rockefeller Institute; he also has numerous earned and honorary D.Sc. degrees from institutions as diverse as the University of Miami and the University of Cagliari in Sardinia. Dr. Edelman's early studies of the structure and diversity of antibodies led to his Nobel award; he then began research into the mechanisms involved in the regulation of primary cellular processes, particularly the control of cell growth and the development of multicellular organisms. In work focusing on cell-cell interactions, Dr. Edelman identified cell adhesion molecules, which guide the fundamental processes by which an animal achieves its shape and form and by which nervous systems are built. At the juncture of these two discoveries lies the basis of Dr. Edelman's theory of the development and organization of higher brain functions, a process known as neuronal group selection, which was presented in his 1987 book, *Neural Darwinism.* Dr. Edelman is a member of the National Academy of Sciences and the author of several books and more than 400 research publications.

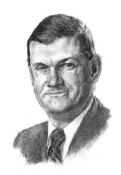

ROBERT G. EVANS, Ph.D., is a professor of economics and a member of the faculty of the Centre for Health Services and Policy Research at the University of British Columbia. He received a B.A. in political economy from the University of Toronto and a Ph.D. in economics from Harvard. He has written extensively on the Canadian health-care system and its economy, and his work has been praised for its extraordinary lucidity and insight. His provocatively-titled publications include *Who Are the Zombie Masters, and What Do They Want?* (1994), *Normative Rabbits From Positive Hats: Mark Pauly on Welfare Economics* (1996), and *Sharing the Burden, Containing the Cost: Fundamental Conflicts in Health Care Finance* (1997). Dr. Evans was a member of the SNS International Panel Review of the Swedish Health Care System in 1991; a consultant at the World Bank/Economic Development Institute Senior Health Policy Seminar in Beijing, China, in 1993; and a member of the LSE Health Team reviewing the Greek Health Services in 1994. He is an honorary life member of both the Canadian College of Health Service Executives and the Canadian Health Economics Research Association.

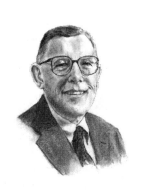

JAMES O. FREEDMAN served as president of Dartmouth College from 1987 to 1998. A native of Manchester, N.H., he rec.ived his B.A., *cum laude,* from Harvard in 1957 and LL.B., *cum laude,* from Yale Law School in 1962. After clerking for Justice Thurgood Marshall, he practiced law for a year before joining the University of Pennsylvania Law School faculty in 1964. He became university ombudsman at Penn in 1973, associate provost in 1978, and law school dean in 1979. In 1982, he was appointed president of the University of Iowa. Freedman's primary teaching and scholarly interests have been administrative law and higher education. He is the author of *Crisis and Legitimacy: The Administrative Process and American Government,* of *Idealism and Liberal Education,* and of numerous articles and reviews. In addition, he chaired the Pennsylvania Legislative Reappointment Commission in 1981, was a member of the City of Philadelphia Board of Ethics from 1980 to 1982, and chaired the Iowa Governor's Task Force on Foreign Language Studies and International Education in 1983. He has served as a professor of law at the Salzburg Seminar in American Studies and as a visiting professor at many institutions, including Cambridge University. In 1991 he received the William O. Douglas First Amendment Freedom Award of the Anti-Defamation League of B'nai B'rith, and in 1996 the Frederic W. Ness Book Award of the Association of American Colleges and Universities. He also holds seven honorary degrees.

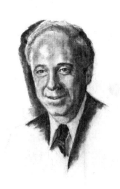

JOSEPH L. GOLDSTEIN, M.D., who shared the Nobel Prize in Physiology or Medicine in 1985 with Michael S. Brown, chairs the Department of Molecular Genetics at the University of Texas Southwestern Medical Center at Dallas. He is also the Paul J. Thomas Professor of Medicine and Genetics and a Regental Professor of the University of Texas. Dr. Goldstein received a B.S. degree from Washington and Lee University and an M.D. from the University of Texas Southwestern Medical School. His work with Dr. Brown, which identified the receptors that control cholesterol metabolism, also earned the Albert B. Lasker Award in Basic Medical Research in 1985 and the National Medal of Science in 1988. Dr. Goldstein spent two years in the Laboratory of Biomedical Genetics at the National Heart Institute in

Bethesda; at the time, the laboratory's director was Dr. Marshall Nirenberg, who was a Nobel Laureate in 1968. Considered a genius in medical school and described as "the most brilliant student I ever had" by Dr. Arno G. Motulsky, with whom he worked at the University of Washington in Seattle in the area of the genetic aspects of heart disease, Dr. Goldstein formed a close working and personal relationship with Dr. Brown while they were both interns at Massachusetts General Hospital.

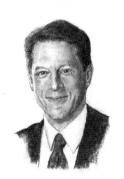

AL GORE is the 45th vice president of the United States. A 1969 graduate of Harvard who also attended Vanderbilt University Divinity School and Vanderbilt Law School, Gore was elected to the U.S. House of Representatives in 1976 and to the Senate in 1984. In 1990, he became the first candidate in modern history, Republican or Democrat, to win all 95 of Tennessee's counties in a senatorial election. As a member of Congress, Gore was active in arms control, consumer and tax issues, and health affairs. He conducted hearings that led to the passage of the National Organ Transplant Act, was a lead sponsor of legislation strengthening warning labels on cigarettes, and was a principal sponsor of the measure that placed warning labels on alcoholic beverages. Gore also served as chair of the U.S. Senate delegation to the Earth Summit in 1992. In his book *Earth in the Balance: Ecology and the Human Spirit,* he outlined an international plan to confront global environmental problems —the topic of his presentation at the Bicentennial Symposium.

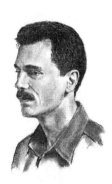

THOMAS HOMER-DIXON, Ph.D., is director of the University of Toronto's Peace and Conflict Studies Program and an assistant professor of political science at Toronto. He earned his doctorate in political science from the Massachusetts Institute of Technology in 1989. Since then, he has used the disciplines of environmental studies, demographics, economics, and the study of violent civil conflict to examine the role of population growth, environmental degradation, and conflict in developing nations. "Humans cannot survive unless we harvest the earth's resources and exploit our environment, and yet we will not survive for long unless we use our resources sparingly. My whole approach is pragmatic," Homer-Dixon has said. Among his past activities have been working as a surveyor for logging companies in the British Columbia interior and as a laborer on a natural-gas rig. More recently, he advised Vice President Al Gore and the heads of the CIA and USAID on the effects of population growth, environmental resource exhaustion, and conflict in Third World countries. Dr. Homer-Dixon is also an associate fellow of the Canadian Institute for Advanced Research and the principal investigator of the project "Environmental Scarcity, State Capacity, and Civil Violence," which is sponsored by the Peace and Conflict Studies Program and the American Academy of Arts and Sciences.

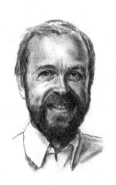

PHILIP KITCHER, Ph.D., is the Presidential Professor of Philosophy at the University of California, San Diego (UCSD). His fields of specialization include ethical issues in contemporary biology, the history and philosophy of biology, scientific explanation, realism, naturalistic epistemology, and the history and philosophy of mathematics. His books include *Abusing Science: The Case Against Creationism* (1982); *The Nature of Mathematic Knowledge* (1983); *Vaulting Ambition: Sociobiology and the Quest for Human Nature* (1985); *The Advancement of Science* (1993); and *The Lives to Come: The Genetic Revolution and Human Possibilities* (1996). He has also written extensively on Kant and is currently editor-in-chief of the journal *Philosophy of Science*. Dr. Kitcher received first class honours in mathematics/history and the philosophy of science from Christ's College, Cambridge, in 1969, and a Ph.D. in the history and philosophy of science from Princeton University in 1974. He was a Guggenheim Fellow in 1988-89; received the UCSD Alumni Distinguished Teaching Award in 1993; was a senior fellow of the Library of Congress (on bioethics issues in molecular genetics) in 1993-94; and is currently vice president of the American Philosophic Association's Pacific Division.

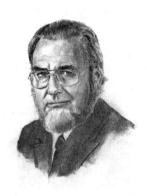

C. EVERETT KOOP, M.D., Sc.D., surgeon general of the United States from 1981 to 1989, is a 1937 graduate of Dartmouth College. He returned to Hanover as the Elizabeth DeCamp McInerny Professor of Surgery in 1992, in order to found the C. Everett Koop Institute at Dartmouth, which is working to reform medical education for the 21st century. Dr. Koop received his M.D. from Cornell University Medical College in 1941 and went on to become a prominent pediatric surgeon at the University of Pennsylvania, where he also earned an Sc.D.; he was also surgeon-in-chief of the Children's Hospital of Philadelphia for more than 30 years. He is a chevalier in the French Foreign Legion of Honor and a fellow of the Royal College of Surgeons in England and of the Royal Society of Medicine. As surgeon general, Dr. Koop gained prominence for his plainspoken campaigns to inform the American public about the dangers of smoking and the transmission of AIDS. He detailed those experiences and others in his 1991 autobiography, *Koop: The Memoirs of*

America's Family Doctor. He continues to be a national figure, speaking out on topics such as obesity, smoking, and patient empowerment in health care. The recipient of numerous honors and awards, including 38 honorary doctorates, Dr. Koop was presented with the Presidential Medal of Freedom, the nation's highest civilian award, in 1995.

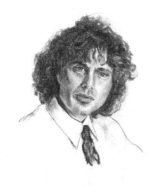

STEVEN PINKER, Ph.D., is the director of the McDonnell-Pew Center for Cognitive Neuroscience at the Massachusetts Institute of Technology, where he is also a professor in the Department of Brain and Cognitive Sciences. His work focuses on cognition and language development in children. Dr. Pinker received a B.A. in psychology from McGill University in 1976 and a Ph.D. in experimental psychology from Harvard in 1979. He has published numerous works, including *Language Learnability and Language Development* (1984/1996); *Visual Cognition* (1985); and two works for general audiences, *The Language Instinct* (1994) and *How the Mind Works* (1997). He has won the William James Book Award of the American Psychological Association (APA) and the Trolana Prize of the National Academy of Sciences; is a fellow of the APA and the American Association for the Advancement of Science; and was honored with a listing on the *New York Times Book Review* Editor's Choice "Ten Best Books of 1994." Dr. Pinker has made many appearances on radio and television, including on *Fresh Air*, *Talk of the Nation*, *Firing Line*, and *Scientific American Frontiers*.

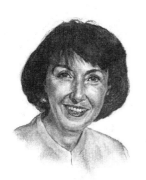

RUTH B. PURTILO, Ph.D., is director of the Creighton University Center for Health Policy and Ethics in Omaha, Nebraska, where she is also the C.C. and Mabel L. Criss Professor in the Health Sciences. Dr. Purtilo holds a B.S. degree from the University of Minnesota and an M.T.S. degree from Harvard Divinity School; she also earned a doctorate in ethics at Harvard. A fellow of the Hastings Center, Purtilo and her husband, Vard Johnson, are codirectors of "Fighting Chance for Children, Inc." She is the author of, among other works, *Ethical Dimensions in the Health Professions* (1993); *Health Professional-Patient Interaction*, which has sold more than 150,000 copies since its initial publication in 1990; and *Survey of Human Diseases* (1989). Her work has focused on patients with physical disabilities, those with AIDS, and "difficult" patients. She was ethicist-in-residence at the Massachusetts General Hospital (MGH) from 1987 to 1991, as well as the Henry Knox Sherrill Professor of Medical Ethics and director of the Program in Ethics at the MGH Institute of Health Professions. Dr. Purtilo has also been a fellow of the Joseph

P. Kennedy Foundation and the National Endowment for the Humanities and has served as an ethics consultant to many agencies and groups in the United States and more than 20 countries worldwide.

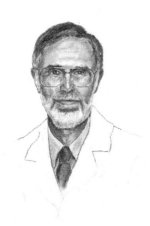

MARCUS E. RAICHLE, M.D., is a professor of radiology, neurology, and neurobiology at Washington University School of Medicine and codirector of the Division of Radiological Sciences at Washington University's Mallinckrodt Institute of Radiology. He was elected to the National Academy of Sciences in 1996, in recognition of his pioneering work in the use of positron emission tomography (PET) to map specific brain areas used in tasks such as seeing, hearing, reading, and remembering, as well as in emotion. His research has led to a better understanding of those areas of the normal human brain responsible for language, thought-processing, and emotion. Using PET to monitor blood flow and metabolism in the human brain, Dr. Raichle and his colleagues have shown how the brain responds when subjects are asked to perform mental tasks such as memorizing words or thinking sad thoughts. In addition, Dr. Raichle and his colleagues have mapped areas of the brain involved in attention, analyzed chemical receptors in the brain, investigated the physiology of major depression and anxiety, and evaluated patients at risk for stroke. Dr. Raichle received his B.A. and M.D. degrees from the University of Washington in Seattle.

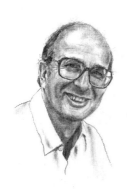

PASKO T. RAKIC, M.D., Sc.D., chairs the Section of Neurobiology at the Yale University School of Medicine. He was born in the former Yugoslavia, where he received his M.D. and an Sc.D. in developmental biology and genetics. In 1969 he emigrated to the United States to join the faculty of Harvard University, and in 1978 he moved to his current position at Yale. Dr. Rakic's research on cellular events is at the interface between gene discovery, on the one hand, and normal and pathological function, on the other. His studies in developmental neurobiology have made it possible to analyze the principles and mechanisms of mammalian brain development, including the complex primate cerebral cortex, at a cellular and molecular level. Furthermore, his studies of the primate visual system provided some of the most striking evidence for the principle of remodeling in the development of synaptic circuitry. This work has also allowed extrapolation of basic research findings in nonhuman primates to the development of normal and abnormal human brains. His publications are widely recognized, including one on the concept of the differential surface-mediated glial guidance by which some classes of neurons move and acquire their final positions in the brain. Dr. Rakic was president of the Society for Neuroscience in 1995-96, is a member of the National Academy of Sciences and of the American Academy of Arts and Sciences, and has received numerous international honors and awards.

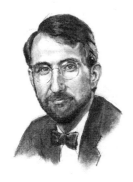

WILLIAM L. ROPER, M.D., M.P.H., dean of the School of Public Health at the University of North Carolina at Chapel Hill since 1997, served as director of the Centers for Disease Control and Prevention from 1990 to 1993 and as administrator of the federal Health Care Financing Administration, which oversees the Medicare and Medicaid programs, from 1986 to 1989. From 1993 until 1997, he was with Prudential HealthCare, first as president of the Prudential Center for Health Care Research and then later as the company's senior vice president and chief medical officer. He has also worked on the White House staff as deputy assistant to the president for domestic policy and as special assistant to the president on health policy. Dr. Roper received his B.S., M.D., and M.P.H. degrees from the University of Alabama and completed his residency in pediatrics at the University of Colorado Medical Center. In his post at Chapel Hill, he also holds appointments as a professor of health policy and administration and as a professor of pediatrics.

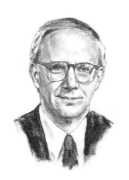

MICHAEL S. TEITELBAUM, D.PHIL., a demographer at the Alfred P. Sloan Foundation, also serves as one of nine members and as vice chair of the U.S. Commission on Immigration Reform (known as the Jordan Commission). He was educated at Reed College and at Oxford University, where he was a Rhodes Scholar. He has been a member of the faculties of Oxford and Princeton; the staff director of the Select Committee on Population of the U.S. House of Representatives; a member of the U.S. Commission for the Study of International Migration and Cooperative Economic Development; and an officer of the Population Association of America. Dr. Teitelbaum is a regular speaker on immigration and demographic change and a frequent invited witness before Congressional committees. His books include *Threatened Peoples, Threatened Borders* (1995); *The Fear of Population Decline* (1985); *Latin Migration North: The Problem for U.S. Foreign Policy* (1985); and, with J.M. Winter, *Broken Boundaries: Migration, Fertility and National Identity Since 1960* (1998). He is also a member of the Council on Foreign Relations and a fellow of the American Association for the Advancement of Science.

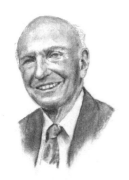

S. MARSH TENNEY, M.D., is considered the "refounder" of Dartmouth Medical School. He received an A.B. from Dartmouth College in 1943, graduated from Dartmouth Medical School's preclinical program in 1944, and has been associated with the School in various capacities, including as dean and twice as acting dean, since 1956. He received an M.D. from Cornell in 1946 and was on the faculty of the University of Rochester before returning to Dartmouth as chair of physiology and associate dean for research and planning. In the latter role, he was charged with accomplishing a major facilities expansion, significant growth in the faculty and student body, and the creation of a research enterprise, paving the way for the School's reintroduction of a full M.D. program after a 60-year hiatus during which it offered only a two-year basic science program. Dr. Tenney's research has focused on the problems of cardiorespiratory physiology, especially adaptive mechanisms to hypoxia; his laboratory studies have been complemented by field work in the California Sierras and the Andes. He holds an honorary Sc.D. from the University of Rochester; he has been a Markle Scholar and chair of the Physiology Study Section and of the Board of Scientific Counselors of the National Institutes of Health; he is a member of the Institute of Medicine and a fellow of the American Academy of Arts and Sciences; and his work has been published in over 200 papers. He is currently the Nathan Smith Professor of Physiology Emeritus, holding a chair named for Dartmouth Medical School's founder.

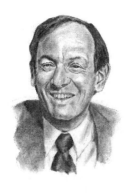

HEINZ VALTIN, M.D., former chair of physiology at Dartmouth Medical School, headed the Bicentennial Symposium Planning Committee as well as another committee that planned the other observances of the School's bicentennial year. He is known internationally for his textbooks on renal function and for his research on diabetes insipidus. He developed two animal models now used throughout the world: the Brattleboro Rat, which has neurogenic diabetes insipidus, and a strain of mouse with nephrogenic diabetes insipidus. Born in Germany, Dr. Valtin emigrated to the U.S. in 1938. He received an A.B. from Swarthmore College in 1949 and an M.D. from Cornell in 1953. After completion of his residency in internal medicine and a fellowship at St. Andrews University in Scotland, he came to Dartmouth as an instructor of physiology in 1957. His textbook *Renal Function* has been the most widely used monograph in renal physiology for more than 20 years; he has also published three additional books on renal function. He received a citation for Distinction in Neurohypophysial Research from the International Conference on the Neurohypophysis, had a lecture named in his honor at the Fourth International Conference on Vasopressin, and is the recipient of the Purkinje Medal of the Czechoslovak Physiological Society, the Pavlov Medal of the Physiological Society of the U.S.S.R., the American Physiological Society's Arthur C. Guyton Award for Distinguished Teaching in Physiology, and the Robert W. Berliner Award for Excellence in Renal Physiology. He is now Dartmouth Medical School's Andrew C. Vail Professor Emeritus and Constantine and Joyce Hampers Professor Emeritus.

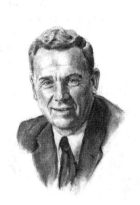

ANDREW G. WALLACE, M.D., served as dean of Dartmouth Medical School and vice president for health affairs of Dartmouth College from 1990 to 1998. A cardiologist, he spent most of his early career at Duke University, where he received both his B.S. and M.D. degrees and completed his housestaff training in internal medicine. He was appointed an assistant professor of medicine in 1964 and chief of cardiology in 1969. In 1981, he became vice chancellor of health affairs at Duke and chief executive officer of Duke Hospital. Dr. Wallace, whose research interests are in cardiac electrophysiology, cardiac rehabilitation, and exercise physiology, served on the Special Medical Advisory Group of the Department of Veterans Affairs from 1992 to 1996 and as its chair from 1994 to 1996; on the National Heart, Lung, and Blood Institute's Cardiology Advisory Committee; and on the Pharmacology and Experimental Therapeutics Study Section of the National Institutes of Health. He has also written and contributed to a wide array of books and journals. In recent years he has held a number of posts with the Association of American Medical Colleges (AAMC), including chair of its Advisory Panel on the Mission and Organization of Medical Schools and of a committee overseeing the transition to a computerized residency application process; he is also a member of the AAMC's Executive Council and the administrative board of its Council of Deans. In 1997, he was elected to the Institute of Medicine of the National Academy of Sciences.

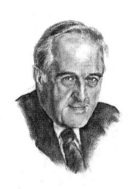

SIR DAVID WEATHERALL, M.D., is the Regius Professor of Medicine at Oxford University. He received his medical degree from Liverpool University in 1965 and after several junior hospital posts, and a period of National Service in Malaya, spent four years at Johns Hopkins Hospital. His main research interests have been in the application of molecular biology to clinical medicine, particularly the genetic disorders of hemoglobin. Dr. Weatherall has published 10 books, including *Science and the Quiet Art: The Role of Medical Research in Health Care* (1995) and *The Thalassaemia Syndromes* (1965), which was designated a "Citation Classic" by *Current Contents* in 1987 for its 1,400 citations in other publications. Dr. Weatherall established the Institute of Molecular Medicine at Oxford in 1989, and he currently serves as its honorary director. In 1987, Dr. Weatherall was knighted, and in 1993 he was elected president of the British Association for the Advancement of Science. He is also a fellow of the Royal Society as well as a foreign associate of the National Academy of Sciences in the United States, and he holds 18 honorary degrees.

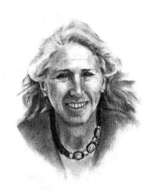

NANCY WEXLER, Ph.D., is the Higgins Professor of Neuropsychology in the Departments of Neurology and Psychiatry at the College of Physicians and Surgeons of Columbia University, as well as the president of the Hereditary Disease Foundation. Involved in public policy, individual counseling, microgenetic data, and federal health administration, she is most widely known for her important scientific contribution on Huntington's disease. A 16-year study of the world's largest family with Huntington's disease, in Venezuela, and the collection of over 4,000 blood samples led to the identification of the Huntington's disease gene. These same blood samples have helped in the mapping of other disease genes, including those for familial Alzheimer's disease, kidney cancer, two kinds of neurofibromatosis, and manic depression. One result of this work was the development of a presymptomatic test for Huntington's disease that can tell who is carrying the fatal gene prior to the onset of symptoms. Wexler received an A.B. from Radcliffe in 1967 and a Ph.D. in clinical psychology from the University of Michigan in 1974. She has held numerous public policy positions, including chair of the Joint NIH/DOE Ethical, Legal, and Social Issues Working Group of the National Center for Human Genome Research and as a member of the board of directors of the American Association for the Advancement of Science. Among the numerous honors and awards she has received is the 1993 Albert Lasker Public Service Award.

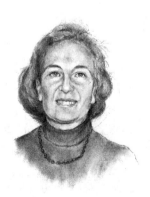

HANIA ZLOTNIK, Ph.D., is chief of the Mortality and Migration Section of the United Nations' Population Division. Trained as a demographer at Princeton University, she has worked on the problems of estimating population fertility, mortality, and migration. As a member of the Committee on International Migration of the International Union for the Scientific Study on Population, she edited a volume of the *International Migration Review* that focused on the theory and practice of measuring international migration, and she collaborated on the editing of *International Migration Systems: A Global Approach.* Dr. Zlotnik was also involved in the organization of the 1984 International Conference on Population in Mexico City and of the 1994 International Conference on Population and Development in Cairo. More recently, she has worked on improving the availability and transparency of international migration statistics, on coauthoring *International Migration Statistics: Guidelines for Improving Data Collection*, and on helping to draft the most recent revision of the United Nations' Recommendations on Statistics of International Migration.

Symposium Commentators

CHARLES N. COLE, Ph.D., a professor of biochemistry at Dartmouth Medical School, has been a member of the Dartmouth faculty since 1983. He was also a founder of the Molecular Genetics Center, a joint initiative of Dartmouth College and Dartmouth Medical School, and served for many years as director of the Molecular and Cellular Biology Program of Dartmouth-Hitchcock Medical Center's Norris Cotton Cancer Center. He has served on several National Institutes of Health study sections and continues to serve as a grant reviewer for the NIH. In addition, he is currently a reviewer for the National Research Council/Howard Hughes Medical Institute, the National Science Foundation, and the Human Frontiers Science Program. He has been a member of the editorial boards of the *Journal of Virology* and of *Virology* and is currently on the editorial board of *Molecular and Cellular Biology*. He has two book chapters and 60 journal articles to his credit. Prior to coming to Dartmouth, he was an assistant professor of human genetics at Yale. He is a cum laude graduate of Oberlin, where he majored in chemistry, and was supported by a National Science Foundation Predoctoral Fellowship during his doctoral work in cell biology at the Massachusetts Institute of Technology. He then went on to do postdoctoral work in biochemistry and molecular biology at Stanford.

MICHAEL S. GAZZANIGA, Ph.D., is director of the Center for Cognitive Neuroscience and the David T. McLaughlin Distinguished Professor at Dartmouth College. He is also president of the Cognitive Neuroscience Institute and founder of the Cognitive Neuroscience Society. He was elected to the American Academy of Arts and Science in 1997 and awarded the C.U. Ariens Kappers Medal for Neuroscience in 1999 by the Royal Netherlands Academy of Arts and Science. The author or co-author of 13 books, including *The Mind's Past* (1998) and *Nature's Mind* (1992), he has also edited six books and has to his credit hundreds of articles, book chapters, and abstracts. He is editor-in-chief of the *Journal of Cognitive Neuroscience*, associate editor of *Cerebral Cortex*, and editor of MIT Press's Monographs in Cognitive Neuroscience series. In addition, he has organized a number of major neuroscience meetings and been chief organizer since 1989 of the McDonnell Summer Institute in Cognitive Neuroscience. Before coming to Dartmouth in 1996, he held faculty positions at, among other institutions, the University of California at Davis, New York University, and Cornell. He did his undergraduate work at Dartmouth College, earned his doctorate in psychobiology at the California Institute of Technology, and did postgraduate study there and at the Institute of Physiology in Pisa, Italy.

RONALD M. GREEN, Ph.D., is the Eunice and Julian Cohen Professor for the Study of Ethics and Human Values at Dartmouth College and also director of Dartmouth's Institute for the Study of Applied and Professional Ethics. He holds a bachelor's degree from Brown and a doctorate in religious ethics from Harvard, where the topic of his thesis was population growth and justice. He is the author of more than 90 articles and five books on ethical theory, religious ethics, and applied ethics, including in the field of medicine. In 1994 he served on the National Institutes of Health Human Embryo Research Panel and during 1996–97 was a consultant to the NIH's National Institute for Human Genome Research, where he aided in the establishment the Office of Genome Ethics. He is currently a member of the Bioethics Committee of the March of Dimes Birth Defects Foundation, president of the Society of Christian Ethics, and secretary of the American Academy of Religion. He is a member of the editorial boards of the *Journal of Religious Ethics* and the *Business Ethics Quarterly*. In 1980, he received Dartmouth College's Distinguished Teaching Award, given annually to a single member of the faculty based on a vote of the entire senior class.

JEFFREY J. HUTSLER, Ph.D., is a research assistant professor at Dartmouth College's Center for Cognitive Neuroscience and Department of Psychology. Also the assistant director of graduate studies for the Program in Cognitive Neuroscience, he serves as well on Dartmouth's M.D.-Ph.D. Committee and chairs the Cognitive Neuroscience Graduate Committee. He has made research presentations at Smith College, the Max Planck Institute for Brain Research in Germany, and several branches of the University of California system, and he has a number of abstracts and journal articles to his credit. Prior to coming to Dartmouth, he was a postdoctoral fellow at the Center for Neuroscience and a research associate at the University of California at Davis. He graduated magna cum laude with a B.A. in psychology from San Jose State University and earned his master's and doctoral degrees in physiological psychology, with the support of two U.C. Regents Fellowships, at the University of California at Davis.

HAROLD C. SOX, JR., M.D., joined the Dartmouth Medical School faculty in 1988 as the Joseph M. Huber Professor of Medicine and chair of the Department of Medicine. He also directs Dartmouth's Robert Wood Johnson Foundation Generalist Physician Initiative. Dr. Sox served as president of the American College of Physicians and the American Society for Internal Medicine during 1998–99. He also chaired the most recent U.S. Preventive Services Task Force and has been a member of the Institute of Medicine since 1993. He is an associate editor of *Scientific American Medicine* and his own publications include three books—*Medical Decision Making, Common Diagnostic Tests: Selection and Interpretation,* and *Graduate Education in Internal Medicine: A Guide to Curriculum.* He received his B.S. from Stanford and his M.D. from Harvard and did his internship and residency in medicine at Massachusetts General Hospital. He then spent two years doing immunology research at the National Institutes of Health and three years at Dartmouth-Hitchcock Medical Center, where he served as chief medical resident and began his study of medical decision-making. After 15 years on the faculty at Stanford, where he was chief of general internal medicine and director of ambulatory care at the Palo Alto Veterans Affairs Medical Center, he returned to Dartmouth.

Index of Contributors